MW00581992

BEAT
BACK
CANCER
naturally

DOMINIC A. BRANDY, MD

BEAT
BACK
CANCER
naturally

5 Scientifically Proven
Natural and Plant-Based
Ways to Prevent, Survive
and Thrive with Cancer

Dedication

This book is dedicated to my amazing wife, Trina, who inspired me when she courageously fought her own battle against Hodgkin's lymphoma at the young age of 28. She is now 56 years old and is my cheerleader in my own battle. She encourages me, helps me stick to the 5 natural ways and critiques me when I need it. She is truly my rock.

TABLE OF CONTENTS

ACKNOWLEDGMENTS

Even though I have never met him, I must thank and acknowledge Dr. Michael Greger for enlightening me after I had read more than 300 books on health and nutrition and after attending numerous anti-aging conferences in my 38-year career of practicing aesthetic and anti-aging medicine. I am thankful every day that his book *How Not to Die* was the first book to pop up on my Kindle while I was on a 2-week cruise that was exactly 2 months before my world was rocked with the diagnosis of multiple myeloma. Three days into reading his book, the scientific evidence was so overwhelming and so well presented by Dr. Greger that I started eating whole food, plant-based and have not touched meat or dairy since and have not missed any of it one bit. Furthermore, Dr. Greger's amazing website *nutritionfacts.org* has helped me gain scientifically based information on a daily basis by watching or listening to at least one of his 5-minute videos every day. I encourage all of you to do the same.

I also want to acknowledge other writers on natural medicine like Dr. Russell Blaylock, Nathan Pritikin, Dr. Caldwell Esselstyn, Dr. Dean Ornish, Dr. Michael McDougall, Dr. Joel Fuhrman, Dr. Neal Barnard, Dr. Alan Goldhamer and Dan Buettner, who have given me an additional base of scientific evidence that I can then share with others who are battling this formidable disease called "cancer."

Also, many thanks to fellow Pittsburgher, Dr. Sally Lipsky, for inspiring me to actually sit down and write a book that many were encouraging me to do. She also referred me to writing coach Lynda Goldman, who taught me that if you break your book down into small increments, it actually isn't as overwhelming as you might think. Thank you, Lynda.

And, of course, I must thank my wife, Trina, for always being an encouragement and my rock. Thank you for joining me in my dietary change and always coming up with new and interesting recipes that have made our dietary experience so much more varied and interesting than ever before. We have eaten plants that I never knew existed, and it has made us both healthier, happier and closer.

I also want to acknowledge the cancer patients who come to my lectures. They inspire me as they use the information that I impart to create a better quality of life for themselves and their families as they battle this daunting enemy.

Finally, I want to thank the advisory board members of Natural Insights into Cancer, LLC . . . Stephen Woodward, Dean Caliguire, Joe Caliguire, Tammy Wyatt, Mit Patel and my wife, Trina Brandy. They encouraged me to write this book and have helped me organize large seminars and smaller monthly meetings that have helped change people's lives.

FOREWORD

A diagnosis of cancer can be shocking, confusing, and scary. In 2017, Dominic Brandy, an accomplished physician, discovered he had an aggressive form of cancer. In this book, Dr. Brandy openly shares his experiences as he journeyed from shock of diagnosis to physically and emotionally grueling treatment and an unknown future. Using his own cancer experiences as a springboard, he informs and guides readers about how to optimize healing and thrive after cancer.

Notably, Dr. Brandy's decades of reading and understanding scientific literature served him well as he dove into the vast array of medical literature to create a natural regimen that he employs alongside conventional treatment. With trustworthy detail, Dr. Brandy explains how he uses a whole-food, plant-based diet, targeted supplements, exercise, stress reduction, and adequate sleep to maximize healing and overall well-being. As a late-stage cancer survivor myself, I marvel at the thoroughness of this book. I've followed a whole food, plant-based diet for years yet learned much from the book's contents.

Readers: don't expect to receive this information from your physicians or other medical practitioners. As such, I recommend you take advantage of Dr. Brandy's bountiful knowledge. Let him guide you, chapter by chapter, as you strengthen your body's ability to fight, heal from, and prevent cancer (as well as a host of other diseases, including cardiovascular, autoimmune, high blood pressure, and type 2 diabetes).

By following Dr. Brandy's road map, you'll gain an incredible sense of empowerment and control over cancer. Like me, you'll thank the author for sharing his remarkable depth and breadth of knowledge—and in a genuinely friendly, down-to-earth style.

If you currently are a cancer patient or cancer survivor not wanting to relapse—this is the book for you. Dr. Brandy provides you with a valuable, potentially life-saving gift. Read it, treasure it, and pass it along to others.

— SALLY LIPSKY, PhD
author *Beyond Cancer: The Powerful Effect of Plant-Based Eating*

PART ONE

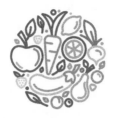

INTRODUCTION

My Personal Cancer Story

Before I begin, I think that it is important for you to understand my cancer story . . . where I started, where I went, where I presently am.

I was born and raised near Pittsburgh, Pennsylvania, in a small, middle-income town called Crafton. It was a wonderful upbringing with a great mom and dad, a brother and 3 sisters. Our diet was the Standard American Diet along with bologna and salami sandwiches, lots of red meat and ice cream. I'll always remember my dad coming home from work, eating dinner, and then sitting on the couch watching television while eating a whole half gallon of neopolitan—strawberry, chocolate, vanilla—flavored ice cream. My mom and dad were both Italian American, so I vividly remember every Sunday afternoon having spaghetti with a delicious meat sauce, meatballs, and a nice, big salad made out of iceberg lettuce (the lettuce du jour of the time). Every Sunday evening, for dinner, we had salami sandwiches on Mancini bread (they added lard for an amazing flavor). What a way to end the week!

On a good-health note, my mother started ordering *Prevention* magazine when I was around 10 years old. I do remember that *Prevention* came every month, and I would read it cover to cover. Health and nutrition was a topic that truly captivated me, even at a very young age.

As I entered the University of Pittsburgh and commuted every day, my lunch choices were strictly mine, and I do remember making it a point to eat a giant salad every day with as many different vegetables as possible and trying to eat at least one piece of fruit at the end of each day. I also took a multi-vitamin daily.

Then it was off to medical school in Philadelphia (Hahnemann College then—Drexel University now). While attending there, I clearly remember my mother mailing me her *Prevention* magazine every month. So *Prevention* magazine was a big part of my life as a child but even as a high school, college and medical student. This was the first time that I did not live at home, so every food choice was mine. This was also the first time that I had to cook my own meals. And, to say the least, it wasn't very pretty. The only thing that I remember clearly is that almost every evening I had a large salad with some frozen fish sticks that I threw into the oven.

As I went through residency and entered into medical practice, reading nutritional books became a part of my life. I always had one going, and, when on vacation, reading 2 cover to cover was a must-do. When I was 30 years old, I started to read Nathan Pritikin's books, which promoted a very low-fat, low-cholesterol diet but included meat products. After Pritikin, I read *The Atkin's Diet, The Zone Diet, The Paleo Diet, The Keto Diet, The Mediterranean Diet, The Fit for Life Diet.* You name the diet, I read a book about it. And after reading all of those books, I was genuinely confused. It wasn't until 2 years ago, when I read *How Not to Die* by Dr. Michael Greger and started watching his 5-minute videos on *nutritionfacts.org*, that all of the confusion was finally cleared up.

After I finished medical training, I practiced emergency medicine for 7 years, but my specialty would end up being aesthetic medicine, which included cosmetic surgery, botox and filler injections, skin-enhancing laser procedures and non-invasive body sculpting methods. Twenty years ago, I added an anti-aging division, which dealt with bio-identical hormone replacement, stem cell treatments and dietary counseling. Back then, my dietary advice always included having some kind of meat with every meal, because I'd bought into the "protein equals meat" fabrication.

Life was great. My children were developing into beautiful adults. My practice was booming. In August of 2016, I added Snapchat and Instagram to my practice and took on the social media name "The Real Dr Skin" (*@realdrskin* on Instagram and Snapchat). My daughter, Olivia, was the person who filmed the surgery every day on Snapchat. We were having a lot of fun together, planning our quiz question of the day, our intro, different memes and skits to keep our viewership (35,000+ viewers) entertained while still educating them. After one year of social media, we were finding that 60% of our patients were coming from all over the world to have me perform their mommy makeovers, breast augmentations and facelifts. Life was indeed amazing!

The second week of September, 2017, my life would take a major turn. My wife and I were just starting a 2-week Viking ocean cruise that would take us from Bergen, Norway to Montreal, Canada. As I explained before, on vacation I would always read a couple of health and nutrition books, and this trip was no different. The first day of the cruise, I went on my Kindle and came across the title *How Not to Die*, by Dr. Michael Greger. The title, to say the least, was extremely tantalizing, so I delved into a sea of knowledge that would forever change my life.

The first chapter that I immediately jumped to was chapter 9, on "How Not to Die from Blood Cancers" because my brother had just been diagnosed with a precursor of multiple myeloma called MGUS (monoclonal gammopathy of undetermined significance). When it was named that many years ago, it was not known what the signifi-cance was, but today we know that MGUS progresses to smoldering myeloma, which then progresses to full-blown multiple myeloma. In that chapter, one study really popped out at me. It was performed at Oxford University, studying 60,000+ individuals over a 12-plus-year period, evaluating their cancer rates in relation to their diets. This 12-plus-year analysis revealed that those who ate vegetarian had half the rate of cancer compared to meat eaters. This relationship was even more pronounced with blood cancers. Another study later in the book revealed a similar larger study of 545,000+ individuals followed over 10 years that came to the same conclusion.

As I read through the chapters about heart disease, diabetes, Parkinson's, high blood pressure, kidney disease and other cancers, it became very clear to me that people who ate a whole food, plant-based diet had a much lower incidence of nearly every chronic disease when compared to those who consumed lots of animal products. As a physi-cian, the thing that really impressed me was the fact that every chapter had a minimum of 100 excellent scientific references, and many of the chapters had more than 200. Because of the enormous amount of good scientific data, 3 days into reading this book, I decided that I was going to start eating whole food, plant-based. And I wasn't going to do this gradually. Some people who make this change give up chicken one month and maybe shrimp the next. It was all in for me because the scientific evidence was so overwhelming.

Now remember . . . all of this was happening while I was on a 2-week Viking Cruise that was taking us from Norway to Montreal. The beautiful seafood and meat preparations, the morning omelettes and the incredible desserts would just have to be left to my fellow passengers. It didn't bother me, though. I was determined to follow this new lifestyle because I was 100% sure that this new way of life would provide me with a longer life with much more energy and less chronic disease. So here we were on this amazing cruise with all of this magnificent food, and it was time to tell my wife, Trina, the news that I was now on a new path in life. And you can imagine her reaction. At first, she was skeptical about what I was reading. Then she was blown away that I was actually following through . . . not partaking of the chicken, seafood, omelettes and desserts on the rest of the cruise! But she knew my personality, and if I made a decision to do something, it was as well as done.

After a week and a half of eating whole food, plant-based, I found that it was really not that hard to do. Of course, we were eating at a buffet for each meal, so the extensive amount of choices made it not that difficult. Trina kept eating her Standard American Diet (SAD), so I was foreseeing that coming home might be a problem.

We arrived home on September 21, 2017, and it was during that first week back to work that I experienced a weird pop in my right collarbone region while performing a liposuction. I had a little discomfort there, but I thought it was possibly a little tendonitis from all of the liposuctions I had done in my career. As the days went on, however, the discomfort was getting worse, and I was starting to get a little concerned. Trina and I were scheduled to go to Portland, Oregon, for a week's vacation during the last week of October, so I figured that, after one week of rest, while also taking a cortisone steroid pack called a "Medrol Dose Pack," I would be good to go when I got back to Pittsburgh.

But to my dismay, the discomfort got worse as the week progressed. The pain was actually keeping me up at night, which it had never done before. I vividly remember telling Trina, "Trina, I think I have bone cancer." She laughed and said, "There is no way—you are the healthiest person I know." Feeling a sense of relief, I agreed, hoping that she was right.

We arrived home right before Halloween, and I remember on Halloween, itself, having a great and fun day on our Snapchat channel @realdrskin. We all dressed up in costumes and made our 35,000+

viewers extremely happy. All seemed great with my surgical practice and my life except for the pain in my right collarbone that was progressively getting worse and worse and was definitely affecting me during surgery. I remember very clearly on Thursday, November 9, 2017, thinking to myself, during what would be the last case I would ever do, *I don't think I can do this anymore.* The pain was just getting so severe.

Friday and Saturday I had patient consultations, and then, on Sunday, November 12, while watching an episode of "The Walking Dead" with my wife, I accidentally knocked over a water container from our coffee table. I lunged wildly to catch it, and, as I did, I heard a loud "pop" and then experienced excruciating pain right where I had been having discomfort for the past 2 months. I immediately asked Trina to go to our local CVS to buy me a shoulder splint because the pain got worse with even minor movements.

I had work the next day. Fortunately, I was just seeing post-op patients and not performing surgery. When I walked into my office on that Monday morning, my staff was completely blown away. Their surgeon, whose hair was always meticulously in place, was totally disheveled (because I couldn't even slightly lift up my right arm to comb my hair), and his usual calm and collected nature was anxious and fearful, not sure what was ahead for him.

That Monday evening, Trina and I headed over to Med Express (a local urgent-care center) to get an X-ray to get verification as to what, exactly, was going on. To my amazement, the doctor refused an X-ray because I hadn't fallen on it. As a former director of an emergency department, I was 100% sure I had fractured my collarbone, and I demanded that it be performed. My anger, I believe, scared him a bit, so off I went to the X-ray department. When the X-ray was completed, the X-ray technician placed the finished product on the board with me in the room. I saw the X-ray before the doctor did, and it was very clear to me that the right collarbone was completely displaced. The X-ray painted a perfect picture of the pain and disability that I was experiencing.

The next day, Tuesday, I called an orthopedic surgeon friend of mine and asked if he could fit me in that day to check out my situation. I remember him going through the scientific literature on his computer, looking for cases of stress fractures in the collarbone region. He could only find 4, and they were all exercise induced. I was hoping and praying that the many liposuctions that I had performed over the past many years was the cause. To be 100% sure about what was going on, my orthopedic surgeon ordered an MRI for the next day.

Wednesday evening is when I experienced my first MRI, and I must tell you, it was quite the experience. They laid me into this tubular structure and told me not to move for 30 minutes. Now that is a tall order for a man who can't keep still for 2 minutes. Thankfully, they asked me if I wanted earphones to distract me from the crazy noises coming from that dreadful machine. I picked some jazz fusion, thinking it would calm me down, but the music had so much static that it actually annoyed me more than the MRI machine. Anyway, I kept my eyes completely closed for 30 minutes, not wanting to see how close the top of this tubular structure was to my head. When the MRI technician said we were done, I must say that was one of the biggest sighs of relief that I had in a long time. She told me the report would be ready in 2 days . . . Friday.

That Friday evening, November 17, 2017, my life would be changed forever. My orthopedic gave me a call around 7:00 PM. He said, "Nick, I have some bad news for you. You most likely have multiple myeloma or possibly a metastasis from another cancer." The words still sting in my heart. For those of you reading this book who have been diagnosed with cancer, you know the exact feeling. For those of you who haven't, I hope you never get this message. But if you do, it will totally rock your world. After I got the news, my wife and I sat together, hugged and wiped away each other's tears. Then my children and my brother came over to my house, and we all cried together not knowing what lay before me.

That Friday evening, I couldn't resist going on the Internet, where I started reading all of the horror stories about myeloma. From my personal experience, I would strongly recommend to anyone getting a cancer diagnosis, please don't do this. It will put you in a downward mental spiral because half the information is wrong, and many of the statistics are 10 years old.

On Monday, my immediate concern, besides my cancer, was my cosmetic plastic surgical practice. Remember, I could not even lift up my right arm, so there was no way that I could perform surgery. So my surgical staff and I had a long meeting, trying to figure out what to do with the 3-month log of patients on the books. What should we tell them? Would I be OK enough to change their appointments to 3 months later? Would my shoulder be OK to operate? Would the chemo treatments debilitate me so much that I could never perform surgery again? Would I even be alive? What we decided to do was to tell the patients that I broke my collarbone and would be ready to go back to surgery in 3 months, so we started canceling everyone and moving them back 3 months to a new surgery date.

An amazing thing happened shortly after this staff meeting that was an unbelievable blessing. I told my Facebook followers what had just transpired. I posted a copy of my X-ray and explained that I had either multiple myeloma or a metastasis from another cancer. The well-wishes were overwhelming and, I must say, inspired me to kick whatever I had going on in me. One of my Facebook followers, Amy Taylor, who I did not even personally know at the time, sent me a message on Facebook Messenger saying that her boyfriend, Dr. Craig Oser, a local plastic surgeon, would be willing to lend a hand if I needed help during this perilous time. I immediately responded to her, at which time she gave me his cell-phone number, and I quickly got in touch with him. We met at my office, where we discussed the possibility of him coming in to do a couple of cases to see how he liked my surgical facility and staff. Also, I wanted to see if my staff liked him, and I wanted to see the quality of his results.

One last snag, however . . . remember that, in August of 2016, I'd started using Snapchat and Instagram as a means of attracting patients. At the time of my collarbone breaking, our Instagram account had 35,000+ followers and our Snapchat 35,000+ viewers per day. We were getting 60% of our patients from these 2 social media venues, so it was absolutely critical that Dr. Oser was willing to be filmed each day by my daughter, Olivia, who was the person responsible for making the Snapchat days educational but also a little entertaining. To my surprise, Dr. Oser was willing to do the Snapchat filming, so we were off to the races.

Dr. Oser had his own, thriving, primarily reconstructive practice, so the trick now was to find a schedule that worked for him. Once we nailed down a half day on Mondays, full Tuesdays and every other Saturday my staff started the task of telling my former patients that I'd been diagnosed with cancer and that I was probably not ever coming back to do surgery. I must say this was extremely difficult . . . seeing what I had built over 38 years being suddenly turned over to someone else.

Now back to my cancer. So after the MRI, I went to my internist, Dr. Ginnie Balderston (who is also my next-door neighbor) for some blood tests. She also scheduled me to see an orthopedic oncologist, who wasn't 100% sure that it was cancer, and so he ordered a biopsy of the collarbone area at the break. At this point, there was a ray of hope that maybe I didn't have cancer after all and that the initial MRI report was possibly a mishap.

Furthermore, right before I went in for the bone biopsy, Dr. Balderston called me and told me that, so far, all of my lab work looked normal. Another glimmer of hope. So I kissed Trina, and off to the operating room I went for my bone biopsy. The nurse gave me a little touch of sedation, they numbed the area with a little local anesthetic, and before I knew it, the procedure was over. They took me to the recovery room for an hour and then back to the prep room, where Trina was waiting for me.

At this point, I was feeling optimistic that possibly the original MRI reading was wrong and that the remainder of the lab work would show no myeloma. But all of those hopes quickly vanished when, while in the recovery area after my biopsy, I received another call from Dr. Balderston telling me that the last important piece of data, my M-spike, was positive for multiple myeloma. Additionally, in 2 days following my biopsy, the report came back as multiple myeloma. So the fun was soon to begin.

Dr. Balderston referred me to a myeloma specialist at UPMC medical center in Pittsburgh. I met with my oncologist, Dr. Agha, and he ran a series of elaborate blood studies, 35 X-rays of my entire body, a PET scan and bone-marrow biopsy (which hurt like hell) to determine how invasive and exactly what type of myeloma I had. All the studies came back, and they showed that my myeloma was as an IgA, light Kappa chain multiple myeloma with 14% invasion of my bone marrow. When I saw the report, I immediately went to the Internet and quickly found out that there are 3 basic types of multiple myeloma . . . IgG, IgA, and IgM. IgG is by far the most common, with an average life span of 6–8 years. IgM was the least common with an average life expectancy of 12 years. My IgA was in the middle as far as incidence, but it was by far the most aggressive, with an average life expectancy of 2 years.

When I read this information, I must say my emotional life was in a major turmoil. I did not sleep well for a month. I was constantly in my bible memorizing bible verses to help get me through this horrible situation, and I was talking to people who had been through multiple myeloma to give me a sense of what was to come. One of these people, Lynn Taylor, told me to immediately get an appointment with a psychologist who deals exclusively with cancer patients and their caregivers. I did some local research and found a cancer psychologist, Dr. Susan Stollings, who helped me tremendously. My biggest fear was not about dying but what I would have to go through to get to death. I think that is the biggest fear of all cancer patients at first diagnosis.

After 3 visits with Dr. Stollings, I was feeling so much better. She told me that 95% of cancer patients during the last 3 months of life are not depressed. They have accepted the fact that they are going to die, and they are at peace with idea of meeting their Creator. Conversely, there are 5% of people who go down kicking to the very end. I was not sure which group I would fit into, but at least I knew most people were able to accept the fact that they were going to die and did it peacefully.

My other fear was pain. Because myeloma is present in all of the bone marrow, many myeloma patients die with severe pain in all of their bones. That idea really scared me, and Dr. Stollings explained to me that there are combinations of pain medications from very strong and very sedating to less strong and less sedating that could manage my pain regardless of the intensity.

After these visits, I was feeling much better and ready for what I was about to face—the treatment of my disease. On my second visit to Dr. Agha, I was told that my IgA myeloma was the most aggressive form of myeloma and that I really needed to have a regimen of 3 drugs . . . lenalidomide, bortezomib, and dexamethasone. Lenalidomide is an immunomodulator that is taken orally 21 days on and 7 days off. Bortezomib is a proteosome inhibitor that is given by injection under the skin 2 days per week, and dexamethasone, a potent anti-inflammatory, is taken orally once per week. My reading about bortezomib was that approximately 60% of patients develop a severe peripheral neuropathy of the feet and hands. Because I wasn't 100% sure if I was going to give up surgery and because I was 100% sure that my whole food, plant-based way of eating was going to help attack this cancer, I refused the bortezomib.

I could tell that Dr. Agha was not happy with my decision. He told me that I really needed to get into as deep of a remission as possible and that, because of my IgA diagnosis, he did not think this was possible with just the oral lenalidomide and dexamethasone. He took me into a room where there was another myeloma patient, who he had apparently asked to allay my fears about the bortezomib. I came back from conversing with that man and told Dr. Agha that I still did not want the bortezomib. Dr. Agha then offered cutting back the concentration of the dose and even doing it once per week instead of twice per week, but I still refused. So, we started with lenalidomide 25 mg, 21 days on and 7 days off, and dexamethasone 20 mg orally once per week.

Lenalidomide is a specialty drug that is a relative of a drug from the 1950s drug called "thalidomide" that caused a rash of severe birth defects in newborns. Did you ever hear of the "thalidomide babies"? Because of that fact, I was required to call into a specialty pharmacy to answer several questions like:

1. Have you had sex with a woman of child-bearing age?
2. Do you wear a condom when you have sex?

On and on the questions went, until they finally asked me when and where I wanted my medication delivered. So on January 5, 2018, a huge package was delivered to my house with a rather large book that described all the bad things that lenalidomide could do to my body. Amidst the book and a slew of written materials, there was hidden the little bottle of capsules that were going to save my life. I looked at the bottle, and I must admit I was scared to death as to what lay before me. Would I have major complications from it? Would I lose all of my energy? Would I be nauseated? Would I get constipation or diarrhea? Would my blood counts significantly drop?

I stared at that little bottle and even took a picture of it amidst its accompanying paper friends. I still have that picture stored in my iPhone and every once in a while take a look at it to remember just how far I have come.

January 8, 2018, was my first capsule. I was petrified. Because lenalidomide makes one sleepy, I was advised by Dr. Agha's team to take the medication before bed. I took the medication, and I must say I slept like a log—probably the best night's sleep that I had had in a year. That good night's sleep made me feel really good the following day, so my fears were somewhat allayed. It reminded me of how I felt when I played high school football. I was so fearful before the game, but as soon as the whistle blew and I received my first hit, all fears were wiped away. That was the way I felt now. It was time for battle, and I was going to do everything in my power to defeat this monster.

All was good until the third day. My scalp started to itch intensely. When I scratched, there was no relief at all, which made it very anxiety provoking. I called my oncology team, and they said that this itching was due to the tumors being rapidly destroyed, which causes a surge of histamine release. They told me to take loratadine to get rid of the problem. I took the loratadine, and, the next day, it was still there but not as intense. The following day, the itching had completely subsided, which brought to me a feeling that I had just crossed my first obstacle.

The second obstacle was soon to come. When I was going through my initial X-rays, PET scan and lab work, it was noted on my X-ray report that I had severe osteoporosis. That really surprised me because I exercised daily, did weight training every other day, and used a testosterone cream daily to keep my levels in the mid-range. Talking to my doctor, it was explained that the cancerous tumor cells of myeloma release a chemical that causes the bone-making cells (osteoblasts) to become less active, while causing the bone-breaking cells (osteoclasts) to become overly active. He said that this was very common amongst myeloma patients, but gave me no instructions about activities that I should preclude.

One of the exercises that I always did during my weight-training sessions was 100 crunches with a 60-pound weight behind my head. On January 22 (14 days after I took my first lenalidomide), I felt a pain in my mid-back after doing my 100 crunches. I then noticed when going down the steps, that, each time I took a step downward, I would feel a little jolt of discomfort in that same spot. I called my nurse navigator, who felt that everything was fine and told me to just take some ibuprofen.

I started the ibuprofen, but I experienced no improvement, and it seemed that my mid-back discomfort was getting worse instead of better. On January 30 (22 days after my first lenalidomide dose), I was walking downstairs to my garage to get into my car and head over to the hospital to get my first post-treatment cycle blood draw, when I developed a severe pain in my mid-back. It was the exact same place that had been nagging me for the past week. I drove to the hospital, parked my car, and, when I tried to get out of the car, my back went into a severe spasm. I could barely walk into the hospital to get my lab work. When I arrived at check-in, I told the oncology staff that I needed a back X-ray ASAP to see what was going on.

While I was in the X-ray room, they drew my lab work. The X-ray was done, and I awaited the preliminary report from the radiologist; it stated that I had a compression fracture of my T-11 vertebra. This news, I must say, was one of the low points of my myeloma journey. I was given an appointment with a neurosurgeon to evaluate the severity of the fracture.

Two days later, on February 1, I received the first results from my lab work, and the results, to me, were not impressive. My IgA and Kappa light chains had come down a little, but my M-Spike had barely budged. These results came to me by computer before my oncologist even saw them, and, not being a myeloma specialist, I was scared . . . really scared. For some reason, I was expecting an enormous improvement in my values because I was on a whole food, plant-based diet and taking a fair number of targeted supplements. I called my oncologist's office the next day, and the nurse navigator explained that the improvements that I achieved were actually good and that my M-spike would be one of the last values to budge. I breathed a sigh of relief but realized I had a long battle ahead of me and needed to start researching every possible natural means to fight this supposedly incurable cancer. This is when I started going to *pubmed.gov* on a daily basis to research natural diets, herbs, phytonutrients, foods, vitamins and minerals that could help me in my battle.

On February 5, I went to the neurosurgeon's office, and he ordered an MRI to see the extent of the fracture that I had on my T-11 vertebra. On February 7, an MRI was performed, and the result showed that I, indeed, had an acute fracture of my T-11 vertebra, but it was not severe enough for a procedure called a "kyphoplasty," whereby they would have injected cement into the compressed area to inflate the vertebra back into normal shape so that it would no longer compress my nerves. That at least was some good news. I was told that I could exercise on my elliptical, which also gave me a sense of relief, because, for the last week and a half, I had been very inactive, and that was driving me crazy. The hardest part of having a vertebral stress fracture was getting out of bed in the morning. When going from no pressure on my vertebrae to suddenly a lot of pressure . . . there was an immediate jolt of pain. I learned to keep a chair near my bed. I would roll from my back to my side, keeping all pressure on my elbow; then I would grab the top of the chair with both hands and very gradually allow the pressure to slowly increase on my T-11 vertebra.

To help restore my bone density, I was now required to receive monthly zoledronic acid infusions. I was also told not to lift any heavy objects so that my vertebra could begin the healing process. Zoledronic acid is a bisphosphonate that causes the bone to build. As I researched this drug, I learned that many people get severe pain and flu-like symptoms after the infusions. I also learned that the half-life (the time for half of the drug to be metabolized) of zoledronic acid was 10 years. That meant that it would take 55 years to get all of the drug out of my system. I also found out that it is very toxic to the kidney, 4% of patients get death of the jawbone, and 2% get a weird oblique hip fracture that does not occur in nature.

This information was very dismaying to me, but I felt I needed to do something to build up this bone deterioration that myeloma had caused.

I had my first zoledronic acid infusion on February 9. The infusion took about a half hour, and everything seemed to have gone fine. It wasn't until that night at around 2:00 AM that the fun began. I was awakened suddenly with severe pain in my sternum (the middle of my chest). It scared the living hell out of me, and I couldn't get back to sleep for the rest of the night. The next day was even worse; I felt like I had a severe flu with myalgias for 24 hours. Therefore my first experience with zoledronic acid was not enjoyable, to say the least. The subsequent ones were even worse, which made me reject any further treatments after I had received 3. Then I discovered the natural element strontium citrate, which has done wonders for my bone density and with no side effects. I will discuss this at length in the chapter on targeted supplements.

February 12 was the lowest emotional point of my journey to the present. I was now already one week into my second cycle of lenalidomide 25 mg and dexamethasone 20 mg. Normally, during consultations for cosmetic surgery, I would photoshop my patients to give them an idea of what kind of result they could expect. Dr. Oser had now been cleaning up my backlog of patients for a month, and I had offered to come in during his consultation day to do photoshops on patients who might want to see what their final outcome might look like. I sat in one of our surgical prep rooms far from where the consultations were being done. I sat with back pain as I awaited what I thought was going to be an onslaught of photoshops. I waited and waited and waited, feeling more depressed as the day went along. Here I was, once the most sought-after cosmetic surgeon in Pittsburgh, now sitting in a little room far from where the consults were being done, in pain, with an incurable cancer, with no one even coming over to say "Hi" to me and zero requests for photoshops. I started to cry in that little room all by myself. The last

3 months had transformed my life into what I thought was a totally worthless one with a future that was completely obscure.

What would I be doing a year from now? Would I even be alive? What kind of work would I be doing? What would happen to the practice I'd spent 38 years developing? Would this back pain ever go away?

Valentine's Day was here. It was on a Wednesday, and Trina and I decided to go to the Sewickley Spa to get a couples massage and then go out for dinner. The problem was . . . I had a fracture right smack in the middle of the massage zone. I told the massage therapist to avoid the middle of my back. I didn't explain why because, to be quite honest with you, I couldn't even come up with a fake explanation. Several times, as we were chatting away, she got close to my T-11 vertebra and I would say, "just a little higher please" . . . "would you go a little lower please, thank you" . . . "a little easier on the pressure, thanks." I must say it wasn't the most pleasant massage I have ever had because of my constant worry of her accidentally breaking my spine in two. But I must say the whole experience of getting the massage and spending the day with my wife did put me in a good frame of mind.

From that Valentine's Day forward, everything took an emotional and physical step forward. My back started to feel better day by day. I made it a point to exercise every single day, as my reading was showing me that even 6 minutes of exercise would increase my immune activity by 50%. I prayed every morning, not only for myself, but for others who had physical and emotional battles far worse than mine. I came to realize my position at my office was different from what it had been for 38 years, so I focused on making our @realdrskin Snapchat and Instagram the best it could be. I chaired our social media committee, so this gave me a new focus. I would also virtually screen all of Dr. Oser's prospective social media patients from my home. I would first photoshop their images and draw up a schematic plan. The images would be sent to the patient. I would then do 4 virtual screening consultations using my iPhone from my home on Tuesday and Thursday evenings and Saturday mornings. Every morning I would go to *pubmed.gov* and search for herbs, phytonutrients and supplements that had been shown in double-blind studies to have a positive effect against cancer cells. Things were starting to look up, and I was getting into a new routine.

I also made it a point, while I did my resistance-band exercise program every morning, to watch or listen to three 5-minute videos by Dr. Greger on *nutritionfacts.org*. Every year Dr. Greger's staff of 20 scientists reviews every single article in the clinical nutritional literature. In 2018 they reviewed 190,000 articles (3,600 per week). They then take this science and produce thousands of 5–8 minute videos that are packed with pure science and which are made quite entertaining by Dr. Greger's narration ability.

Watching or listening to at least one of these videos per day is an activity that I strongly recommend to individuals trying to make the switch to a whole food, plant-based diet (WFPBD). When converting from the Standard American Diet (SAD diet) to a WFPBD diet, you need to be constantly educated about the amazing benefits of eating whole plant foods, because the uneducated culture will continually be pulling you in the opposite direction. Learning what the scientific evidence says will keep you motivated, and, before you know it, you will be living an amazingly healthy lifestyle and seeing improvements in your energy levels, your appearance and your emotional state. And if you have cancer, you should start seeing improvements in your cancer biomarkers.

That is what happened to me. After my first set of myeloma lab results, my biomarkers kept gradually getting better month by month. By month 6, I had achieved a complete response with just 2 oral medications and without the bortezomib, which would have required me to go to the hospital 2 times per week for injections under my skin and which probably would have resulted in me living with peripheral neuropathy for the rest of my life.

When I walked into Dr. Agha's office at my 6-month appointment, he had a huge grin on his face and threw a graph sheet in front of me showing the continual improvement of my biomarkers to the point of a complete response. I told him that I had been on a strict whole food, plant-based diet, exercised daily, and had been taking a whole array of supplements, which you will learn about in this book. He said that what I was doing was definitely helping because it was extremely rare to get to a complete response with IgA myeloma without the bortezomib injections as part of the treatment protocol.

The next goal was to start lowering the strength of the lenalidomide 25 mg, because lenalidomide is known to cause genetic mutations, which can then lead to acute myelogenous leukemia and other secondary cancers. We first lowered it to 20 mg, and all the biomarkers held. We went to 15 mg and the same thing . . . the biomarkers held. We went to 10 mg, and the biomarkers held again. When we went down to 5 mg, the biomarkers went up a little, so Dr. Agha raised me back up to 10 mg. At the time of this writing, I am at 10 mg, with all biomarkers in check.

In September of 2018 (10 months after I cracked my collarbone), I heard about the chairwoman of the Pittsburgh Myeloma Support Group, Yvonne Yaksic. I had heard through the grapevine that she was a 13-year survivor of myeloma, so I contacted her to see if we could have lunch together. Over lunch we chatted for more than 3 hours as I was trying to learn everything single thing about her 13-year survival. One thing that I did learn is that her 13-year journey had not been an easy one. A stem cell transplant, a broken hip bone from the zoledronic acid infusions, a rod in her back from broken vertebrae, and extreme emotional ups and downs during her journey.

I told her about how I had achieved a complete response just on lenalidomide and dexamethasone, and she seemed intrigued by all of the natural approaches that I was taking. That is when she asked me to speak at the Pittsburgh Myeloma Support group on November 13, 2018. I had no lecture together, but in the month of October, I threw together 200 slides to create a lecture detailing what a whole food, plant-based diet, targeted supplements, daily exercise, adequate sleep and stress reduction could do against cancer. I was going to use this lecture as a directive from Above as to whether I should take this message to the broader public.

The lecture was unbelievably well received, and one attendee emailed me the day after the lecture:

"My wife is carrying the syllabus around like a bible. I've been coming to those meetings for 2 ½ years, and that was the most positive, empowering meeting ever. You really were a clearinghouse of information. You took complicated concepts and made them understandable. Life changing."

I had the strong sense that these cancer patients and their caregivers were in desperate desire of information about natural steps that they could do aside from the radiation, chemo infusions, pills and potions. Their oncologists seemed to be totally immersed in the conventional medical world of the pharmaceutical industry and knew little about nutrition. I know as a medical doctor graduating from medical school in 1979 that we had a total of 2 weeks of nutritional training, and it was truly on the level of a high school health class . . . the food groups, what each vitamin did, what severe vitamin deficiencies cause, etc., etc. Recently, my sister's daughter graduated from medical school, and, when I asked her about the amount and quality of her nutritional training, it was the same as mine . . . almost zero.

I am not denigrating the achievements of conventional medicine, because I do firmly believe that, when you have billions of cancer cells in your body trying to quickly destroy your health and your life, you need conventional treatments to destroy the bulk of that cancer. The daughter cancer cells are usually easily taken out by conventional treatments, but it is the cancer stem cell, which is slower-growing, that really does need the help of a metabolic approach which involves diet, phytonutrients, herbs, targeted supplements, exercise, adequate sleep and stress reduction. We will discuss these at length in this book as I empower you beyond the radiation, pills, potions and infusions.

Because of the positive, exuberant response of the Myeloma Support Group, I decided to form a non-profit LLC, which I titled "Natural Insights into Cancer, LLC." The goal of this company would be to educate as many people as possible about the natural ways to combat the dreaded disease of cancer. After I formed this non-profit LLC, I booked a room at The Pittsburgh Plaza Hotel for January 9, 2019. Mit Patel, who was the owner of the hotel and also the husband of my physician assistant, Jenny Patel, said that I could use the hotel for free because he believed so much in what I was trying to do. That was a sigh of relief because I could keep the entry fee very low at $10.00. On the marketing end, I had the graphic designer for my medical practice, Peg Warnock, create a social media post advertising this event. Then I started posting it on my personal Facebook page and on my Instagram and Snapchat sites.

During the month of December, I posted the event weekly, and more followers than I could imagine stated that they were very interested in attending. One of the reasons that I think so many were interested is that I had been posting my monthly biomarker results on my Facebook page, and many people were fascinated on how my results gradually got better with 2 oral medications, that I was having minimal side effects, and that my meds were starting to be decreased each month. I also was keeping them informed on the fact that I was eating a whole food, plant-based diet.

One of my followers, Michelle Wright, who is a celebrity on one of our local TV stations, asked me if I would be willing to do a story about my cancer and how I was using natural methods to help me keep it under control. She felt that, right after the new year, my whole food, plant-based diet with exercise might not only be a good way to tell my story, but also a way to encourage their viewers to adopt some healthy lifestyle changes for the new year.

She and her crew came over to the house on Wednesday, January 3, 2018 (6 days before the scheduled event on January 9). They spent a couple of hours filming me adding my nutrient-dense, freeze-dried powders to my coffee, making my morning smoothie, exercising on my elliptical and answering questions in my sunroom. She said it would air on Friday evening. On Friday around noon, she contacted me and said that the story would not air because of other important news that popped up. She told me possibly on the weekend, but the weekend passed, and it did not appear. I was becoming a little concerned because I felt that the story would help draw a lot of people to the January 9 lecture that I was going to deliver.

On Monday, January 7, the story finally aired on the evening news, and it was so well done I couldn't have asked for more. I posted it on my Facebook page and on my new website *www.naturalinsightsintocancer.com*, and the response was overwhelming. Even to this day, random people will come up to me and ask me if I am the doctor who was on the news who had cancer. They also invariably ask me, "How are you doing?" And I invariably respond, "Great!"

Now was the day of the event . . . Wednesday, January 9. We had about 80 RSVPs from Facebook, my website, Eventbrite, and my email address *info@naturalinsightsintocancer.com*. As the crowd started to pour in, I was sure that we were going to go beyond that number. They just kept coming and coming. My wife, Trina, had to approach the hotel staff to get extra chairs as we were approaching the start of the lecture at 7:00 PM. I mingled with the crowd from 6 to 7 o'clock and asked many of them about their cancer diagnoses and if they were incorporating any dietary or natural methods to augment their conventional treatment, and every one of them said, "No." I asked them if their doctors had recommended any dietary changes, seeing as how the National Cancer Institute recommends 9 servings of fruits and vegetables for the prevention of cancer. Again, everyone of them said, "No." So I knew I had before me an incredible opportunity to educate.

I must admit I was quite nervous because of the amazing opportunity that lay before me, and I did not want to blow it. I started my lecture talking about the Viking cruise Trina and I had taken 2 months before my collarbone broke and how the book *How Not to Die* by Dr. Greger got me eating whole food, plant-based. I always emphasize that, because I did not start eating whole food, plant-based on a reaction to a cancer diagnosis. I started eating this way because the book was so intense on the science, and the science was showing over and over again that those eating a whole food, plant-based diet had less cancer, heart disease, diabetes, hypertension, metabolic disease, and all-cause mortality.

I realize some of you may be agnostic about God, but I do believe that the way this book popped up on my Kindle 4 months before I would take my first chemo pill was divinely inspired. In fact, I recommend to all cancer patients ready to undergo cancer treatment to start eating at least 12 servings of fruits and vegetables one month before undergoing chemotherapy or radiation to prepare for the coming onslaught to their normal cells.

During the lecture, I reviewed the work of Dr. Dean Ornish, who had done an elegant study that demonstrated that early-prostate-cancer patients showed reversal of their cancer when put on a whole food, plant-based diet. The WFPB diet group had their PSA levels (biomarker for prostate cancer) decrease by 4% while the Standard American Diet (SAD diet) group had their PSA levels increase by 6% . . . a 10% difference. These reversals were also nicely demonstrated on PET scans.

I then presented another amazing study performed on this same group of patients that revealed, on heat-map analysis, that more than

500 genes were positively affected by a whole food, plant-based diet. It validated that 48 good genes were up regulated and 453 bad genes were down regulated. This means that more than 500 genes were made to act in a more positive way. And this was after only 3 months on a whole food, plant-based diet. The way that lifestyle choices affect the way that genes act is called "epigenetics," and this study demonstrated beautifully and concretely what a whole food, plant-based diet can do to the expression of one's genes.

I then went through the positives of exercise and how critical the 25,000+ phytonutrients found in fruits, vegetable, whole grain, legumes, mushrooms, nuts and seeds were for the prevention and relapse of cancer.

I discussed all the negatives of animal products, which we will go over in detail throughout this book. Everyone was encouraged to read the book *The China Study*, by T. Colin Campbell. This was the largest epidemiological study ever performed on populations in China over a 20-year period that established that those who ate a high amount of animal products had much higher levels of all-cause mortality compared to those who ate primarily a plant-strong diet.

I then talked about how genetic mutations cause cancer and cancer relapses and how antioxidants can help prevent and repair these mutations. Plants have 63X the antioxidant power compared to animal products, which makes another strong case for eating more plants. Other important topics were the very detrimental effects of animal proteins, the importance of sleep, stress reduction, social interaction and prayer. I ended the lecture reviewing targeted supplements that have demonstrated anti-cancer properties and then gave some spiritual encouragement for the finale.

My final slide made me and several of the audience who were struggling from cancer cry as I read it. It was from one of my morning Chuck Swindoll devotions and read as follows:

Cancer is limited:

- It cannot cripple love,
- It cannot corrode faith,
- It cannot eat away peace,
- It cannot destroy confidence,
- It cannot destroy friendship,
- It cannot shut out memories,
- It cannot silence courage,
- It cannot invade the soul,
- It cannot reduce eternal life,
- It cannot quench the Spirit,
- It cannot lessen the power of the resurrection.

You cannot deny that you have the disease, but you shouldn't despair about it taking control. Whoever you are, whatever your circumstances, call for God's daily delivery of wisdom, strength and grace. Each morning, slam the door on despair. If you don't, it will slip in and rob you. And you'll soon find peace missing.

After this final slide, I said, "Thank you," and the crowd rose up and gave me a standing ovation. I was totally taken by surprise and touched deeply. In the more than 200 lectures that I had given to physicians and lay people alike, I had never received a standing ovation. To this day, I really don't know why it happened. Was the lecture that good? I don't think so. Were they just feeling sorry for me because I was diagnosed with an incurable blood cancer and was not only battling it successfully with conventional and natural means but sharing the information with the general public? Was it because their oncologists were giving them very little information on how they could be empowered beyond the pills, radiation and infusions?

Looking back, I think it was probably a combination of all the above. Additionally, I let them know that I was making no money for my efforts and that my sole goal was to educate as many people as possible about the power of plants, phytonutrients, exercise, sleep, stress reduction and prayer in the battle against the world's most dreaded disease.

Immediately after the lecture, I took one-on-one questions after the group Q and A, and many cancer patients came up to me asking questions about their specific cancer treatment. One that stuck in my mind was a woman who had the same diagnosis as me . . . multiple myeloma. We were talking about how she came to her diagnosis and the treatment protocol she was on, and then the discussion went to diet. She was obviously extremely overweight, and she told me that she had asked her oncologist if she should adjust her diet in any way. The doctor's reply was, "Just keep eating the way you are . . . the drugs will take care of everything." She told me that she was actually shocked by his response, knowing deep in her heart that he was wrong. She knew that the way that she'd been eating to get to her obese state could not possibly be good for the battle before her. She felt relieved that I had taken the time to do the research and present an approach that would get her weight down while helping her in her fight against billions of cancer cells that were trying to take her life.

During the lecture, I had given the audience my email address and told them that, if they had any questions, to feel free to contact me and that I would surely get back to them with an answer. To my surprise, I was inundated with questions and requests for my slide presentation. Because of this intense interest, I decided to have smaller monthly meetings at my medical spas. It is one thing to hear one lecture, get all jacked up about it, immediately start eating whole food, plant-based, but then, one month later find it unsustainable and return to the same rut of eating the Standard American Diet (SAD). I knew that monthly meetings which would include a *nutritionfacts.org* video, a 30-minute lecture, a cooking demonstration, and a question-and-answer session would be the only way to keep people on track and to help them change their lives.

The monthly meetings were a tremendous success and to this day draw 50–70 people every month. The reason I start off with a 5-minute *nutritionfacts.org* video is because I believe that you need not only monthly education but also daily education. As I previously stated, I personally watch or listen to three 5-minute *nutritionfacts.org* videos while I do my daily morning resistance-band routine, and it not only keeps improving my knowledge base, but keeps me motivated and positive that this lifestyle is helping me fight my cancer.

In March of 2019, I started an Instagram site called *@cancerveggiedoc* where I post whole food, plant-based recipe videos, interesting cancer facts and photos of me in action fighting this relentless enemy. I strongly encourage you to follow this wonderful site. Then on July 31, 2019, I put together another large meeting, with 4 speakers besides myself. It was amazingly well attended. With this book, I hope to expand the number of people I can educate because the message needs to be spread.

Enjoy the information that lies before you. If you are a cancer patient, I am positive it is going to help your prognosis and quality of life. If you are a caregiver or an individual just wanting to prevent the development of cancer, I know that, if you follow the basic principles of this book, you will have a healthier, happier life with lots of energy to share with your loved ones.

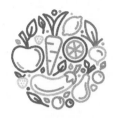

CHAPTER 1

The Way Cancer Starts and Progresses

Since President Nixon officially declared war on cancer through the National Cancer Act in 1971, billions and billions of dollars have spent trying to kill this dreaded disease. When you honestly look at statistics since 1971, for most of the major cancers, the death rates have not budged a whole lot. A few cancers like childhood leukemias and multiple myeloma (which I have) have had a significant jump in overall survival, but my cancer is still considered incurable. Conversely, other cancer death rates are fairly unchanged, and, if they seem improved on paper, it is many times because of earlier diagnosis. If you diagnose a specific cancer one year earlier in 2019 due to better diagnostic technology and compare the overall survival to 1971, the survival rate is going to look one year longer. So many times it is not so much the wondrous technologies that are done on the back end, but it is the earlier diagnosis by the wondrous technology on the front end that leads to the appearance of better survival rates from current treatment protocols.

Over the past couple of decades, there have been more and more discoveries about how cancer starts. One of those discoveries is the realization that mutated stem cells appear to be at the center of everything that is going on with a given cancer. The cancer stem cell is the first cell that receives many mutations to its genes from the onslaught of free radicals that we generate in our bodies secondary to carcinogens, chronic diseases, medications, our horrible diets, chronic stress, inadequate sleep and bad habits like smoking and drinking. The list could go on and on for the entirety of this page.

The mutated stem cell then loses its ability to stop dividing uncontrollably and starts creating daughter cells at an incredibly fast rate. Most chemotherapeutic agents and radiation treatments easily knock off the daughter cells because they are dividing at a very quick speed. Because most chemotherapeutic agents are working at the DNA level, the more rapidly the daughter cell is dividing, the more likely the chemo or radiation will obliterate that cancer cell. That is why certain parts of the body are frequently affected by chemotherapy more than other parts.

For example, cancer patients usually experience hair loss, because hair follicles divide at a very rapid rate. Patients get severe nausea and diarrhea because the cells of your digestive tract also divide at a very rapid rate. So not only are the daughter cancer cells being destroyed, but so are normal cells. That is why this book will help you develop ways to limit the damage to your good cells and help your body kill the cancer stem cells, which are the cells that are extremely difficult to destroy with conventional therapies. And not destroying them adequately is the basis for many cancer relapses.

Most cancer stem cells do not get killed during conventional chemo and radiation treatments, which explains why approximately 70% of cancer patients end up relapsing and why there is an extremely poor cure rate for metastatic cancer. More and more studies are showing that the 25,000+ phytonutrients found in many types of natural whole foods can kill cancer stem cells and their daughter cells, which can enhance the results of conventional treatments and do it with no added side effects or complications.

In this book I will not be encouraging anyone not to go through some kind of conventional therapy. When you are first diagnosed with billions of cancer cells dividing wildly in your body, I feel strongly that you need conventional therapy along with a whole food, plant-based diet, daily exercise, targeted supplements, stress reduction and adequate sleep. Even though there are many people who have been totally cured with a whole food, plant-based diet, combined with exercise and lifestyle changes, there have not been enough controlled double-blind studies for anyone to recommend forgoing conventional treatment. I do, however, advocate patients to ask their oncologist to see if he or she can use the lowest chemo or radiation dose as possible at the beginning of their treatment to see how their dietary and lifestyle changes are affecting the results. That is exactly what I did with my oncologist, and it left me with minimal side effects from the treatment and with a complete response as my reward. I rejected a triple drug regimen for my very aggressive IgA multiple myeloma and instead insisted upon a weaker, double oral medication approach because I felt confident that my whole food, plant-based diet, along with lifestyle changes, was going to have a positive effect on my cancer. Most of the people I know who have gone through the aggressive high-dose triple drug regimen (that I rejected) have developed a peripheral neuropathy and some other significant side effects. The knowledge that we now have about a whole array of new targets for cancer control and cure (conventional and natural) is an exciting prospect for the future.

Normally, the cells in our body live, divide by mitosis, and perish in a predictable way. At a very basic level, cancer occurs when certain cells keep dividing uncontrollably and our body cannot stop this out-of-control process. We will discuss them one by one so that you have a clear understanding of the multitude of processes that start and keep a cancer flourishing even against the onslaught of chemotherapy and radiation that we frequently throw against it. The first thing we need to understand is the concept of genetic mutations, which is at cancer's root.

GENETIC MUTATION . . . THE ROOT OF ALL EVIL

Most experts in the field of cancer would agree that all cancers start with genes that have gone awry. We know that cells that divide more rapidly tend to develop cancers more often than cells that normally divide slowly. The most rapidly dividing cells in our bodies are in our bone marrow and lymph nodes, and these are where the majority of cancers occur . . . mine included (multiple myeloma). Conversely, brain neurons divide very slowly after our teenage years and is why brain cancers are relatively rare in adults.

Why do rapidly dividing cells have a higher risk of turning into cancer? It is because with each cell division there is a risk that the cell's DNA will be damaged by free radicals (we will discuss this shortly) and carcinogens. When the DNA helix opens up during the cell-division process, the DNA is exposed to free-radical damage. When the stem cell's DNA is damaged, that mutated DNA will then be carried over to the new cells that have just been formed. As this process occurs over and over again, more and more mutated genes accumulate in that cell to the point that the cell cannot control the growth-regulating instructions that come from our proto-oncogenes.

PROTO-ONCOGENES

To be able to understand how genetic mutations are at the root of cancer, we need to know about proto-oncogenes and how they become oncogenes. First off, what is a proto-oncogene? A proto-oncogene is a gene in your DNA that controls cell replication, cell suicide, growth and division. When it is mutated, however, it has the potential to start cancer [1]. Upon the exposure to free radicals and carcinogens, this proto-oncogene becomes a harmful oncogene that can start the whole sequence of cancer development. Most in the field of cancer agree that oncogene formation and its activation are one of the first things that happen in cancer initiation [2].

Most normal cells will experience a programmed rapid cell death (apoptosis) when critical functions of a cell go haywire. As previously alluded to, when a proto-oncogene is mutated, it becomes an abnormal oncogene, which will cause cells that normally would have committed cell suicide (apoptosis) not only to survive but to proliferate. [3]. Usually you need many of these mutated proto-onocogenes, along with several mutated tumor-suppressor genes (genes that normally suppress tumor activity) to act together to cause cancer. Several cancer drugs actually attack the proteins that are encoded by these oncogenes [2],[4],[5],[6].

Examples of proto-oncogenes are MYC, RAS, WNT, ERK and TRK. The MYC proto-oncogene, for example, is involved with Burkitt's lymphoma, which starts with a chromosomal translocation mutation (one part of the gene moves to another part of the gene or to a completely different gene). When this MYC proto-oncogene is now mutated by having a wrong sequence in its DNA, it will start forming a multitude of inaccurate protein enzymes and a loss of regulation, which causes the stem cell and its subsequent daughter cells to grow uncontrollably. These kind of translocation mutations are also associated with several types of leukemias.

Another important gene regulator are microRNAs (miRNAs), which are small (21-25) units of RNA that keep the bad oncogenes from doing their deadly activity [7]. These miRNAs can also get mutated, which leads them to start activating bad oncogenes instead of doing their normal job of deactivation [8]. As you can see, there is a lot of destructive activity occurring on many different fronts in the environment of inflammation that triggers cancer.

FREE RADICALS AND HOW THEY DAMAGE THE DNA

Many of us know that various viruses, chemicals, bad diets, radiation, smoking, drinking alcohol and chronic infection can cause cancer, but what is the basic mechanism behind these inducers of cancerous activity? What they all seem to have in common is massive overproduction of what are called free radicals.

So what is a free radical? To start with . . . most scientists agree that we all age primarily due to free-radical damage that accumulates in our bodies with time [9]. If you go back to your chemistry class, a free radical is any atom or molecule that has an unpaired electron in its outer shell [10]. And if you also think back to your chemistry class, you probably remember that electrons always like to be paired and not unpaired. Examples of free-radical molecules in the body are superoxide, hydrogen peroxide, hydroxyl radical, singlet oxygen, hydroperoxy radical, lipid peroxide radical, nitric oxide and peroxynitrite.

What happens in the normal processes of metabolism is that there are trillions of molecules that are released each day that do not have paired electrons. We call these "free radicals," and we know that they are extremely unstable because they need to have another electron for stability. Inside a cell, these free radicals can destroy most structures that they come in contact with through the process of oxidation. Did you ever leave a peeled apple out overnight and see what happens to it? It turns brown, right? That is oxidation in action. Same thing happens to your car over time . . . it rusts through the process of oxidation. Well, a similar process occurs in your body.

Inside your cells, these free radicals will go wherever they can to grab onto to another electron so that they can become stabilized.

Unfortunately, in the process, they will oxidize the fats found in our cell membranes, the proteins in our enzymes, and, most importantly, our DNA. When these free radicals collide with our fats, proteins and DNA, they can set off a chain reaction, because, as they grab onto to one electron from one molecule, the molecule that just had its electron stolen now becomes a free radical, and the process can go on and on until an antioxidant comes in to save the day.

This is where our cells' innate antioxidants come into play. The way an antioxidant works is that it can donate an electron to a free radical while at the same time maintain its stability. Normally, each cell has 3 important antioxidants called "superoxide dismutase," "catalase" and "glutathione peroxidase," which can immediately neutralize free radicals [11]. These 3 antioxidants squelch trillions of free radicals per day and can usually keep the free-radical damage in your body at negligible levels. Catalase, for example, has been shown to be able to neutralize 40 million free radicals in one second!

As we age, the number of these very important intracellular antioxidants decreases, and our ability to absorb antioxidants from our digestive systems also decreases, so with aging, we actually grow older at a faster rate. Have you ever noticed that someone going from 30 to 40 years of age doesn't seem to age as quickly as someone going from 60 to 70? A lot of it has to do with our increasing inability to squelch the free-radical activity going on constantly in our bodies.

That is why the science shows over and over again that those who eat a whole food, plant-based diet usually have approximately half the cancer risk as meat eaters. Plants have been shown, on average, to have 63X the antioxidant power when compared to animal products. That is also why the National Cancer Institute recommends 9 servings of fruits and vegetables for the prevention of cancer. The studies show over and over again that plants have protective effects against cancer. I will repeat again and again in this book the extreme importance of the 25,000+ phytonutrients in fruits, vegetables, legumes, whole grains, mushrooms, nuts and seeds that constantly and effectively battle the free-radical-oxidative rampage to our DNA.

What can we do to lessen the free-radical load to our bodies? Since we know that 95% of free-radical production comes from our metabolism, it would make sense that the less food we intake, the less free-radical production we would see. And this is exactly what we see when we perform animal studies. Animals that are put on high-caloric diets routinely have higher cancer rates and overall shorter life spans. So decreasing the amount of calories that we eat on a daily basis is one way to decrease our free-radical load and our cancer risk. Plant foods are calorically low and nutritionally high. Animal products are calorically high and nutritionally low. It would, therefore, make sense to increase the amount of plant foods and decrease the amount of animal products.

What are other ways to overload the system with free radicals? Smoking is definitely the worst. Some studies show that just one puff of a cigarette can create 8 hours of free-radical activity in our bodies. Most people don't realize that there are more than 4,000 toxic chemicals in cigarettes, such as benzene, formaldehyde, cyanide and cadmium that wreak havoc on our bodies. Because of the massive free-radical production from cigarettes, smokers live around 15 years less than non-smokers according to census reports. Smoking is one of the greatest testaments for how free radicals can cause massive destruction to our bodies and do it in a rapid fashion.

Extreme exercise is another way to create free-radical overload. Exercise for up to 45 minutes per day is excellent for our bodies, as I will detail later in this book, but when the exercise starts becoming too lengthy and overly strenuous, an overload of free radicals can appear. Recent studies have validated that extreme athletes with inadequate antioxidant intake have an increased risk of all diseases, including cancer.

Other factors that massively increase our free-radical production are high amounts of animal products, saturated fats and cholesterol, fried foods, excessive alcohol intake, too much UV radiation, many medications, toxins in our environment, chronic stress and lack of sleep. We also know that most chronic diseases are associated with extensive free-radical production. For example, the chronic diseases of diabetes, arthritis, lupus and most autoimmune diseases produce hefty amounts of free radicals [12]. And of course, cancer, the main interest of this book, creates an enormous quantity of free radicals itself, which helps perpetuate its deadly course. The more we learn about all of these diseases, the more we realize that it is their free-radical production that causes most of their complications and higher cancer risk.

In one study, published in the journal *Cancer*, investigating 15,626 cancer patients in one region of the United States, they found that 68.7% of these people had a chronic disease and that 32.6% had 2 chronic diseases [13]. The study also found that the cancers were diagnosed 12 years (on average) after the onset of the chronic disease, which insinuates that it is the daily onslaught of free-radical production from the chronic disease, damaging DNA day after day, that eventually leads to cancer. In smokers, during this same study, the time between onset of the chronic disease and cancer was even shorter, most likely due to the tremendous amount of additional free radicals generated from smoking.

We also know that the continual assault of free radicals to our DNA from the conventional cancer treatments can be the very thing that leads to relapses and a more-aggressive cancer. During an interview about myeloma relapse, Dr. Nikhil Munshi, a famous genomic-myeloma scientist, stated that, at the time of diagnosis, a myeloma patient probably has about 5,000 genetic mutations in his or her myeloma cells and that, at the time of relapse, there are about 12,000 mutations. We know that chemotherapy and radiation create a blitz of free-radical formation. So the thing that is killing the cancer is also the thing that is making the cancer more resistant to the treatment. This is why, during conventional cancer treatments, it is critical to eat as many plant foods as possible because of their high antioxidant content and free-radical protection. It is also important to ask your oncologist if you can start off with the lowest dose possible if you are eating a whole food, plant-based diet. If you are not eating whole food, plant-based, I would just go along with your oncologist's recommendation. This is a decision that you and your oncologist need to make together.

GENETIC ABILITY TO HANDLE FREE RADICALS

We have all seen or heard about someone who smoked 3 packs of cigarettes, drank a fifth of whiskey per day, and lived to be 100 years old. How can that be? Remember earlier in this chapter when we talked about the 3 basic antioxidants present in each cell? They are superoxide dismutase, catalase and glutathione peroxidase. Genetically, these are at high, medium or low levels in various individuals, thereby affecting a person's capability to neutralize free radicals. And a poorer ability to neutralize free radicals equals a greater chance of acquiring cancer.

There are no available tests to check the innate levels of these antioxidants in your cells. We only know that if you eat nutrient-dense, high-antioxidant plant foods, you can significantly reduce your chance of getting cancer, and, if you already have it, you can slow its growth [14]. Additionally, these antioxidants will protect your normal cells as you are undergoing conventional chemotherapy or radiation.

Besides the innate antioxidant levels in our cells, we are each endowed with certain abilities to genetically repair our mutated DNA, which is imperative to our very survival. Each day as we are bombarded with trillions of free radicals, there are repair enzymes that are continually repairing the translocation, deletion and insertion mutations that are occurring to our DNA. It is estimated that we receive 800+ incidents of DNA damage per hour, which equals 19,200+ per day! The vast majority of these mutations are repaired, but, if they are not repaired, the cell is instructed to commit cell suicide by healthy proto-oncogenes. It is the few that are not repaired and do not commit cell suicide that can lead to the growth of cancer. As we age, this ability to repair the damaged DNA decreases dramatically and is why, once we hit 65 years of age, the incidence of cancer starts to skyrocket. One of the reasons this happens is that the 100+ genes responsible for making the DNA-repair enzymes also get mutated.

Two of these DNA-repair genes many of you have probably heard of before. They are the breast cancer 1 (BRCA 1) and breast cancer 2 (BRCA 2) repair genes. Angelina Jolie had both breasts removed pro-phylactically because both of these DNA-repair genes were found to be mutated. When these are mutated, those individuals have a greater chance of developing breast cancer and is why these 2 mutations account for almost 50% of all premenopausal breast cancers [15]. And the more we learn about similar defects in DNA-repair mechanisms, the more we are learning that it is much more common than we originally suspected. So, one of the easiest proactive things that we can do is to eat as many high-antioxidant foods as possible to protect us from the DNA damage in the first place and to avoid activities that form free radicals, such as smoking, high amounts of saturated fat and cholesterol, fried foods, seared meats, eating too much food, UV-radiation overload, high stress levels, excessive alcohol consumption and toxins present in our environment.

Another area where we can get exposed to increased free-radical activity is from simple diagnostic tests like X-rays, CT scans and mam-mograms. Mammography screening, for example, is associated with a 19% overall reduction of breast cancer mortality [16]. However, some studies have shown a 3% per year increased risk of breast cancer from the mammogram itself. Recent radiologic studies have also provided compelling evidence that the low-energy X-rays used in mammography are approximately 4X—but possibly as much as 6X—more effective at causing DNA mutations than higher-energy X-rays [17]. Therefore, the net benefit of screening depends greatly on the baseline breast cancer risk. So the very people with the increased genetic risk of breast cancer are the very same people who are at greater risk of developing cancer from the mammogram itself . . . a dilemma that needs to be discussed thoroughly with your healthcare provider. We will discuss more in the chapter on radiation therapy.

INFLAMMATION

It was observed more than 150 years ago that all advanced tumors had the characteristics of an infectious boil. More recent studies have confirmed these observations, that even in the very early stages of cancer evolution, the hallmarks of intense inflammation are present [18]. It is becoming more and more obvious to researchers that this inflammatory microenvironment is a critical element for not only the initiation of cancers but also for its progression. It is also becoming evident that the mere activation of cellular proliferation—as was previously thought—is incapable of cancer development [19]. While scientists still accept the notion that multiple mutations are required for the creation of cancer, there is a tremendous amount of evidence that the inflammatory generation of high concentrations of free radicals are critical for tumor initiation, progression, invasion and metastasis.

As I alluded to before, individuals who have chronic diseases (with their accompanying chronic inflammation) such as diabetes, lupus, ulcerative colitis and rheumatoid arthritis have been shown to have much higher rates of cancer when compared to the general population [20]. We also know that many chronic bacterial and viral infections eventually lead to the formation of cancers. For instance, hepatitis B and C (liver cancer), schistosomiasis (bladder cancer), HPV virus (cervical cancer), Bovine leukemia virus (breast cancer), H. Pylori (stomach cancer) and Epstein-Barr virus (lymphoma) all have been linked to cancer formation.

Without inflammation, however, these viruses and bacteria cannot induce a malignancy [21,22,23].

Additionally, the inflammation created by certain toxic chemicals has been demonstrated in several studies to promote cancer in the laboratory setting with animals [24]. Conversely, anti-inflammatory drugs have been shown to slow and even reverse tumor growth in many different types of cancers. In fact, dexamethasone, which is an extremely potent anti-inflammatory drug, is a part of my myeloma treatment and is added to many chemotherapeutic regimens.

So how does inflammation play a critical role in every phase of tumor development? We know that inflammation creates instability of the genes, new-blood-vessel growth for cancer (angiogenesis), activation of cell proliferation, increase in tumor-inducing growth factors, the increase in receptors to accept those growth factors, massive increase in free radicals and the induction of pro-inflammatory enzymes. There is also increased activity of NFkB (a protein complex that regulates the immune response to infection) and STAT3 (a protein complex involved with cell growth and cell suicide) [25,26]. These all are active promoters of cancer growth.

We also know that the more intense the inflammation, the more aggressive and metastatic the cancer [27]. Conditions that can exacerbate inflammation are carcinogens, radiation, chemotherapy, a Standard American Diet, chronic stress, inadequate sleep and incessant viral or bacterial infections [28,29].

CELL SIGNALING

When cells are functioning normally, they are communicating with each other through what scientists call "gap-junction intracellular communication." When cells are communicating properly with one another, they keep each other's growth from getting out of control. If one cell starts to grow to quickly, its neighboring cells will send signals to quiet down this out-of-control activity through chemical messengers. The current consensus appears to be that the loss of this gap-junction intercellular communication is an early event in malignancy, with total gap-junction deterioration occurring in the event of metastasis [30].

Genetic mutations, once again, are the culprits in ruining this control system. Mutations to the DNA responsible for controlling these cell-signaling systems cause the cell to no longer produce enough chemical messengers to keep cell growth under control. Thankfully, there are some phytonutrients that we will learn about later in this book that can help restore proper cell signaling, which is critical to keeping cancer growth under control.

IRON AND COPPER

Because cancer cells are dividing at such a rapid rate, they have an enormous requirement for iron and copper. In fact, cancer has been demonstrated to steal iron and copper from an individual's normal iron stores to keep cancer-cell division perpetuating.

One of the first animal studies looking at iron utilization of cancer cells took human liver cancer cells, placed them into mice, and found that, if you gave them an iron-chelating agent (deferoxamine) to block iron uptake by the tumor, the cancer started to digress [31].

Since that time, there have been several studies using breast cancer cell lines that establish that deferoxamine has an anti-cancer effect [32,33,34]. In advanced liver cancer, it is currently being used to prevent cancer cell recurrence and to preserve liver function [35].

One of the primary sources of iron in the Western diet is meat. Meat has a highly absorbable form of iron called "heme iron." In one observational study, those who ate the most red meat had much higher cancer rates when compared to those who avoided meat. Besides high heme-iron content, other possible mechanistic factors proposed were nitrosamine compounds (NOCs), heterocyclic amines (HCAs), polycyclic aromatic hydrocarbons (PAHs), increased carcinogenic bile acids and infectious agents. This research project revealed cancer rates that were astonishingly high in the meat eaters. For example, lung cancer was 3X higher and, in smokers who ate red meat, 5X higher. A very interesting note is that individuals in this study who ate significant amounts of green and yellow vegetables, in addition to the red meat, had a 60% lower cancer rate compared to those who ate meat and did not eat green and yellow vegetables. This demonstrates the powerful effect of vegetables to inhibit cancer directly and also to chelate iron from the cancer cell.

It is also important to realize that, even though green vegetables have a concentration of iron quite similar to meat, only a small amount of the iron is absorbed from vegetables, whereas the majority of the iron from meat is absorbed. It is, therefore, critical that cancer patients keep their iron intake to a bare minimum by eating primarily a whole food, plant-based diet and definitely avoiding any iron supplements.

IGF-1

Another factor that is coming more and more into focus is the fact that IGF-1 (Insulin-like Growth Factor-1) levels seem to correlate with cancer rates as we age.

When we are born, IGF-1 is a growth hormone that is needed by the body to allow us to reach our full growth potential as an adult. The pituitary gland secretes human growth hormone (HGH), which then instructs the liver to produce IGF-1 (Insulin-like Growth Factor-1). If you look at an IGF-1 graph, you would see that those growth-hormone levels continue to rise until they peak at around our late teens. From that point forward, the IGF-1 levels gradually decline year after year.

I believe that this gradual lowering of IGF-1 is critical, because, as we age, we gradually accumulate a multitude of mutations that make us prone to cancer development. IGF-1 is a promoter of cell growth and replication. High IGF-1 levels in the presence of many mutated chromosomes is a deadly combination. So if you would simultaneously look at graphs of IGF-1 and mutation development . . . mutations would be going up and the IGF-1 would be going down. This inverse relationship occurs, in my view, for the preservation of life. In fact, many studies have shown a link between higher IGF-1 levels in adulthood and cancer [36,37,38].

Another interesting fact supporting the correlation between IGF-1 and cancer is that if you look at a very small group of dwarves in Ecuador, called "Laron dwarves," you will find a zero incidence of cancer. Interestingly, these dwarves have a genetic mutation that does not allow them to make IGF-1. In this group of people, no IGF-1 equals no cancer.

In regard to how IGF-1 levels relate to diet, there was one study conducted that looked at the levels of IGF-1 in meat eaters compared to vegans. The vegans' average IGF-1 level was 139 pmol/L, while the meat eaters averaged 201pmol/L. Other studies have shown this same correlation. This is a significant difference in IGF-1 levels and is another finding that should encourage those with cancer (and those who want to prevent it) to stick with eating a whole food, plant-based diet or, at the very least, significantly decrease their meat and dairy consumption.

Why does IGF-1 increase in meat eaters? There is no definitive answer, but it has been hypothesized that, when the liver is presented with a complete protein, like what is found in meat—but not in plants—the liver begins to manufacture IGF-1. The liver is sent a signal by the complete protein that growth is about to take place, and this signal starts the manufacture of this growth-promoting hormone. Interestingly, this signal does not occur with plant protein, because it is not a complete protein, due to the fact that an individual plant food will not contain all 9 essential amino acids.

METHIONINE

In a study published in 1974, it was demonstrated that cancer cells absolutely require the amino acid methionine for their very existence [39]. Normal cells, on the other hand, could exist just fine without the methionine.

This initial scientific paper went pretty much unnoticed for 20 years, until scientists discovered the actual biochemical defects that are present in cancer cells which make them methionine dependent [40]. What they found was that there is an extremely important part of cancer cell division, called the "S/G2 phase," that has an absolute requirement for methionine. Without enough methionine present, the cancer cell dies.

Another scientific paper published in 2001 in the *Journal of the American College of Nutrition* asked the question as to whether or not methionine restriction could increase the effectiveness of chemotherapy of advanced cancers [41]. They put the concept into practice by feeding patients a diet that was very low in methionine. And what kind of diet would that be? You guessed it . . . a whole food, plant-based diet. The foods highest in methionine are fish, with chicken being second, and after that eggs, red meat and dairy. The foods with the least amount of methionine are fruits, vegetables, whole grains, legumes, nuts and seeds.

What they found was that a methionine-restricted diet was safe and appeared to cause improvement in many biomarkers for cancer. One patient had a 25% decrease in the PSA marker for prostate cancer after only 12 weeks on the diet. Another patient with renal-cell cancer had radiological improvement from methionine restriction.

So with the known fact that methionine restriction can have positive effects on cancer progression, pharmaceutical companies have gone all in looking for drugs that deplete methionine. In one study a pharmaceutical company developed a methionine-depleting drug called "methioninase," which was found to have a complementary positive effect against cancer when combined with conventional chemotherapy [42].

A simpler strategy, without taking a drug that has toxic side effects, is to adopt a whole food, plant-based diet. You get the benefit of methionine restriction with all of the other advantages of the health-promoting phytonutrients.

mTOR ACTIVATION

It is generally accepted in the scientific community that, when you calorically restrict animals, they achieve significant life extension [43]. This may be due to fewer free radicals being produced by fewer oxidation reactions, but studies also point to caloric restriction's deactivation of a gene called the mTOR gene, which is in control of many of the cell-growth and replication processes of the body.

When you are young, mTOR promotes healthy growth. But after development, mTOR speeds up the aging process. If this gene is highly activated in older individuals with their normal increase in DNA mutations, this can cause the growth of cancer. In fact, it received its name mTOR (mammalian target of rapamycin) because an anti-rejection drug called "rapamycin" was found to kill the cancer "Kaposi's sarcoma" and seemed to do it by inhibiting mTOR. This drug, rapamycin, was thought to be the cancer cure everyone was looking for, but it was found to have too many negative side effects . . . one being immunosuppression. So, it never found its way into general cancer therapeutics.

As scientists began investigating how caloric restriction enhances longevity, they discovered that protein restriction can achieve the same effect and maybe do it even better. A comprehensive meta-analysis of dietary restriction found that decreased protein intake [44] had a better effect on longevity than did caloric restriction and was much easier for the participants to adequately carry through.

Additionally, protein restriction may even be more effective than full caloric restriction because it suppresses both mTOR and IGF-1[45]. Remember how IGF-1 stimulates cancer growth?

LEUCINE

Do all amino acids have the same stimulatory effect on mTOR? The answer is a resounding "No." The amino acid that shines as the king of mTOR activation is leucine [45]. So, where is leucine found in high concentrations? You guessed it . . . fish, chicken, beef, dairy and eggs. The least amount is found in fruits, vegetables, whole grains, legumes, nuts and seeds. Another reason to eat a whole food, plant-based diet.

DAIRY PRODUCTS

I highly recommend that you read the book *The China Study*, by Dr. T. Colin Campbell and his son, Dr. Thomas M. Campbell II. It was first published in the United States and has sold more than 1 million copies, making it one of the world's best-selling books on nutrition.

The book is based on the China-Cornell-Oxford Project, which took 20 years to complete. This was a massive undertaking investigating the health habits of people living in rural and urban China over a 20-year period. It was described by the *New York Times* as "The Grand Prix of epidemiology," conducted by the Chinese Academy of Preventive Medicine, Cornell University and the University of Oxford.

One of the first experiments that Dr. T. Colin Powell did was to utilize an aflatoxin that was known to cause liver cancer in mice. He added 20% casein (the primary protein in cow's milk) to the diet of the mice, along with the aflatoxin, and the liver cancer formed quickly and was aggressive. He then changed the casein concentration of the milk to 5%, and immediately the tumors started to regress. Back and forth he went, and the same result occurred. The higher the casein content . . . the more aggressive the tumors. The lower the concentration . . . the less aggressive the tumors. This astounding result is what prompted him to start the massive China study to observe how dairy, eggs, and meat products, including fish, affect the development of not only cancer, but of heart disease, stroke, diabetes, metabolic disease, hypertension and all-cause mortality.

This extensive study observed the mortality rates from cancer and other chronic diseases from 1973 to 1975 in 65 counties in China. The data was then correlated with 1983–1984 dietary surveys and blood work from 100 people in each county. The research was conducted in those counties because they had genetically similar populations that tended, over many generations, to live and eat the same way and in the same place. The study's conclusion was that the counties with highest consumption of animal-based foods in 1983–1984 were more likely to have higher death rates from "Western" diseases compared to 1973–1975, while the opposite was true for counties that ate more plant foods.

These results verified Dr. Colin T. Campbell's original casein study, which demonstrated that the casein in milk is a very strong promoter of cancer cell growth. Remember that cows grow 40X faster than humans. Therefore, as one would expect, there are a number of very powerful growth factors present in cow's milk that are not present in human breast milk.

The other important fact is that the human species is the only species that continues to drink milk after infancy, and we (to put the icing on the cake) drink the milk of a different species—milk that is loaded with casein, growth hormones and excessive protein, which stimulates IGF-1 and mTOR. It is also loaded with saturated fat and cholesterol, bovine leukemia virus and high pesticide levels, except for organic cow's skim milk.

I personally use organic almond and soy milk because it not only helps prevent cancer, but is also tasty. There are also other plant-milk products that you can try, such as oat milk, pea milk, cashew and coconut milk. I am, however, not a big fan of coconut milk because it is loaded with saturated fat.

REFINED SUGAR

Refined sugar is another source of cancer activation. Let's first go back to Dr. Otto Warburg's research from back in 1926 [46].

As you may remember from earlier in this chapter, cancer is initiated by a multitude of mutations to proto-oncogenes, which then become deadly oncogenes, which then, along with mutated tumor-suppression genes, allow the cancer to start, progress and metastasize. As tumors progress, they develop an oxygen-deficient (hypoxic) microenviroment that normal cells cannot thrive in. The cancer cells have, therefore, adapted their form of respiration to what is called "Warburg's aerobic glycolysis." I am going to call it "anaerobic glycolysis" for the remainder of this book because anaerobic means "without oxygen" and aerobic means "with oxygen."

Aerobic oxidative phosphorylation is the way that each of our normal cells respires, creating 36 ATP molecules (our energy molecules) from just one glucose molecule. A cancer cell's anaerobic glycolysis, on the other hand, creates only 2 ATP molecules from one glucose molecule. So you can see that cancer's form of respiration (which is essentially fermentation) is very crude and requires a great deal of sugar just to keep its flames burning.

For those of you who have received a PET (positive emission tomography) scan, this crude form of cancer respiration is taken advantage of so that cancers can be detected by scanning technology. First, a radioactive form of glucose is injected into a vein, and a scanner takes a picture of where the glucose is being used by the body. Cancer cells show up brighter in the picture because cancer needs an enormous quantity of sugar just to keep itself alive.

Because of the information initially brought to us by Dr. Otto Warburg and our subsequent research on sugar metabolism in cancer, it is critical to stay away from refined sugars and processed foods with high sugars. Cookies, cakes, refined breads, white rice, refined pasta and table sugar all fall into that category. Fruits, however, do not fall into that category because of the high fiber content that stops the quick release of glucose into the bloodstream. I personally drink a smoothie with blackberries, strawberries, raspberries, blueberries, banana, mango, apple, Kale, flaxseeds, chia seeds, dragon fruit powder, noni-fruit powder, guava/matcha powder, AMLA powder, and camucamu powder one hour before I get my monthly blood work, and I have never had a blood-sugar level above 85 mg/dl. To put that into perspective, with a glucose-tolerance test, doctors allow the blood sugar to go up to 140 mg/dl up to 4 hours after eating, and that is considered normal. A fasting blood sugar's highest allowed level is 100 mg/dl, which I am not even close to with my large fruit smoothie one hour before my lab work.

INDUCING ANGIOGENESIS
(NEW BLOOD VESSEL GROWTH)

Currently, it is believed by scientists that a tumor mass cannot exist at a volume greater than 0.5 mm^3 without enough blood supply. This is the volume of the tip of a ballpoint pen. This tells us that angiogenesis (the formation of new blood vessels) is critical for the spread and growth of cancer.

By age 70, cancers are detected in virtually everyone's thyroid gland. By age 50, approximately 50% of men have cancer detected in their prostate glands, and, by 40 years of age, 40% of women have detectable cancer cells in their breast tissue. However, these cancer cells stay dormant because they cannot grow beyond the 0.5 mm^3 in size due to inadequate blood supply and the immune system's normal ability to keep that growth in check.

I don't want to scare you—but to reach the size of the tip of a ballpoint pen, it requires about 90 million cancer cells. To try to survive past that size, the tumor cells will migrate toward existing vessels, a process known as "vessel co-option." Beyond this size, however, their metabolic requirements exceed the supply of nutrients obtained by passive diffusion from nearby vessels. To be able to grow past this pinpoint size, the tumor starts releasing a chemical called "VEGF" (vascular endothelial growth factor). This and other secreted angiogenic factors stimulate migration, proliferation and new blood vessel formation by endothelial cells (cells that form the inside of blood vessels) in adjacent, established blood vessels. The newly vascularized tumor no longer depends on diffusion of oxygen and nutrients from nearby vessels, which allows progressive tumor growth.

Thankfully, phytonutrients found in many of the foods that we eat can block this process of angiogenesis. Flavonoids are one class of phytochemicals that have been tested in the lab and in animals and have been validated to have potent anti-angiogenesis properties [47]. One of these, called "fisetin," is found in strawberries, grapes, peaches and apples and has been found to have a strong anti-angiogenesis effect against many cancers [48].

In a TED talk by Dr. William Li, entitled *Can We Eat to Starve Cancer?* he reviewed a list of both foods and generic drugs that have potent anti-angiogenesis properties. You should check out that amazing lecture on YouTube. Among the foods and drugs shown during this fascinating, scientifically based lecture were simvastatin, soy extract, artichokes, doxycycline, parsley, berries, garlic, grapes, cruciferous vegetables, citrus fruit, dexamethasone, glucosamine, pravastatin, lavender, green tea, glucosamine, turmeric, black tea, lenalidomide, catopril and Vitamin E.

BAD FATS

If you remember from a previous section on inflammation, cancer starts and proliferates in a microenvironment of inflammation. With this knowledge, we need to look at the 2 primary types of fats that we must ingest for survival. These are called essential fats, and there are 2 primary types . . . omega-6 fats and omega-3 fats.

Omega-6 fats are very inflammatory, while omega-3 fats are extremely anti-inflammatory. The ideal omega-6 to omega-3 ratio is believed to be somewhere between 1:1 and 4:1, depending on the author you read. These ratios may seem to be widely different, but when you realize that the average Western diet has a very pro-inflammatory ratio of anywhere between 20:1 and 40:1, depending upon the survey, there is huge room for improvement.

In the year 2000, the omega-6 to omega-3 ratio was anywhere from 2:1 to 4:1 in butter, pork, beef and eggs, but as these animals began being fed grains instead of being allowed to feed on natural grasses, this ratio dramatically changed. Also, many of the vegetable oils that many Westerners use for cooking have omega-6 to omega-3 ratios greater than 1,000:1. Furthermore, as foods have become more processed, the amount of omega-6 fats eaten by the average Westerner has skyrocketed. As a result, most Americans and Europeans eat an extremely inflammatory diet that leads to cancer and many of the chronic diseases that are rampant in Western society.

Therefore, it is important to eat as many foods that are high in omega-3 fats. These would be walnuts, edamame, flax seeds, chia seeds and fatty fish, such as salmon. Because I do espouse a whole food, plant-based diet, I do avoid fatty fish, but I do take a very purified fish oil supplement called *Omax3 Professional Strength Ultra-Purified*. I take 3 gel caps in the morning and 3 at night, which keeps my omega-6 to omega-3 ratio at around 2:1. A test by Quest Diagnostics can give you your omega-6 to omega-3 ratio . . . so ask your doctor to perform this inexpensive lab test.

Three capsules of *Omax3 Professional Strength Ultra-Purified* in the morning gives me 2,265 mg of EPA (eicosapentaenoic acid) omega-3 fat and 564 mg of DHA (docosahexaenoic acid). I also supplement with one *Omax Cognitive* in the morning, which gives me an extra boost of 800 mg of DHA, which some studies show has a strong anti-cancer effect. These supplements can be purchased on Amazon. I have done a lot of research on the company that makes this brand of fish oil supplement, and I am very confident that all toxins have been removed from the product. The gel caps also contain vitamin E, which keeps the oil from getting rancid, and they are completely enclosed in a blister pack.

Some proponents of eating strictly vegan say that you should get your omega-3 fatty acids only from plant sources. The form of omega-3s in flax seeds, chia seeds, walnuts and other plant sources is alpha-linolenic acid, which must must be converted in the body to the utilizable forms . . . EPA and DHA. The problem with the reliance on this conversion is that some people genetically do not carry out this biochemical reaction very well. Therefore, I recommend to those eating a strict whole food, plant-based diet to take the *Omax3* supplements and or an algae-based omega-3 supplement, if there is an aversion to all animal products.

CHOLESTEROL

Increasing evidence demonstrates that cholesterol and its carriers, the lipoproteins, play a role in the development of breast cancer and other cancers [49], and scientists are deriving compelling evidence from laboratory studies that cholesterol is capable of regulating the proliferation, migration and signaling pathways in breast cancer.

Studies also show that transformed cancer cells take up LDL (bad cholesterol) at higher rates and express more LDL receptors than normal cells. They have also shown that lipoproteins are capable of stimulating growth of cancer cells in vitro.

In the largest study to date published in the *International Journal of Cancer*, involving around 1.2 million participants and 79,000 cancers, there was demonstrated a causal relationship between cholesterol levels and the incidence of cancer with prostate, colon and breast being the greatest [50]. These individuals were observed for 14 years, until cancer diagnosis or death.

Another meta-analysis article in the journal *Science*, involving approximately 1.1 million participants and reviewing 95 cohort studies looked at the relationship of statin use and cancer incidence [51]. The collation of these 95 studies found that there was an association between statin use and decreased cancer incidence. This association remained consistent after being stratified by publication type, tumor location, study design, sample size, initiation of statins, disease stage, research country, follow-up duration, or research hospital involved.

In Jane McLelland's excellent book *How to Starve Cancer*, she describes 3 energy sources for cancer . . . glucose, cholesterol and glutamine. The general belief in the oncology community is that cancer uses only sugar through Warburg's anaerobic glycolysis, but when delving further into the scientific literature, you will find that cancer has an ability to shift between energy sources when one or the other is not available. And in some cancers, like prostate, colon and breast, they primarily utilize cholesterol as an energy source right from the beginning. That observation correlates with the above study showing that breast, prostate and colon cancer have a strong correlation to statin use . . . the greater the statin use, the less the cancer incidence.

In order to starve the cancer stem cell from all 3 angles, a whole food, plant-based diet is the perfect approach in my view. Because you are eating only complex carbs with high fiber content, the blood-sugar levels never get into abnormal range. The protein content is typically around 10% of total calories, which starves the glutamine-fermentation pathway, and the fat and cholesterol content is around 10%, which starves the cholesterol pathway.

Researchers have also found in recent years that estrogen-receptor-positive breast cancers can be stimulated even without estrogen being present

[52]. Researchers reported that a metabolite of cholesterol, 27-hydroxycholesterol (27HC), is a potent stimulator of the estrogen receptor. Cholesterol is converted into 27HC in the liver by the enzyme CYP27A1. Normally 27HC is metabolized by a different enzyme, but patients with very aggressive breast cancers make much less of this proper enzyme, so they accumulate higher levels of 27HC. So, get those cholesterol levels down in coordination with your doctor. Your goals should be a total cholesterol under 150, an LDL cholesterol under 80, and triglycerides under 80.

Some non-prescription supplements that can help you achieve your goal of lower cholesterol are ones that affect cholesterol synthesis. These are panthethine (400–1200 mg daily); Chinese red yeast (600–1200 mg per day); garlic standardized extract (1500–3000 mg daily) and AMLA (Indian Gooseberry) (500–1000 mg daily).

You can also lower cholesterol levels by inhibiting absorption from the gastrointestinal tract. This can be done by eating at least 30 grams of dietary fiber per day, increasing whole plant prebiotic food (feeds and proliferates probiotic bacteria), increasing plant sterols through a plant-strong diet, and increasing isoflavones from soy products.

Finally you can enhance cholesterol elimination with artichoke leaf; standardized extract: 500–1,000 mg daily.

DECREASED OXYGEN

Decreased oxygen, called "hypoxia," plays a significant role in cancer induction as well as maintenance and metastasis. With solid tumors, the decreased oxygen can be due to inflammation itself, from the individual's medical condition, or from the tumor outgrowing its blood supply. When there are low oxygen levels, there is an enzyme released called "HIF-1-α" (hypoxia-inducible factor 1-alpha) that increases the release of pro-inflammatory signaling chemicals (cytokines) and growth factors from tumor and immune cells.

One of the most important of these pro-inflammatory signaling chemicals (cytokines) is called "Tumor Necrosis Factor-alpha" (TNF-α), which causes the insertion of a signal-cell receptor called "CXCR4" into the membranes of tumor cells. Studies show that the more CXCR4 that is inserted into the tumor cell membrane . . . the more invasion and metastasis of cancers [53].

To simply summarize . . . tumors thrive and multiply in a low-oxygen environment. One of the best ways to increase oxygen levels in the tumor environment is to routinely exercise. In one study, it was demonstrated that there was a 90% decrease in "tumor hypoxia" (low oxygen) among rats that engaged in long-term, moderate-intensity treadmill exercise [54]. This means that the tumor-oxygen levels inside of the tumors increased by 90%, which cancer cells hate. We will discuss more about this in the chapter on the power of exercise.

ACIDIC MICROENVIRONMENT

Whether at the primary or metastatic site, an acidic pH seems to stimulate invasive behavior and increased survival [55,56]. An acidic pH has been shown to induce the expression and activity of a number of systems involved in the tumor-remodeling regions surrounding the tumors. These include enzymes called matrix metalloproteinases such as collagenase (MMP1) or gelatinases (MMP-2 or MMP-9) [57,58]. A metalloproteinase, like collagenase, for example, actually eats away the collagen in the areas surrounding the tumor so that it can progress to a new area. Furthermore, low pH can stimulate angiogenesis (new-blood-vessel growth) through induction of vascular endothelial growth factor (VEGF) or the cytokine interleukin-8 [59], or it may stimulate invasion simply by inducing cell suicide (apoptosis) in the surrounding normal cells [60])] and causing cancer-cell-suicide resistance [61].

Because of these complicated scientific facts, I try to keep my urine pH between 6.5 and 7.5 and use *Hydrion pH 5.5-8.0 Strips* (Amazon) to measure my urine pH throughout the day to keep me on track. I use an *Acid/Base Food Chart* (at the end of this book) to help me with this endeavor. When the pH is leaning more acidic, I eat more foods on the alkaline side of the chart. If I am leaning too alkaline, I eat more foods on the acidic side of the chart. Most people in the Western hemisphere have a very acidic urine pH due to the fact that high-protein foods are quite acidic and most plant foods are alkaline. And, as we know, most Westerners have high meat consumption and low plant consumption. Furthermore, as we age, our urine pH becomes more acidic due to various factors like diminished kidney function and pockets of chronic inflammation. When I test individuals, most are between 5.5 and 6.5. Therefore, very rarely will you be trying to acidify your urine pH. To further help me in this endeavor, I personally also use a water purifier that also alkalinizes. These can be purchased from *www.alkalinepgh.com*.

DECREASED IMMUNE FUNCTION

The immune-surveillance theory postulates that, at any one time, there are numerous cells (precancerous and malignant) that have the potential to become a tumor if not detected and destroyed by the immune system. Fortunately, in the presence of a healthy immune system, immune cells (white blood cells, natural killer cells and macrophages) protect us by detecting and eliminating those harmful cells as soon as they are identified.

Our immune system is also constantly protecting us from viruses that can cause cancer, such as Epstein-Barr virus, human papilloma virus, hepatitis B and C viruses, human herpes virus, human T-cell leukemia virus and bovine leukemia virus. If our immune system is weakened or suppressed, precancerous cells, cancer cells and cancer-causing viruses are able to wreak havoc and eventually lead to the development of an out-of-control cancer growth.

Also important to note is that cancer cells can sometimes trick our immune system by camouflaging themselves. They do this by covering themselves with camouflaging proteins that deceive immune cells into thinking that they are normal cells. This essentially makes these cancer cells undetectable to the immune system. Checkpoint inhibitors like pembrolizumab actually work by blocking these cloaking proteins, making the cancer detectable by the immune system.

Other times, the immune system is weakened and unable to do its job adequately, so cancer cells are missed and are able to grow. People who suffer from immunodeficiency diseases such as AIDS, or those who have received an organ transplant and must take lifelong immune-suppressing steroids to prevent organ rejection are at a very high risk for developing cancer because their immune defenses are compromised.

There are ways to keep our immune systems as healthy as possible. Studies show that one of the simplest and cost-free ways to do this is by exercising on a daily basis. Just 6 minutes of exercise increases immune activity by 50%. Many studies show that people who exercise experience fewer cancer relapses, cancer occurrences, and cancer deaths. These kind of studies will be reviewed in chapter 8 . . . "the power of exercise."

SUMMARY

As you can see, cancer development and progression is a very complex process. And trust me, I have just touched the tip of the iceberg. I could go on and on. My goal was to give you a foundation about how cancer starts and progresses. I know this chapter was quite technical at times, but the processes that cancer goes through are quite intricate and needed to be explained so that you have a good basic understanding. Once you have that knowledge, you will better understand how our bodies can fight back with the power of plants, targeted supplements, exercise, fasting, stress reduction and adequate sleep.

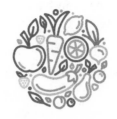

CHAPTER 2

Chemotherapy . . . The Pros and The Cons

Over the years cancer has become correlated with the word "chemotherapy." When the average person thinks of chemotherapy, their first thought is hair loss, nausea, vomiting, loss of energy and the possibility of a long, drawn-out, painful death. And although chemotherapy has definite benefits for certain cancers, it is my view that, at times, it is used at too high doses at the beginning of treatment. Also, anyone undergoing chemotherapy needs to discuss with their oncologist not only the benefits of the chemotherapy, but also the fact that chemotherapy itself causes secondary cancers through the creation of multiple mutations.

The other thing that cancer patients need to understand is that there is a big difference between cancer cure and cancer control. Most oncologists say that, if your cancer does not come back in 5 years, you are cured. It is my opinion and the opinion of many oncologists that 10 years should be called "a cure," and, even at that time frame, cancer stem cells are most likely lying in a dormant state. That is why this book is so important for those trying to prevent a relapse. Remember that approximately 70% of individuals with cancers who get into a remission will relapse.

You also need to ask your oncologist if he or she is trying to wipe out your cancer, trying only to control it, or attempting solely to relieve symptoms like pain. For example, my cancer, multiple myeloma, is considered incurable, so I knew from the very beginning of my treatment that the primary goal was to control the growth and shrink the cancer into a state of not progressing. In essence, my oncologist was treating it like a chronic disease. I also knew that the chemo drugs that I would be taking would cause mutations and that these mutations would likely cause my chemo drug to become resistant, at which time a new drug therapy would be initiated.

My wife, on the other hand, had Hodgkin's lymphoma at the age of 28 and understood from the very beginning of her treatment that this cancer could be wiped out by her chemo/radiation regimen, and the statistics were very high that it would not come back. Conversely, she was informed that, in 10–20 years, she could develop secondary cancers and possible heart, lung, and thyroid issues from the mutations that her high-dose chemotherapy and radiation would cause. In fact, 25 years after her treatment, she has developed heart-conduction problems from the radiation and chemotherapy that was administered long ago.

COMMON MISCONCEPTIONS

As I communicated in the last chapter, for many cancers, the survival rates have not budged a whole lot for many cancers since President Nixon's original declaration of war on cancer in 1971. However, the medical establishment makes it seem as if much progress has been made. As I also discussed, one of the primary reasons that it appears that treatments are improving for some cancers is that cancer is now being diagnosed at an earlier stage of the disease because of advanced technology. Therefore, this is giving the false impression that people are living longer due to their treatment.

Another common bit of misinformation is to compare high-dose versus lower-dose treatments and conclude that the high-dose treatments work better because more patients survive longer. The naked truth, however, is that patients are chosen into the high-dose groups because they are in better physical shape. If they are not in good physical condition, they will not be able to survive the higher-dose drug regimen. Furthermore, some patients in high-dose groups will have such horrible side effects that they will withdraw from the study. The result will be that only the healthiest patients (the very ones who would live longer even with no treatment) are the ones who will be left standing in the high-dose treatment group. This artificially makes the treatment look more effective than that of the low-dose group. The data, therefore, can create a misconception to the general public.

The bottom line is that the data can disguise the fact that some forms of chemotherapy and radiation may actually be causing some patients to die earlier. I am not saying that conventional chemotherapy and radiation are bad, because they definitely kill cancer cancer cells and are needed for most people with cancer, but there are certain types of patients who may actually do better with a whole food, plant-based diet combined with a targeted supplement program and lifestyle changes. We, however, will probably never know because there are no studies (and probably never will be) that compare chemotherapy and radiation treatments to other treatments, such as a plant-based diet/supplement/exercise/fasting/stress-reduction/sleep-enhancement program, surgical treatment alone, or no treatment at all. Also, studies never take into consideration the advancements in general medical care of the person with cancer. When all of these factors are taken into consideration, certain types of patients may well do better without chemotherapy, especially for cancers that have been shown to respond either poorly or not at all to conventional treatments.

PREVENTION OF RECURRENCE

If a tumor is fairly well localized and there is no evidence of invasion into local tissues, sometimes your oncologist will recommend chemotherapy and/or radiation to eliminate any stray cancer cells that might lie around the area. Several studies have shown that such adjunctive chemotherapy and/or radiation may reduce the incidence of tumor spread or recurrence. The problem with these studies is that the results have never been compared to those of a whole food, plant-based diet along with targeted supplements, exercise, stress-reduction and sleep-enhancement techniques. It is my opinion that this kind of approach may be as effective, and possibly even more effective, than chemotherapy or radiation when trying to avoid spread and recurrences in these types of situations. In fact, my friend Dr. Sally Lipsky, author of the book *Beyond Cancer*, chose a whole food, plant-based nutritional approach after her initial treatments for ovarian cancer and has been clean from ovarian cancer for more than 12 years. I also have an employee who had stage-4 ovarian cancer who took the same approach and is now 5 years post-treatment and living an amazing life.

NUTRITIONAL APPROACH WITH CHEMO

If you decide to use a whole food, plant-based diet/supplement/exercise/fasting/stress-reduction/sleep-enhancement program with your chemotherapy, I think that it is extremely important to start before the treatments begin. If you remember in the introduction of this book, I came across the book *How Not to Die* 2 months before

I was diagnosed with multiple myeloma. After reading the book, I immediately started eating a whole food, plant-based diet because the science was so overwhelming. When I look back, I consider coming across that book, at the time that I did, as one of the greatest blessings I have ever received in my life because it prepared my body for the diagnostic radiation and chemo drugs that were coming my way. And it has truly allowed me not only to survive, but to thrive through my treatments.

I feel strongly that a plant-based diet works best if started before the conventional treatments, but it will also be effective if started afterward. Regardless of when you start, a whole food, plant-based diet with a targeted supplement program will greatly enhance the effectiveness of the conventional therapy and reduce complications. In fact, a good nutritional plant-strong program, because of its high antioxidant levels, will also significantly decrease mutation formation instead of promoting it.

ONE WARNING . . . if you mention taking targeted supplements along with your whole food, plant-based diet, don't expect your oncologist to jump up with joy. I know, from the experience of attending medical school, that we doctors get almost zero education on nutrition, and the nutritional education we do get is on the level of a high school health class. In general, it has been demonstrated that high-quality, targeted supplements do not have a negative effect on cancer treatment. In fact, Dr. Keith Block's excellent meta-analysis of 965 studies, published in the *International Journal of Cancer*, looked at how antioxidant supplements affected cancer outcomes. What he discovered was a positive effect on treatment outcome and less damage to normal cells [1]. Also, patients were found in several of these studies to be better able to complete their chemotherapy at the recommended dose and did not need to have dose reductions because of complications or side effects. Another meta-analysis of 280 peer-reviewed studies came to the same conclusion, with the additional finding that many of the supplement groups had better final outcomes [2]. The only cancer drug that has been found to possibly be negatively affected by antioxidants is bortezomib, which we will discuss later in this book.

COMPLICATIONS OF CHEMOTHERAPY

As we have previously learned, many chemotherapeutic drugs destroy not only rapidly dividing cancer cells but also rapidly dividing normal cells. It is also important to note that many chemotherapeutic drugs can damage cells that do not divide, like the neurons in the nervous system. In addition, chemotherapy drugs are usually quite toxic to the liver cells, which play a critical role in metabolizing the toxic drugs being given to the cancer patient, but in also getting rid of the toxins released by the dying tumor cells. If the patient's nutritional status is poor at the time of their treatment, they will very likely incur toxic reactions, which can further impair their immune system. The more the immune system is suppressed, the greater the debilitation of the body and the more likely the treatment will fail. In addition, a person made toxic by these drugs will be more likely to suffer recurrences of the cancer. Regrettably, the nutritional considerations are ignored by many oncologists.

An additional fact to understand is that some chemotherapy agents are much more toxic than others. In general, the alkylating agents like melphalan are among the most toxic. More than 20 different chemotherapy drugs have been demonstrated to cause cancer in humans [3]. In another study, patients who survived ovarian cancer for one year and who took the drug melphalan were 100X more likely to develop non-lymphocytic leukemia or pre-leukemia than the patients who received no chemotherapy [4]. In general, it has been found that the risk gets higher with higher drug doses, longer treatment time and higher dose-intensity (more drug given over a short period of time).

Studies have shown that leukemia risk begins to rise about 2 years after treatment with alkylating agents, becomes highest after 5 to 10 years, and then declines.

COMBINING CHEMOTHERAPY

As with most toxic chemicals, when chemotherapy drugs are combined as a "cocktail," the total toxicity of the combined drugs will typically exceed the toxicities of the individual drugs added together. This is called synergy . . . 2 + 2 = 7. In my study of Dr. James Berenson, a myeloma specialist with the highest myeloma-survival rates in the country, I have found that one of the keys to his success is that he significantly lowers the dose of all the drugs when using combination therapy. This keeps the total toxicity to a minimum and improves the quality of life for his patients.

To get an idea of how toxic a combination regimen can be, let's take a look at a study that I was exposed to in Dr. Russell Blaylock's excellent book *Natural Strategies for Cancer Patients*. In the book, he described a study analyzing the drug combination called ICE (ifosfamide, carboplatin, and etoposide). In this study, the incidence of complications was found to be extraordinarily high, even for the lowest doses used [5]. For example, damage to the mouth mucous membranes and gastrointestinal tract receiving the low-dose combination was 67% and 39%, respectively. Fifty percent of patients receiving the moderate dose had neurotoxicity and lung damage. The high-dose patients had even higher toxicity, with 61% getting liver toxicity, 81% hearing deterioration, 70% kidney impairment, and 92% pulmonary damage. Especially disheartening was the finding that 94% of patients developed heart-muscle destruction, and the most horrifying was that 8% of the patients actually died from the treatment. And even more distressing than 8% of patients dying was the author's conclusion that the drug combination was well tolerated, with acceptable side effects and organ toxicity. How could this possibly be called "acceptable risk," especially with a 8% mortality rate? This, however, is very common thinking in the conventional cancer community.

Besides the synergistic toxicities, science exists that these chemotherapy combinations can sometimes cause cancers to grow and spread much quicker than would normally occur. In one study on relapsing breast cancer, described in Dr. Blaylock's book, it was shown that the women who received chemotherapy had advancement of their cancer much earlier than the women given just hormone treatment [6]. Additionally, the effectiveness of the treatments differed considerably, with 47% of the women treated with just hormone therapy showing a positive response versus only 23% of the chemotherapy group. The probability that chemotherapy makes tumors more invasive, impedes the immune system, and destroys vital organs was reviewed in the medical literature as far back as 1987 [7]. After this review, it is my impression that chemotherapy, in some cases, makes cancer more aggressive and more likely to metastasize.

TYPES OF CHEMOTHERAPY

We talked about chemotherapy in general. Now let's review some of the various chemotherapies used by oncologists and give you an idea about how they work.

Alkylating Agents

Alkylating agents work very similar to radiation and are called "cell cycle non-specific" because they can work on any part of the cell cycle and do their work by attaching to DNA at several points, which results in breakage of the DNA. Once enough DNA breaks occur, the cancer cell cannot survive. The problem with this mechanism of action is that the alkylating agent is also attaching to normal-cell DNA and causing DNA breaks there, too. Our hope is that our normal repair mechanisms can repair all of this DNA damage. But remember that most people who get cancer do not have the greatest DNA-repair mechanisms, so, much of the DNA damage goes uncorrected. This is one reason that alkylating agents have the highest incidence of secondary cancers after a variable latent period.

It is well known in the research community that alkylating agents can create cancer very quickly in research animals. And as I mentioned before, the longer the exposure and the stronger the dose, the greater the probability of these cancers developing. Besides cancers, these alkylating agents have also been shown to cause chronic degenerative diseases through the same mechanism of genetic damage to once-normal cells. This genetic damage also occurs to the DNA of the mitochondria, which are the energy-producing organelles inside of the cell. The genetic-repair mechanisms of mitochondria are very poor and might explain the poor energy levels of individuals receiving this type of chemo.

Below are the types of alkylating agents.

- Mustard gas derivatives: mechlorethamine, cyclophosphamide, chlorambucil, melphalan and ifosfamide
- Ethylenimines: thiotepa and hexamethylmelamine
- Alkylsulfonates: busulfan
- Hydrazines and Triazines: altretamine, procarbazine, dacarbazine and temozolomide
- Nitrosureas: carmustine, lomustine and streptozocin. Nitrosureas are unique because, unlike most types of chemotherapeutic treatments, they can cross the blood-brain barrier.
- Metal salts: carboplatin, cisplatin and oxaliplatin

Plant Alkaloids

Plant alkaloids are chemicals that are derived from certain types of plants. The vinca alkaloids are made from the periwinkle plant

Catharanthus rosea. The taxanes are developed from the bark of the Pacific Yew tree *Taxus.* The vinca alkaloids and taxanes are also known as anti-microtubule agents. They inhibit cell division by binding to a protein called "tubulin." This protein normally forms the microscopic strands that pull the chromosomes toward the new cell during cell division.

Below are plant alkaloids:

- Vinca alkaloids: vincristine, vinblastine, and vinorelbine
- Taxanes: paclitaxel and docetaxel

Topoisomerase Inhibitors

Toposiomerase inhibitors are a class of drugs that also interrupt cell division. Normally, when cells divide, their DNA strands are pulled apart. These DNA strands must be temporarily broken, however, so that other DNA strands can pass through. Special repair enzymes (toposiomerase 1 and 2) fix these temporary breaks so that all keeps functioning normally.

Topoisomerase inhibitors do not allow the toposiomerase enzyme to function properly, which leads to death of the cancer cell. Unfortunately, like all other chemotherapeutic drugs, it does the same thing in normal cells. Thankfully, not all normal cells are dividing when these drugs are given. The cells that do divide quickly (gastro-intestinal cells, hair follicles, skin cells) will be primarily affected by this class of chemo drugs, with the less actively dividing cells being somewhat spared.

The 2 basic types of topoisomerase inhibitors are the podophyllo-toxins and the *Camptothecan* analogs. The podophyllotoxins are derived from the "May Plant." *Camptothecan* analogs are derived from the Asian "Happy Tree" (*Camptotheca aciminata*). Notice that almost all of the aforementioned chemo drugs are derived from plants.

Below are topoisomerase inhibitors:

- Podophyllotoxins: etoposide, amsacrine, tenisopide and etoposide phosphate. Also called "topoisomerase 2 inhibitors."
- *Camptothecan* analogs: irinotecan and topotecan. Also called "topoisomerase 1 inhibitors."

Anti-tumor Antibiotics

Anti-tumor antibiotics are chemo drugs that started off as antibiotics but were discovered to be way too toxic. They kill cancer cells by creating large amounts of free radicals and are considered "cell-cycle specific" because they interfere with cell division at specific points in the process. These drugs are made from natural products produced by the species of the soil fungus *Streptomyces*.

There are several types of anti-tumor antibiotics:

- Anthracyclines: doxorubicin, danorubicin, epirubicin, mitoxantrone and idarubicin
- Chromomycins: dactinomycin and plicamycin
- Miscellaneous: mitomycin and bleomycin

Anti-metabolites

Anti-metabolites are types of chemo drugs that are very similar to normal substances within the cell. They imitate a major cellular metabolite, thereby interfering with the cancer-cell functioning. The problem, however, is that they also interfere with normal-cell functioning. Methotrexate is a good example of an anti-metabolite in that it closely resembles folate, but the body cannot use methotrexate at the specific point of cell division that folate would have been utilized. The cell, therefore, dies during that point of cell division. Anti-metabolites are named in accordance to the specific metabolite that they interfere with:

- Folate antagonist: methotrexate
- Pyrimidine antagonist: 5-flourouracil, foxuridine, cytarabine, capecitabine and gemcitabine
- Purine antagonist: 6-mercaptopurine and 6-thioguanine
- Adenosine deaminase inhibitor: cladribine, fludarabine, nelarabine and pentostatin

Immunotherapy

Cancer immunotherapy attempts to stimulate the immune system to destroy cancer. One of the oldest forms of immunotherapy is the use of the BCG vaccine, which was originally used to vaccinate against tuberculosis and was discovered later to be a treatment for bladder cancer [8].

Topical immunotherapy uses an immune-activating cream called "imiquimod," which produces a chemical called "interferon," which causes the patient's natural killer T-cells to destroy warts, actinic keratoses, basal-cell cancer, vaginal cancer, squamous-cell skin cancer, skin lymphoma, and even superficial malignant melanoma [9].

Immunomodulators

This is an array of various synthetic and natural preparations. The drugs in this class are used against multiple myeloma, myelodysplastic syndrome, and acute myeloid leukemia. They are:

- lenalidomide (the drug that I am presently taking)
- thalidomide
- pomalidomide
- apremilast

These drugs work on several fronts, from activating natural killer cells to inhibiting angiogenesis (new cancer blood-vessel growth), to directly killing the cancer cells by an unknown mechanism.

As with every single drug discussed in this section, the side effects with these immunomodulators can be significant, but not to the degree of alkylating agents and other chemo drugs. Some of the side effects include decreased energy, skin rashes, lowering of the blood counts, liver damage, lung clots, increased stroke and heart-attack risk, and mutations to a developing fetus. That is why, when I get my monthly lenalidomide from a specialty pharmacy, I must complete an exhaustive survey about my sexual activity before they will dispense the drug to my home.

Knowing that this drug is causing many mutations in my body makes me very diligent about sticking with a whole food, plant-based diet. I know that plants have 63X the antioxidant power compared to meat products. I also know that eating a whole food, plant-based diet is keeping me away from meat pesticides, bovine leukemia virus, growth hormones, estrogens, saturated fat and cholesterol. Multiple myeloma is known for the fact that a drug regimen will work for a given period of time, but almost always gives way to a relapse. And it is the accumulation of additional mutations to various cancer genes that allows the cancer to develop resistance and start continuing its deadly activity.

Checkpoint Inhibitors

As most of you know by this point in the book, our immune system protects us from disease by killing bacteria, viruses and early cancer cells. There are 2 primary type of immune cells . . . B-cells and T-cells. B-cells work primarily by making antibodies. T-cells actually engulf the invader.

As I revealed in the previous chapter, cancer cells can sometimes trick our immune system by camouflaging themselves. They do this by covering themselves with camouflaging proteins that deceive immune cells into thinking that they are normal cells. This essentially makes these cancer cells undetectable to the immune system. Checkpoint inhibitors actually work by blocking these cloaking proteins, making the cancer detectable by the immune system. Drugs that block checkpoint proteins are called "checkpoint inhibitors." They stop the proteins on the cancer cells from pushing the stop button. This turns the immune system back on, and the T-cells are able to find and attack the cancer cells.

The checkpoint inhibitors block different checkpoint proteins, including:

- CTLA-4 (cytotoxic T lymphocyte associated protein 4)
- PD-1 (programmed cell death protein 1)
- PD-L1 (programmed death ligand 1)
- CTLA-4 and PD-1 are found on T-cells. PD-L1 are on cancer cells.

PD-1 INHIBITORS include:

- nivolumab
- pembrolizumab. To find out if you can have pembrolizumab for non-small-cell lung cancer, you need to have your cancer cells tested. To have this PD-1 inhibitor for lung cancer, you need to have large amounts of the PD-L1 protein on your cancer cells. This is called "PD-L1 positive cancer."

This testing does not apply to all checkpoint inhibitors, so you need to ask your oncologist if this is for you.

Nivolumab and pembrolizumab are treatments for some people with:

- melanoma skin cancer
- Hodgkin's lymphoma
- non-small-cell lung cancer
- cancer of the urinary tract
- cancer of the kidney (renal pelvis)

CTLA-4 Inhibitors

⊚ Ipilimumab is the primary one in this category and is a treatment for advanced melanoma.

PD-L1 Inhibitors

⊚ Atezolizumab is a treatment for some people with lung cancer and urothelial cancers. It is also in clinical trials for other cancers, including breast cancer.

These drugs boost all the immune cells, not just the ones that target cancer, so the overactive T-cells can cause side effects like tiredness, feeling or being sick, itchy skin, skin rash, loss of appetite, diarrhea, breathlessness and a dry cough, caused by inflammation of the lungs. These drugs can also disrupt the normal working of the liver, kidneys and hormone making glands (such as the thyroid).

CAR T-Cell Therapy

Another type of immunotherapy that is getting a lot of attention is CAR T-Cell (Chimeric Antigen Receptor T-cell) therapy. At the time of this writing, it is FDA approved for B-cell non-Hodgkin's lymphoma and acute lymphoblastic leukemia, with many clinical trials going on for other blood cancers like the one I have, multiple myeloma.

With this fascinating technology, T-cells are removed from the patient's blood, and an artificial receptor (called a chimeric antigen receptor) is added to their surface. The receptor on these T-cells functions as a type of "heat-seeking missile" which allows the modified cells to home in on the exact cancer cells in question and produce chemicals that kill the cancer. Before infusing these cells back into the patient, they are cultured in a lab so that thousands of these modified T-cells are available. After infusion, these T-cells begin multiplying in the body as they attack their specific cancer.

At this point in time, the response rates have been very high in the cancers being treated, but 70–90% of patients experience something called a "cytokine storm," which is an extreme inflammatory reaction that can last 5–7 days. Early on in the clinical trials, this was sometimes deadly, but a rheumatoid arthritis drug called "tocilizumab" has been found to reverse the storm fairly quickly.

Another significant possible side effect that affects the brain is called "CRES" (CAR T-cell Related Encephalopathy Syndrome), which can occur at around 5 days after infusion and causes patients not to be able to speak at all for a few days. To say the least, this is very disheartening for patients and their families, but it typically lasts between 2 and 4 days and is completely reversible.

Miscellaneous Therapies

Several miscellaneous types of chemotherapy are the following:

⊚ Ribonucleotide reductase inhibitor: hydroxyurea
⊚ Adrenocortical steroid inhibitor: aminoglutethimide and metyrapone
⊚ Enzymes: asparaginase and pegaspargase
⊚ Retinoids: bexarotene, isotretinoin, tretinoin

Other than these aforementioned types of chemotherapy, many other types of chemo treatments exist, such as targeted therapy, monoclonal antibodies, proteosome inhibitors and hormone therapy.

CHEMOTHERAPY SIDE EFFECTS AND COMPLICATIONS

As most of you are well aware by now, chemotherapy has many possible side effects. I am going to briefly touch on the most common ones and give you some ideas on how to either prevent or better cope with them.

Fatigue

Fatigue is the most common complaint of cancer therapy. Patients describe fatigue as feeling tiredness, with no energy. Fatigue in cancer patients is so common that it has a variety of names, such as "cancer fatigue," "cancer-related fatigue," and "cancer treatment-related fatigue." Cancer-related fatigue tends to be different from fatigue in a healthy person. Typically, when a healthy person is tired out by their daily activities, their fatigue can be relieved by sleep and rest. Cancer-related fatigue is different in that it sometimes cannot be completely relieved by sleep and rest and may last for a long time. Fatigue generally decreases after chemotherapy, but patients may still feel some fatigue for months or even years after therapy ends.

Patients treated with chemotherapy usually feel the most fatigue in the days immediately after each treatment. Then the fatigue gradually decreases until the next treatment. The fatigue usually increases with each cycle, and some studies have shown that patients have the most severe fatigue about midway through the cycles of chemotherapy. Chemotherapy-induced fatigue may also be exacerbated by pain, depression, anxiety, lack of sleep and, very commonly, anemia.

The anemia is caused by almost all chemotherapy drugs that invariably have a depressive effect on bone-marrow stem cells. This causes an inadequate number of red blood cells, which are the oxygen-carrying cells. Therefore, the lower the red-blood-cell level, the lower the oxygen-carrying capacity, which makes the patient feel extremely tired. One of the ways that you can improve this anemia naturally is by eating plant foods that are higher in iron such as green leafy vegetables and beans. The other way is to get on a daily-exercise program. Exercise forces the bone marrow to make more stem cells, which, in turn, will increase the red-blood-cell count. Another method of increasing stem-cell activation is through a 5-day, fast-mimicking diet done periodically [10]. Prolon makes an excellent product that you can use intermittently. You can purchase the 5-day program at *prolonfmd.com.*

If these natural methods do not work, transfusions of red blood cells may be required. These always work to treat the anemia, but there are possible side effects, such as an allergic reaction, infection, graft-versus-host disease, immune-system changes and too much iron in the blood.

Another option for anemia that cannot be solved naturally is to administer drugs that cause the body to make more red blood cells. Two drugs used for this are epoetin alfa and darbepoetin alfa. These medications, however, may shorten survival time, increase the risk of serious heart problems, and cause some cancers to grow faster or relapse. So you need to have a serious discussion about the risks and benefits of these drugs with your doctor before undergoing this kind of treatment.

The bottom line is that poor nutrition is a major cause of fatigue for most cancer patients. That is why I stress over and over in this book that it is very important to start a whole food, plant-based diet/supplement program before treatment starts. When receiving chemotherapy, patients will often have a lower appetite, nausea and, sometimes, vomiting and diarrhea. This makes it difficult to eat food. The chemotherapy can also affect the ability of the gastrointestinal system to absorb nutrients. If you remember from earlier in this book, gastrointestinal cells divide very rapidly, so they are keenly affected by chemotherapy. If you are eating a typical Western diet, the amount of nutrients that you absorb when you do eat will be much less than if you are eating a plant-strong diet.

Nausea and Vomiting

Of all the side effects of chemotherapy, nausea and vomiting are the most feared by cancer patients. Oncologists tend to downplay this, claiming that we now have powerful anti-nausea drugs like ondanestron and granisetron. It, however, still affects a significantly large number of cancer patients. Nausea and vomiting fall into 2 basic categories in cancer patients: acute and delayed. Acute nausea or vomiting develops while the chemotherapy is being administered and usually subsides when it ends, whereas late symptoms can occur for months after the treatments have been completed. Ondanestron and granisetron work quite well for the acute type of sickness, but are not effective for the delayed symptoms. The main risk factors for developing nausea and vomiting with chemotherapy are being female, younger than 50 years of age, a history of motion or morning sickness and being an alcohol teetotaler.

It is important to note that chemotherapy-induced nausea and vomiting is caused in 2 ways. One way is to stimulate the nausea center of the brain, called the "chemoreceptor zone." The second way is by the inflammation of the gastrointestinal tract caused by the chemo. Both of these causes can be significantly reduced by following dietary guidelines and by using targeted supplements. Many phytonutrients have potent anti-inflammatory properties, which translates into patients on a nutritional program having less nausea. In regard to targeted supplements, there are several that soothe the stomach lining by increasing mucus production (something that is lost from chemotherapy). The one that I highly recommend is ginger root extract . . . *Ginger Root Max-V* made by Douglas Labs and available on Amazon. Not only will this supplement calm the stomach, but it will also improve your digestion and decrease bloating. Additionally, it has a powerful anti-cancer effect, which you will learn more about in the chapter on targeted supplements. Fennel powder, cumin extract and cinnamon have also been shown in some studies to have a positive effect against nausea.

When undergoing most chemotherapy regimens, not only are many of the gastrointestinal cells destroyed, but also many of the good probiotic bacteria that live in the gastrointestinal tract. These bacteria are critical to our immune function and overall good health. Some research papers are quoted as stating that up to 80% of our immune system resides in the gut. Therefore, because chemotherapy and antibiotics can destroy many of these good probiotic bacteria in our gut, it is critical to try to preserve these crucial organisms as if they were a precious gem. The best way to restore probiotic bacteria is through plant foods which cause proliferation of these health-promoting organisms. Another way is to take a probiotic supplement. The one I recommend is called **Multi-Probiotic 40 Billion** made by Douglas Labs and available on Amazon. Take 2 in the morning and 2 in the evening. Remember that, once you open the bottle, keep it refrigerated so that the bacteria remain intact.

In my view, a plant-strong diet, targeted supplementation and taking certain precautions is the best holistic way to avoid chemotherapy-related nausea and vomiting. I also think that drinking smoothies is a great way to get an abundance of phytonutrients and fiber while making it easy on your gastrointestinal tract. I recommend getting a high-quality Vitamix for this task.

The natural things that you can do to avoid nausea and vomiting is to:

- Avoid foods that are sweet, fried or fatty. In addition, cool foods may give off less bothersome odors.
- Cook and freeze meals in advance of treatment to avoid cooking when you're not feeling well, or have someone else cook for you.
- Try cool beverages, such as purified water, unsweetened fruit juices or tea. It may help to drink small amounts throughout the day, rather than larger amounts less frequently. I would also recommend avoiding drinking while eating.
- Avoid unpleasant smells. Pay attention to what smells trigger nausea for you, and limit your exposure to these unpleasant smells. Fresh air may help.

- Make yourself comfortable. Rest after eating, but don't lie flat for a couple of hours. Try wearing loose-fitting clothing and distracting yourself with other activities.
- Use relaxation techniques. Examples include meditation and deep breathing.
- Consider complementary therapies such as acupuncture and peppermint aromatherapy, which may help you feel better when used in combination with medications from your doctor. Tell your doctor if you're interested in trying these treatments. He or she may be able to recommend a practitioner who works with people undergoing cancer treatments.
- Avoid food additives like MSG and aspartame.
- Eat a whole food, plant-based diet. As I already stated, drinking smoothies is a great way to get an abundance of plant phytonutrients and fiber while making it easy on your gastrointestinal tract. By eating and drinking a diet composed mostly of fruits and vegetables, you will avoid many of the foods that activate nausea. The increased fiber will also restore and proliferate your good probiotic bacteria. Furthermore, many of the phytonutrients in plants, especially the flavonoids, will diminish inflammation, alkalinize your blood, and directly inhibit the factors known to stimulate nausea and vomiting. You will find that certain plant foods will tend to soothe your digestive tract more than others. Stick with those foods until the nausea is alleviated.

Food Aversion

A thing to be aware of with chemotherapy is the development of food aversions. This is a reaction to foods eaten just prior to the chemotherapy treatment. Some oncologists will tell you to stay away from the foods that you like before starting your chemotherapy treatments because after the treatment, you may not enjoy them. In some patients, even the thought of the food you once enjoyed can initiate a sense of nausea and vomiting. Food aversion can especially be a problem when it includes the whole food, plant-based foods that you need to keep you healthy in this battle against cancer. Taking nutritional supplements and eating a whole food, plant-based diet for a few weeks before you begin treatments may help prevent this reaction. The precautions described for nausea and vomiting also help minimize food aversions.

Sore Mouth and Throat

Many chemotherapy regimens, as well as radiation treatments to the head, neck, or upper-chest area, can cause sore, inflamed tissues of the mouth and throat. Malnutrition, due to an inability to swallow, is one of the main concerns with this problem along with dehydration and bleeding. The cells lining the mouth and esophagus divide very rapidly and thus are very sensitive to these treatments. Several steps should be taken to minimize the occurrence of this problem:

- Eat only foods that are slightly warm or cold.
- Stay away from spicy foods and drinks.
- Do not smoke, chew tobacco, or drink alcohol.
- When brushing your teeth, use a soft toothbrush, and brush gently. If you use dentures or other dental appliances, make sure you have a perfect fit so that they do not rub against your gums or the inside of your mouth.
- Avoid mouthwashes that contain alcohol, peroxide or fluoride.

To prevent infections, Dr. Blaylock, in his book *Natural Strategies for Cancer Patients*, recommends the use of a grapefruit-seed-extract mouthwash. He recommends mixing one drop of liquid-grape-seed extract **Nature's Plus Grape Seed Extract** (Amazon) with 3–4 oz. of water and stirring well with a spoon. Rinse and swish the mixture twice each day to help kill oral bacteria. Gradually increase the dose of the extract to no more than 3 drops as you adapt to the taste. Because grapefruit-seed extract is extremely bitter, you can add the natural sweetener stevia. Grapefruit-seed extract is a very powerful anti-bacterial, anti-fungal and anti-parasitic that alleviates inflamed tissues.

In almost all cases, the mouth and throat soreness will go away in 2–3 weeks following the completion of your treatments. The measures described above will allow you to deal with the displeasure much more effectively.

In regard to prevention, one of the things you can try is to swish ice chips or cold water around in your mouth for the first half-hour of your treatments. The cold limits the amount of the drug that reaches your mouth, reducing your risk of mouth sores.

Another way to possibly prevent the problem is to ask your doctor for a prescription for palifermin, which stimulates the growth of cells on the surface of your mouth. If the cells of your mouth recover quickly, you will be less likely to experience severe mouth sores. Palifermin is approved by the Food and Drug Administration for use in people with blood and bone-marrow cancers who receive bone-marrow transplants.

Hair Loss

Hair loss is one of the biggest fears when cancer patients find out they have cancer. It is the stigma that you are a sick person on the verge of death. The simple answer from most oncologists is to buy a wig. But there are better answers. The reason that chemotherapy treatments cause the hair to fall out is that hair cells divide very rapidly, just like cancer cells. A simple and effective way to help prevent this from happening is to use a strong dose of antioxidant vitamins during the treatments. I, personally, saw my wife keep her hair (although a little thinner) while going through a heavy quadruple chemotherapy regimen for Hodgkin's lymphoma using this approach. If you are trying to keep your hair, I would recommend my daily-maintenance regimen in Chapter 12. My regimen is very intense, so, at the very least, I would take the supplements that are asterisked. I would also recommend adding **Biotin** by Douglas Labs, available on Amazon, to your regimen because of its importance to hair growth. Take 8 mg in the morning and evening.

If you use antioxidant supplements during your treatment, you should also find that your hair will grow back faster and healthier than the hair of other patients. This is because the antioxidants protect the hair-follicle cells from being impaired by the treatments. And don't fear using antioxidants with your treatment, as this should have no negative effect on the final result of your treatments, as previously communicated.

The following are other steps you can take to reduce hair loss:

- Avoid astringent shampoos, especially those containing sodium lauryl sulfate.
- Dry your hair either naturally, with a fan, or with a blow-dryer set on low heat.
- Wash your hair every other day instead of doing it daily.

Another interesting step that you can take for hair-loss prevention is to use cold-cap therapy (CCT), which involves the use of special caps, frozen to a very cold temperature, and worn for a period of time before, during and after each intravenous chemotherapy session. Studies have shown that scalp cooling reduces the blood flow to the scalp and the metabolism of chemotherapy in the hair follicles. This result is less hair loss from chemotherapy.

Although there are many CCT systems on the market, the most commonly available cold-cap system in the U.S. is called the **Penguin Cold Cap**. This cap is filled with gel material that is cooled down to minus 22 degrees Fahrenheit. The caps have to be changed every 30 minutes during the chemotherapy session. Typically, the cap is worn 30–60 minutes before the start of each chemotherapy session. Then, every 30 minutes, throughout the chemotherapy infusion, a new frozen cap is placed on the head. The patient continues to reapply the frozen caps for 30 minutes (for up to 4 hours, depending on the chemotherapy regimen) after the chemotherapy infusion has been completed.

An analysis of 53 studies from 1995 through 2003, published in the *Annals of Oncology*, demonstrated an average success rate of 73% [11].

Blood Cell Depression

The depressed production of blood-forming cells in the bone marrow and other places of the body is an extremely common problem while undergoing chemotherapy. As we learned earlier, chemo treatments suppress the production of the most rapidly dividing cells, normal or cancerous, and increases their rate of death. The body's demand for red blood cells, immune cells, white blood cells, and platelets is so huge that these cells normally divide as rapidly as many cancerous tumors. Believe it or not, billions of these kinds of cells can be created every minute.

The immune cells are produced not only in the bone marrow, but also in the intestinal wall (Peyer's patches), lymph nodes and spleen and collectively are called the "hematopoietic system." When all of these cell types are depressed, the results can include an increased risk of infections, increased metastasis of the cancer, aberrant bleeding, and intense anemia. Almost all of the chemotherapeutic drugs cause varying degrees of depression of the blood-forming organs, with some affecting some cell types more than others. On occasion, the suppression can be so severe that the treatment is required to be stopped, either temporarily or permanently. Studies show that hematopoietic-system suppression is one of the most common reasons cancer patients need to discontinue their chemotherapy treatment. This is very important, since it has been shown that discontinuing chemotherapy treatment, even temporarily, or lowering the dose of the chemotherapy agent, is a common cause for failure of the treatment.

Several nutrients have shown an ability to protect the bone marrow and to stimulate a return of normal cells. Because of the enormous number of cells produced by the hematopoietic system, many nutrients are needed. Even though it is quite intense, I would try to follow as much of my daily-maintenance regimen in Chapter 12 as possible. At the very least, take the supplements asterisked in this chapter. Additionally, if you are having blood-cell depression, I would add *Methyl Folate L-5-MTHF* by Douglas Labs (Amazon) 2X per day because folate plays a major role in hematopoietic-cell reproduction. Large amounts of this vitamin are needed to produce these cells. I would also recommend adding *Niacinate 400* by Douglas Labs (Amazon) because this vitamin plays a major role in DNA synthesis, a process used by the blood cells to reproduce. The niacinamide in the *Niacinate 400* is the form of niacin used by the body. It is safer than niacin and does not cause the intense flushing common with plain niacin.

Take this in the morning and evening. Also make certain that you are taking the under-the-tongue *Methyl B12 Plus* by Douglas Labs (Amazon) daily while trying to up your blood count, as this vitamin plays a major role in blood-cell reproduction.

I also very strongly recommend exercising daily to enhance stem-cell production in the bone marrow. The more vigorous, the more you will stimulate red-blood-cell production from your bone marrow. Also, as you will learn in the chapter on "the power of exercise," it has many additional powerful anti-cancer benefits.

Heart Toxicity

Cardiac toxicity is a common cause of death for cancer patients, either during or following chemotherapy treatments. I know from a personal perspective that these side effects can occur even many years after treatment, as my wife developed heart-conduction problems 25 years after her Hodgkin's lymphoma treatments. It is a problem especially with doxorubicin, an antibiotic that is frequently used to treat various types of cancer, including my wife's Hodgkin's lymphoma. This drug can be associated with irreversible heart-muscle toxicity, which, in its worst form, can progress to fatal congestive heart failure. The horrifying aspect of this drug is that the heart failure may occur during treatment (acute toxicity) or even years later (delayed toxicity), as I described with my wife. A scary and sad fact is that delayed heart failure is most common in young children treated with the drug. This is because the drug poisons the heart muscle during the child's development, not allowing it to reach its required size in later life. According to PDR, as many as 40% of pediatric patients treated with doxorubicin will suffer from subclinical heart dysfunction, and 5–10% will develop overt congestive heart failure.

When used in combination with other chemotherapeutic drugs, doxorubicin can result in even higher incidences of heart damage due to the synergy effect that we discussed previously in this chapter. The amount of damage inflicted is also dose dependent—that is, the higher the dose of the drug, the greater the damage. The delayed type of heart damage is particularly frightful because it does not respond to the heart medications usually used to treat congestive heart failure. Biopsies of the heart muscle in such cases demonstrate swelling of the mitochondria, the main energy source in the heart-muscle cells. Other chemotherapeutic drugs that cause heart toxicity are herceptin, cyclophosphamide, taxol, cytarabine, daunomycin, actinomycin D and mitoxantrone.

In order to protect the heart during treatment, I would recommend following as much of my daily-maintenance regimen as possible. Again, at least take the asterisked supplements in Chapter 12. Of major importance, take the natural mixed vitamin E supplement *Tri-En-All 400* by Douglas Labs available on Amazon. I would take this 3X per day instead of my usual once per day while going through treatment. Several studies show that it can help prevent acute heart damage [12]. It, however, has shown no effectiveness against delayed damage.

In regard to delayed damage, the only supplement that has been shown to have protective effects [13] is coenzyme Q10 (*Ubiquinol-QH* by Douglas Labs on Amazon). That is why I would increase the dosage of *Ubiquinol-QH* from the normal 200 mg 2X per day to 4X per day starting one week before your treatment and continuing that for 3 weeks after the treatment. Once that 3-week period is finished, go to the normal 200 mg twice per day.

Another supplement to make sure you take is the fish oil supplement *Omax3 Professional Strength Ultra-Pure* on Amazon. Take 3 capsules in the morning and 3 in the evening before taking your other supplements. These essential omega-3 fatty acids have been found to protect against arrhythmias that may develop from the chemo-induced heart damage. In addition, they improve blood flow through the coronary arteries and enhance cardiac-muscle function. Ask your doctor to also check your omega-6 to omega-3 ratio on a test that can be done inexpensively through Quest Diagnostics. As I previously mentioned, this ratio should ideally be 2:1. Most Westerners have a ratio of 20:1 to 40:1 based on several studies.

Lung toxicity

The alkylating agent, busulfan, and the anti-tumor antibiotic, bleomycin, are major culprits in regard to lung toxicity. The anti-cancer effect of bleomycin is unique among anti-cancer agents and is thought to involve the production of single- and double-strand breaks in DNA by a complex of bleomycin with iron and oxygen molecules. The mechanism of bleomycin-induced lung injury is not entirely clear, but likely includes components of oxidative damage, relative deficiency of a needed deactivating enzyme called "bleomycin hydrolase," genetic susceptibility and a release of inflammatory cytokines.

For bleomycin, free-radical damage to the lung appears to be a critical component of lung injury, and antioxidants may ameliorate the process [14,15]. Depletion of iron with chelators that bind iron also reduces the toxicity of bleomycin both in vitro (on a petri dish or in a test tube) and in vivo (in animals and patients), probably secondary to decreased production of free radicals [16,17]. This goes along with what we learned about previously concerning high-heme-iron content in meat products and its correlation with high amounts of free-radical damage.

The major limitation of bleomycin and busulfan therapy is the potential for life-threatening interstitial pulmonary fibrosis in up to 10% of patients receiving the drugs [18]. Although it is not that common, if you get this acutely, it is very difficult to treat and is often fatal within 6 months. As with cardiac toxicity, this lung damage can also occur in a delayed fashion up to 10 years after the therapy, with average onset at 4 years.

My wife experienced this pulmonary fibrosis in an acute and a delayed fashion after she received bleomycin for her Hodgkin's lymphoma. So we know firsthand the life-saving effects, but also the debilitating effects of chemotherapy. You typically do not get away scot-free with any of these medications.

Regarding what to do to prevent this from happening, I, again, recommend following my daily-maintenance program in Chapter 12 as much as possible, with the asterisked supplements being the most critical to use. A plant-strong diet is, however, of foremost importance.

Liver damage

As we are learning in this book, in the complex world of cancer therapy, the administration of medications intentionally designed to kill cancer cells will inevitably cause negative consequences. The liver is the primary site of metabolism for many of these drugs, and this liver-drug interaction should be (but many times is not) accounted for while dosing chemotherapy. Preexisting liver disease can impair the process of recovery after injury, and in preparation for chemotherapy, oncologists almost always assess both liver function and potential liver involvement by the cancer [19].

The National Cancer Institute has published common toxicity criteria for adverse events, and liver toxicity is one of the primary focuses of this publication. In this publication, intense liver-function monitoring is advised for patients starting a new chemotherapy regimen. It remains controversial among oncologists how often liver testing should be performed and what constitutes liver dysfunction, but it is widely agreed that the serum liver enzyme activities of "alanine aminotransferase" (ALT), aspartate aminotransferase (AST), alkaline phosphatase (ALP), γ-glutamyltransferase (GGT) and total bilirubin should be closely watched. There is also agreement on the need for dose reduction for agents that are dependent upon liver metabolism for clearance from the circulation. The major chemotherapeutic agents in this group include methotrexate, sorafenib, dactinomycin, ifosfamide, gemcitabine, etoposide, irinotecan, procarbazine, 6-mercaptopurine, cytarabine, crizotinib, and cyclophosphamide. The chemotherapeutic agents that should be used with extreme caution in patient with pre-existing liver disease include the anthracyclines, taxanes, vinca alkaloids, temsirolimus, imatinib, axitinib, lapatinib, erlotinib, nilotinib, pazopanib, ponatinib, and ruxolitinib.

My recommendation for anyone receiving any kind of chemotherapy is to take milk thistle in the morning and the evening. I, personally, use *Milk Thistle Max-V* by Douglas Labs available on Amazon. This supplement contains milk thistle extract (250 mg of Silybum marianum) standardized to provide 200 mg of silymarin flavonoids and 100 mg of non-standardized milk thistle seed. Hundreds of studies demonstrate not only milk thistle's protective effect on the liver, but also its ability to kill cancer cells [20]. That is why it is a must supplement, in my view, for anyone undergoing chemotherapy.

Kidney damage

Nearly 10% of cancer patients treated with chemotherapy or newer targeted drugs may be hospitalized for serious kidney injury. In one study published in the *Journal of the National Cancer Institute*, involving roughly

163,000 patients who started chemotherapy for a new cancer diagnosis, 10,880 were hospitalized with serious kidney damage or for dialysis [21].

Since this is such a common problem with cancer patients, you need to do everything you can to avoid the problem. One of the most important things is to do is to maintain excellent hydration. The other important thing is to avoid drugs that can increase risk to the kidneys like ibuprofen and other non-steroidal anti-inflammatory drugs, certain heart medications and diuretics. In fact, in this study, older patients taking water pills or certain heart medications were at higher risk for serious kidney problems. If you are a cancer patient, you should contact your doctor immediately if you experience decreased urine output, swelling, nausea, vomiting, diarrhea, fatigue or confusion because these are often the early signs of kidney failure.

Also important to note is that cancer patients are more than twice as likely to develop acute kidney problems within the first 90 days of starting cancer treatment. Therefore, if you are a cancer patient, be diligent in the first 90 days of treatment to hydrate, and contact your doctor immediately if you have any of the aforementioned symptoms of early kidney failure. Vigilance is important because cancer patients who develop acute kidney injury during treatment do have reduced odds of survival.

In regard to a supplement, I use *Organic Dandelion Leaf and Root Tea* by Traditional Medicinals on Amazon before bedtime. Dandelion has been validated in an important animal study to have significant protective effects on the kidney [22]. Dandelion tea has also been shown to have the greatest antioxidant power compared to a variety of other well-known high-antioxidant teas.

Nerve damage (Neuropathy)
Chemotherapy-induced peripheral neuropathy (CIPN) affects the lives of up to 40% of cancer patients who receive chemotherapy.

Many times CIPN symptoms can be so bothersome that oncologists need to lower the treatment doses or stop treatment altogether. Most commonly, these CIPN-causing drugs cause symptoms (e.g., pain, burning, stabbing, numbness, tingling, temperature sensitivity) in the hands and feet. In more severe cases, these symptoms move up the arms and legs. It can make it difficult to perform normal day-to-day tasks like buttoning a shirt, sorting coins in a purse, or walking. In severe cases, patients can develop weakness of legs and leg cramps, numbness around your mouth area, constipation, pain during bowel movements, balance problems, hearing loss, jaw pain, trouble swallowing, and trouble passing urine.

The risk and severity of CIPN varies based on the individual drug, combinations of drugs, having received prior chemotherapy, your nutritional status, the duration and dose of your chemotherapy and genetic factors that predispose some individuals to more severe neuropathic symptoms. The drugs most common for causing CIPN are the platinum-based drugs, taxanes, such as paclitaxel, docetaxel, the vinca alkaloids, the podophyllotoxins, epothilones, thalidomide, lenalidomide, bortezomib, interferon, methotrexate, florouracil and cytarabine.

We don't know exactly what causes this peripheral neuropathy, but one proposed theory is that it can develop as a result of damage to the fatty covering of the nerves called the "myelin sheath." This likely occurs from free-radical production from the drugs themselves. Nerves with damaged myelin can't send signals properly. It is believed that numbness occurs when nerves are no longer transmitting a signal. Tingling happens if a false signal is sent. Pain is felt when the electrical information overloads your unprotected nerves. Other areas of the nerve that can be damaged are the microtubules, the dorsal root ganglia, the ion channels, the mitochondria and the small nerve fibers.

Regrettably, the pharmaceutical industry has not been able to develop a drug that has been proven to work well for CIPN. All the drugs we currently use to treat CIPN are actually commonly prescribed for use in other conditions (e.g., depression, pain, muscle spasms). Although these drugs have some effect on reducing CIPN severity, they are not that effective in most patients and often have untoward side effects.

The more commonly used conventional therapies to treat this neuropathy are antidepressants (e.g., duloxetine, venlafaxine, amitriptyline) for tingling and numbness, anti-convulsants (phenytoin, carbamazepine) for pain, muscle-relaxant (baclofen), analgesic (ketamine), steroids, lidocaine patches, narcotics for severe pain and cannabinoids.

The scientifically researched supplements that I recommend if you are receiving a drug with the potential of creating CIPN are:

Super R-Lipoic Acid 240 mg by Life Extension available on Amazon is one that you can try. R-lipoic acid (stabilized form of alpha-lipoic acid) is now a standard recommendation by The Harvard/Dana Farber Cancer Institute for patients receiving neuropathy-inducing drugs. To date, the evidence on the effectiveness of alpha-lipoic acid in neuropathy management is not 100% proven, but there is enough scientific evidence [23] for me to recommend it because peripheral neuropathy can be a horrific side effect of chemotherapy. Symptoms should start to improve in 4–6 weeks. There is some evidence that alpha-lipoic acid may have a negative effect on the proteosome-inhibitor drug, bortezomib. So make sure you first consult with your doctor. There is also one petri-dish study that indicated that alpha-lipoic acid may make myeloma cells more viable [24], so I personally do not take it.

Turmeric/Curcumin with Piperine by aSquared Nutrition on Amazon is a supplement that I take, not only for the fight against cancer, but for the protection against neuropathy. Studies show that it has a positive effect against diabetic peripheral neuropathy and may also have some effectiveness against CIPN. I take 5 capsules in the morning and 5 in the evening along with 5 tablets of ***Bioperine*** (piperine black-pepper extract) by Biosource on Amazon. A very important study published in the journal *Planta Medica* demonstrated that adding piperine to turmeric increases its bioavailability by 2,000% [25]. You should also ingest fat before taking turmeric. I, therefore, take 3 **Omax3 Professional Strength Ultra-Pure** fish-oil gel caps in the morning and 3 in the evening before taking all of my supplements.

Vitamin B6 (pyridoxine) may also help alleviate neuropathy. Clinical trials are underway to determine if vitamin B6 (50 mg, 3 times per day) is effective in preventing CIPN. To date, definitive evidence on the effectiveness of vitamin B6 in CIPN management is still not 100% known. The recommended dose is 50–100 mg per day. The multivitamin that I recommend for those not eating a whole food, plant-based diet is **Ultra Preventive X** by Douglas Labs on Amazon. If you take 4 in the morning, you will be getting 25 mg of B6 per day. I feel that when you are eating a whole food, plant-based diet you are getting enough B6. I, therefore, do not take a multivitamin. But if your diet is not very plant-strong, I would recommend taking the above-mentioned vegetable-based multivitamin.

Some studies suggest that vitamin B12 may also alleviate neuropathy. The natural form of B12 found in food is methylcobalamin, which appears to be the most effective form to protect our nerves. All individuals eating a whole food, plant-based diet should be taking B12 anyway. I personally use **Methyl B12 Plus** by Douglas Labs on Amazon. I take one sublingually daily. This supplement supplies 1,000 mcg of B12 and 400 mg of folate.

A I stated previously, you should take your **Omax3 Professional Strength Ultra-Pure** fish oil supplement so that you can achieve an omega-6 to omega-3 essential-fatty-acid ratio near the 2:1 range. Remember that these essential fatty acids can't be made by our body (they must come from your diet) and are important components of our cellular membranes, including the protective nerve-sheath covering (myelin). It is almost impossible in our Western diet (which is typically very low in EPA and DHA) to consume a high enough amount of these fatty acids to repair and protect your nerves from CIPN. Taking a high-quality omega-3 fatty-acid supplement like *Omax3 Professional Strength Ultra-Pure* is, therefore, strongly recommended. As I formerly discussed, certain vegetables, nuts, and seeds also have an omega-3 fatty acid called "alpha-linolenic acid" (ALA), but this fatty acid is not in the 2 forms (EPA and DHA) that our body uses. ALA can be converted in our body to EPA and DHA, but this conversion is not very efficient in some people. Most nutritional experts agree that consuming foods or supplements containing EPA and DHA are superior to those containing just the ALA form. Some studies show that EPA and DHA may be able to protect against CIPN when taken during chemotherapy [26].

The final supplement that I recommend for the prevention of neuropathy is *Tri-En-All 400* by Douglas Labs on Amazon. This is a natural mixed vitamin E supplement, which means that it contains d-alpha, beta, gamma and delta tocopherols along with 4 health-promoting tocotrienols. In 2 good double-blind scientific studies looking at vitamin E and its effects on cisplatin-induced peripheral neuropathy, vitamin E had a significant preventive effect [27,28].

CHEMOTHERAPY RESISTANCE

Chemotherapy resistance occurs when cancers that have been responding to a therapy suddenly start growing. In other words, the cancer cells have figured out a way to escape the mechanism of action of the chemotherapy drug or regimen. You may hear statements like "the cancer chemotherapy failed." When this occurs, the drug or the drug regimen needs to be changed.

There are several possible reasons for chemotherapy resistance. The science shows that one of the primary reason for this happening is that some of the cells that are not killed by the chemotherapy have their

DNA mutated and then become resistant to the drug. Once they multiply, these new cancer cells may be even more resistant and aggressive compared to the original cancer cells.

Another cause of resistance is something we call "gene amplification." In this process, a cancer cell produces hundreds of copies of a particular gene. This gene then triggers an overproduction of a protein that renders the anti-cancer drug ineffective.

Cancer cells also start to develop an adaptation mechanism that actually pumps the drug out of the cell as fast as it is going in, by using a molecule called "p-glycoprotein." They also can develop resistance by establishing the ability to stop the protein that transports the drug across the cell wall to get into the cell. Another way that these defiant cancer cells develop resistance is by learning how to repair the DNA breaks caused by some anti-cancer drugs.

Furthermore, cancer cells can develop a mechanism that inactivates the drug. Much research is underway to investigate ways of reducing or preventing chemotherapy resistance. In the section on herbs, phytonutrients and supplements, I will show you many studies that are demonstrating that many natural phytonutrients have an ability to decrease chemotherapy resistance.

The development of drug resistance is one reason that drugs are often given in combination. It is thought by oncologists that this may reduce the incidence of developing resistance to any one drug. It has been found that, if a cancer becomes resistant to one drug or group of drugs, it is more likely that the cancer may become resistant to other drugs. This is why many oncologists think that it is important to select the best possible treatment protocol first. In other words, when treating cancer, one should use the best weapon when there is the smallest possibility of chemotherapy resistance.

The idea of hitting a cancer from multiple angles is also my approach to using many different herbs, phytonutrients and supplements. If you look at my daily regimen at the end of this book, you will see that I take more than 30 varied supplements to attack this predator on as many fronts as possible. I also eat as many different types of fruits, vegetables, whole grains, legumes, mushrooms, nuts and seeds as possible.

SUMMARY

As you can see from reading this chapter, cancer is a relentless enemy that needs to be attacked on many different fronts. In my opinion, a whole food, plant-based diet should, ideally, be started a month before therapy, but if this cannot be accomplished beforehand, it certainly should be incorporated during treatment. A plant-strong diet will not, by itself, defeat cancer, but it will provide a high level of antioxidants that will help your body destroy the cancer while protecting you from the toxic aftermath of the treatment itself. Exercise, fasting, stress reduction and adequate sleep are additional adjuncts that we will be discussing extensively in the remainder of this book. These will give you the added power to not only defeat the cancer, but to protect you from the many adverse effects of conventional chemotherapy.

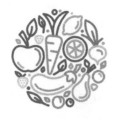

CHAPTER 3

Radiation Therapy . . .
The Pros and The Cons

Most cancer patients, when they first learn that they need radiation treatments, are usually struck with anxiety because they have heard that radiation causes a multitude of problems, such as burns, nausea and vomiting, hair loss, and even additional cancer. Their worries are justified and for good reason. Authorities in the field of radiology and radiation do not even agree on the safety of diagnostic X-rays, which involve much lower doses of radiation than radiation therapy. Today, many oncologists recommend that their patients undergo radiation treatments following surgery or chemotherapy just as an insurance policy so that the cancer won't come back. To me, this is not always the best idea. Despite the fact that we have many good ways to figure out who should have postoperative radiation and who shouldn't, we are not using many of these evaluation tools for some cancer patients. What's even more disconcerting is that many of the side effects and complications associated with radiation treatments can be averted simply by using what we know about certain radio-protectant phytonutrients. Yes, we can avoid many of the complications associated with radiation treatments, including the production of new cancers, by changing to a whole food, plant-based diet and using targeted nutritional supplements.

A History of Radiotherapy

The history of radiation therapy can be traced back to experiments performed soon after the discovery of X-rays in 1895. It was observed very quickly that exposure to radiation produced burns to the skin. After this was observed, doctors began using radiation to treat growths and lesions produced by skin diseases such as basal-cell carcinomas [1]. After it was also observed that radiation killed bacteria, it began being used as an additive to medical treatments for tuberculosis and other bacterial infections [2].

When these treatments ventured away from diagnostics to therapeutics, many problems started to arise. It soon became recognized that X-ray particles could not only kill cancer cells, but also cause cancer. In fact, if you look at the biography of Marie Curie, you will see that she and her scientific partner (and daughter) died of leukemia caused by their repeated exposure to radium. Also, in the early 1900s, radiologists used the skin of their arms to test the strength of radiation from their radiotherapy machines, looking for a dose that would produce a pink reaction (erythema) that looked like sunburn. They called this the "erythema dose," and this was considered an estimate of the proper daily dose of radiation. It's no surprise that many of them developed leukemia from regularly exposing themselves to radiation.

As the strength of X-ray machines was increased, more and more strategies were developed to treat cancer. In the 1930s, high-intensity X-rays were utilized to treat patients with inoperable breast cancer. Even after using extremely high dosages of radiation, later examinations of the breasts on these women revealed surviving cancer cells. Therefore, these early tries at using radiation treatments before surgical removal of breast cancers were short lived because of the discouraging results and plethora of complications.

During the 1950s and 1960s, radiation after surgery was used in breast cancer patients, but since it resulted in little benefit and a multitude of complications, it was used only occasionally. Later studies indicated that using radiation only on the lymph nodes surrounding the cancer did reduce recurrence. Over time, the precision of the technology has been greatly improved.

During the last quarter of the 20th century, radiation physics made it possible to aim radiation more accurately. Conformal radiation therapy (CRT) uses CT images and very specialized computers to create a map of the the location of a cancer in 3 dimensions.

Another form of radiation therapy, called "intensity-modulated radiation therapy" (IMRT), is like CRT, but, in addition to targeting photon beams from many different directions, the strength of the beams can be fine-tuned. This gives the radiation oncologist more control in lowering the radiation reaching normal tissue while delivering a high dose to the cancer.

A similar technique, called "conformal proton-beam radiation therapy," uses proton beams instead of X-rays. Protons are parts of atoms that cause less destruction to the normal tissues that they pass through, but are very effective in killing cells at the end of their path. This means that proton-beam radiation can deliver more radiation to the cancer while possibly reducing damage to nearby normal tissues.

Stereotactic radiosurgery is another method which uses a linear accelerator, or special machines such as the "Gamma Knife" or "CyberKnife" that can deliver a large, precise radiation dose to a small tumor. These are primarily used for brain tumors.

Intra-operative radiation therapy (IORT) is a treatment method that targets radiation during surgery. The radiation is aimed at the cancer or to the nearby tissues after the cancer has been surgically removed. It's more commonly used in abdominal or pelvic cancers and in cancers that tend to recur. IORT minimizes the amount of tissue that's exposed to radiation, because normal tissues can be moved out of the way during surgery and shielded, allowing a higher dose of radiation to the cancer.

An area of evolving research is the development of what are called "radiosensitizers." These are substances that make cancer more sensitive to radiation. The goal of research into these substances is to create agents that will allow the radiation to more easily destroy the tumor without affecting normal tissues.

As you can see, all the goals of the most recent advancements in radiation therapy have been to limit the amount of damage to normal cells surrounding the cancer while still killing the cancer.

Unforeseen injuries

Even with all of these recent innovations, the major problem with radiotherapy for cancer is that it still impairs the normal cells surrounding the cancer. The sad part is that the negative effects of this peripheral radiation damage is not always immediate. Significant delayed damage is usually recognized years later, due to the fact that radiation's negative effects are accumulative. It may take many years for the complications to become evident.

In fact, the resulting complication may not appear for as long as 10–20 years following the radiation exposure. Some cells are more prone to this malignant transformation than others. For instance, bone-marrow cells are more likely to undergo malignant transformation and to do so sooner than lung cells. This is because bone-marrow-blood cells divide more quickly, which makes them more prone to DNA damage. In addition, people with inadequate ability to repair their DNA are more likely to develop cancer following radiation exposure than are those with normal genetic-repair mechanisms. These individuals also have cancers that emerge much earlier. When radiation treatments are combined with chemotherapy, the combination makes cancers crop up even earlier after exposure.

Another adverse effect of radiation that can happen years after the treatments is to end up with something called "radionecrosis" (death of tissue secondary to radiation therapy). This delayed radionecrosis can occur following radiation to the brain, spinal cord or jawbone region. This radiation ingress may have occurred intentionally (during the treatment of a brain, spinal cord or mouth cancer) or unintentionally (when the nervous-system structures or jawbone are in the line of fire). This dead nervous or bone tissue will usually heal with time, but there will be permanent damage to the affected areas.

It is also important to note that radiation can essentially cause damage anywhere in the body where it has been used to treat cancer. For instance, radiation to the urinary bladder can cause pain, incontinence and bleeding which is called "hemorrhagic cystitis." Radiation proctitis or enteritis can occur when there is radiation to the area of the lower gastrointestinal tract. This can cause pain, incontinence, spasms, diarrhea and bleeding. Additional radiation injuries in this area can lead to fistula formation or wounds directly connected to the bowel. Delayed radiation injury to other soft-tissue locations can cause permanent wounds, pain and nerve deficits. Radiation has even been discovered to cause premature atherosclerosis in arteries in the line of fire.

Antioxidants for Protection

Studies have shown that the risk of developing damage to tissues can be greatly reduced simply by giving the patient targeted antioxidants during the treatment and for several months after. The tissue damage occurs because of free-radical damage precipitated by the radiation, so antioxidants are a logical antidote. In fact, the FDA recently approved a very potent antioxidant intravenous drug called "ethiofos" for use during radiation and chemotherapy to protect normal tissues from their damaging effects. The FDA approval was based on an extensive review of the data, which found no reduction in the efficacy of radiation therapy or chemotherapy when the ethiofos was given intravenously during treatments. They also found that the normal cells were protected compared to the control group.

What is so interesting is that the majority of oncologists will tell patients not to take any antioxidants for fear that the treatments will not work as well. But the studies that I have extensively reviewed and discuss in the chapter on targeted supplements demonstrate the opposite. The results are usually just as good, with less damage to the normal cells and with fewer side effects and complications. So, on the one hand, some oncologists are telling their patients not to consume any weak antioxidants such as vitamin E, C, and green tea, but on the other hand, they will administer an FDA-approved, man-made antioxidant, given through an IV, with way more potency.

In regard to the scientific literature's 2 cents regarding this topic, an already referenced meta-analysis of 280 peer-reviewed in vitro and in vivo studies performed since the 1970s, including 50 human studies involving 8,521 patients, 5,081 of whom were given nutrients, has revealed that non-prescription antioxidants and other nutrients do not interfere with therapeutic modalities for cancer. Furthermore, they enhanced the killing effect of therapeutic modalities for cancer, decreased their side effects, and protected normal tissue. In 15 human studies, 3,738 patients who took non-prescription antioxidants and other nutrients actually had increased survival [3]. In a future chapter on dispelling common myths, I will again discuss Dr. Keith Block's meta-analysis of more than 965 articles on this topic that came to the same conclusion [4]. The only drug that may be affected by antioxidants is bortezomib, which we will discuss later in this book.

Radiation Exposure of Diagnostic Studies

Another problem that no one ever talks about is the carefree combining of diagnostic X-rays with radiation therapy. It is important to note that radiation's harmful effects are accumulative when administered over time. A good example is what happens with lung cancer. Before you have your surgery, you typically receive several CT scans, at least one series of chest X-rays, a radioactive bone scan, and several other diagnostic X-rays . . . and all within a short period of time. When all of this radiation is added together, these diagnostic studies calculate to a significant dose of radiation. Finally you receive your radiation treatments, which are then followed up by more radiologic diagnostic studies with the equivalent radiation dose of several hundred chest X-rays.

Just to give you an idea of equivalent radiation of diagnostic radiologic procedures, let's take a look at the radiation exposure of some different tests and daily activities. Radiation exposure is measured in micro-sieverts (uSv):

- A flight from Sydney to LA is 40 uSv.
- A chest X-ray is 60 uSv.
- A mammogram is 400 uSv.
- A head CT scan is 2,000 uSv.
- A chest CT scan is 6,000 uSv.

Those CT scans emit a lot of radiation exposure! That is why I advise cancer patients to try to limit their radiation exposure. Far too often, I will have cancer patients tell me that they are having a little back pain so they want to get a PET scan to make sure it's not cancer. The bottom line is . . . the more DNA mutations caused by any kind of radiation exposure, the greater the chance for the tumor to develop resistance to treatment, which ends up in relapse. And even with this knowledge, it is not uncommon for chest CT scans to be repeated every 3–4 months in cases of lung tumors. Therefore, the cumulative dose of radiation for the average cancer patient, adding up all of the diagnostic X-rays and radiation, is incredibly high. I personally have rejected the suggestion by my oncologist to have a PET scan for a routine follow-up. My question was, "How is this going to change my treatment?" It wasn't going to change anything, so why expose myself to unneeded radiation?

Mammograms

Of particular concern and something I briefly alluded to before is the woman who has had yearly mammograms for 5–10 years before her cancer is diagnosed. The accumulative radiation exposure to both of her breasts, even before diagnosis, can be quite substantial. We know that in cancer-prone women, the risk of breast cancer in the non-diagnosed breast is already higher (even without the radiation exposure), because these women typically have defective DNA-repair mechanisms. Add the accumulative radiation to the undiagnosed breast, and the chances of breast cancer in that breast increase strikingly. Women are rarely, if ever, told this. Most women tremble at the thought of getting their yearly mammogram because of the memory of having their breasts squashed during the study. The radiological technologist, in an attempt to get the best pictures possible, will often compress the breasts as flat as possible, which often brings tears to the woman's eyes. Regrettably, the pain and embarrassment are not the least of her worries..

We are now realizing that the pressure on the breast is so high during a mammogram that, if a cancer is present, spreading it to areas beyond the original tumor is a possibility. Also, doctors are starting to recognize that some patients have higher sensitivity than others to radiation exposure. For example, patients who have a chronic disease, such as diabetes, have normal cells lying outside the cancer that are much more susceptible to the effects of radiation than are the cells of a normal person. Older patients are also at greater risk, as are those who have been administered chemotherapy before or during their radiotherapy. Poor nutrition also dramatically elevates a person's vulnerability to radiation injury. Nutritional deficiencies, even of a single nutrient, can also put patients at increased risk.

An alternative is to ask your doctor for an MRI which does not emit unwanted radiation and does not require extreme pressure to the breast tissue. Nowadays, almost all radiologists are trained in reading an MRI for the detection of breast cancer. The negative is that an MRI costs about $1,000 versus $100 for a mammogram. Ultrasounds and thermograms can also be used to diagnose breast cancer, but ultrasounds can't pick up small cancers, and thermograms are only 60% to 70% accurate in finding lesions.

Radiation and Nutrition

The cells most susceptible to radiation are the cells lining the gastrointes-tinal tract, the cells of the bone marrow, lymph system, spleen, and hair follicles. This is because these cells are all rapidly dividing, which makes them more easily damaged by radiation. Other factors that increase the risk of radiation injury are age (very young or very old), smoking, illicit drug use, chronic disease, low intake of fruits and vegetables, high intake of meat and other sources of heme iron, chronic stress, chemotherapy, impaired DNA-repair system and extreme athletic exertion.

During gastrointestinal radiation treatments, you can end up with an inability to absorb nutrients because of severe inflammation of the bowel wall with resulting bloody, mucus-filled stools. Radiation dam-age to these cells can significantly transform the body's ability to absorb foods, vitamins, and minerals, which can lead to significant malnutrition, despite a healthy diet. The simple fact is . . . if food cannot be properly digested and absorbed, a healthy diet is not going to help much. This problem becomes even more evident when chemotherapy is combined with radiation. This combination therapy can kill off the good probiotic bacteria in the colon, which can result in an overgrowth of harmful microorganisms. When the gut is severely damaged, these harmful pathogens enter the bloodstream, with significant negative consequences to the immune system.

In severe cases of radiation injury to the gastrointestinal tract, the inner lining of the intestine can be damaged to the point that it can culminate in intense abdominal pain, cramping and bloody diarrhea. Fortunately, these complications can be subdued by taking targeted supplements that I will be recommending in a later chapter. Again, I feel that it is very important to start eating a whole food, plant-based diet and taking targeted supplements at least several weeks before beginning your chemotherapy or radiation treatments. The diet and nutrients are still effective during treatment; however, when you start late, you will not get their full protection. In addition, it is much more difficult to repair a damaged gut than to prevent the problem in the first place. It is also important to note that plant phytonutrients act one way with normal cells and in a diametrically opposite way with cancer cells . . . making the cancer cells more sensitive to the radiation and the normal cells more resistant.

A Carotenoid Study

In Dr. Russell Blaylock's book *Natural Strategies for Cancer Patients*, he presented an interesting carotenoid study that nicely displayed the power of antioxidants to protect normal tissue from radiation damage. In this study, the researchers implanted mice with tumor cells [5]. Initially, the study established that a carotenoid-rich diet could significantly improve the survival rate of normal mice exposed to whole-body radiation as compared to mice on a regular diet. On average, the mice consuming the carotenoid-rich diet lived 4X longer than the control mice, who were consuming a regular diet. They then treated the tumor-infested mice with an extravagantly high dose of radiation to the area of cancer growth. The mice on the high-carotenoid diet with radiation exhibited much greater tumor-killing capability compared to those on a regular diet. But what was very surprising was that the mice eating high levels of carotenoids with radiation had all of their tumors regress completely. Conversely, the tumors in the regular-diet group also had tumor regression, but with eventual tumor relapse. All of the mice in the regular-diet group were dead within a year of the radiation treatment. Even more surprising to the scientists was that the mice eating the carotenoid-rich diet barely had any of their surrounding normal cells affected. Conversely, the normal cells surrounding the tumors of the control group without high carotene levels were strikingly damaged by the radiation.

You may have heard in the past that there was a study that demonstrated that beta-carotene supplementation can actually cause lung cancer. This population study was published in the *Journal of Epidemiology* and found that the long-term use of beta-carotene caused an increase in lung cancer. It also found that the use of retinol and lutein supplements for 4 years or longer was associated with increases of lung cancer by 52% and 102%, respectively.

This study has been highly refuted as an extremely flawed study by many reliable sources who have analyzed it. Many who have critiqued this observational study feel that reliance on questionnaire data asking for supplement usage going back 10 years is an exceptionally poor way to gather data. Reacting to the study, Professor Hans Konrad Biesalski, from the Institute of Biological Chemistry and Nutrition at the University of Hohenheim, stated, "It is hardly conceivable that the subjects were able to remember accurately enough in which sequence, how frequently, and in what composition they had taken products containing micronutrients in the previous 4 to 10 years. The validity of the questionnaires used and, above all, the conclusions drawn from them, are, therefore, questionable." He went on to say, "For the first time, it is not the absolute dose that increases the risk of lung cancer, but the length of time of use. This is not surprising since recall of dosages is surely even more dubious than recall of preparations. However, it is the consideration of intake in the more distant past based solely on memory which represents an essential weakness of the VITAL study." He added, "Numerous epidemiological studies confirm a preventive effect for lung cancer from a balanced, carotenoid- and vitamin-rich diet. Clearly, micronutrients alone cannot compensate the consequences of harmful behavior such as smoking." It was also noted that the number of incidents of lung cancer cases in the study was not great enough to stratify the effect of antioxidant effects on non-smokers.

In regard to supplementation use, a different study of 1,129 non-small-cell lung cancer performed at the Mayo Clinic found that vitamin/mineral supplement users had much higher survival rates compared to non-vitamin/mineral users. The median survival was 4.3 years versus 2.0 years for vitamin/mineral users and non-users, respectively [6].

In my extensive review of the literature, it can be generally stated that observational studies such as the beta-carotene study discussed above are not very accurate. Randomized, controlled double-blind studies give much better and more accurate results. To date there have been only 9 of these randomized studies looking at the long-term relationship between synthetic-beta-carotene and synthetic-vitamin-E (d-alpha tocopherol) supplementation and the prevention of cancer [7,8,9,10,11,12,13,14,15]. Five revealed no difference in cancer rates, 2 demonstrated improvement in the supplemented group and 2 demonstrated a higher cancer rate.

Two problems with all 9 of these studies is that a single and synthetic vitamin was used in each of these studies . . . synthetic-beta-carotene and synthetic-vitamin-E (d-alpha tocopherol). You will see in the chapter on targeted supplements that I recommend a mixed-carotenoid supplement and a mixed-vitamin-E supplement. The vitamin E supplement (*Tri-En-All 400* by Douglas Labs on Amazon) consists of not only d-alpha tocopherol, but also beta, gamma and delta tocopherol and the 4 tocotrienals naturally present in vitamin E. This is the way vitamin E exists in nature and the way it should be recommended in patients, because it has been found to be much more effective and safe in its natural form.

Also, in regard to beta-carotene, there is evidence that using beta-carotene with the many other carotenoids in algae and plants is more effective and safe than using beta-carotene alone. So far, more than 40 carotenoids have been identified in the human diet. The most dominant forms against cancer have been found to be the canthaxanthins, beta-carotene, alpha-carotene, lutein and lycopene. This is why I recommend that if you are going to take a beta-carotene supplement, it is best to use carotenoid mixtures from the *Dunaliella salina* algae. These carotenoid phytonutrients work much better in concert than alone. That is why I take a daily supplement called **Full Spectrum Carotene** by Source Naturals on Amazon. I personally take one gel cap in the morning. Because carotenoids are fat soluble, it is also critical to take your purified **Omax3 Professional Strength Ultra-Pure** fish oil capsules before ingesting your **Full Spectrum Carotene**. If not done, the carotenoids will not be absorbed and utilized by the body. Later in the book, you will be receiving information on a slew of other effective, highly studied supplements that you can add to your daily regimen.

Remember, however, that supplements should not be taken in place of a whole food, plant-based diet. And remember to eat 9 varied plant foods per day for cancer prevention and eat at least 12 varied plant foods per day if you are actively fighting cancer. Cancer is an incredibly multifaceted disease that depends on disorders of oxidative damage, inflammation, hyperglycemia, a weakened immune system, stress hormones, genetics abnormalities and a network of other cellular mechanisms that have gone awry. Thinking that you can protect someone from this incredibly formidable disease by giving a single vitamin is totally absurd. Both preventing and fighting cancer, therefore, demands a full-scale assault on an array of cancer-causing lifestyle patterns.

Turmeric

Another way to protect the normal cells from radiation, while giving an additional boost in cancer-killing effectiveness, is to use supplements that block the cyclooxygenase 2 (COX-2) enzyme. COX-2 is a special enzyme that creates inflammation in the body, and, as we have already learned in this book, cancer loves and thrives in an inflammatory environment. All arthritis drugs, called "nonsteroidal anti-inflammatory drugs" (NSAIDs), block this enzyme.

Another important effect of blocking the COX-2 enzyme is to protect normal cells against radiation damage. This has been shown using such arthritis drugs as indomethacin [16]. Many of the plant flavonoids, such as curcumin, quercetin, hesperidin, and kaempferol, also powerfully inhibit this enzyme from functioning properly. Of special interest is turmeric's most potent phytonutrient . . . curcumin. Not only does curcumin block the COX-2 enzyme, offering radiation protection, but it also strongly inhibits the growth, invasion, and metastasis of many cancers. This is truly a targeted therapy, with a major bonus of simultaneously protecting normal cells.

This is why turmeric is the one supplement I tell cancer patients to take if they are on a strict budget. I personally use a called product *Turmeric Curcumin with Piperine* made by aSquared Nutrition that can be purchased on Amazon. I like this product because it is primarily the whole root instead of just curcumin. Some studies show that the other 300+ phytonutrients such as the tumerones and zingerones in the turmeric may be more effective than just the one phytonutrient . . . curcumin. I also recommend taking 4 grams in the morning and 4 grams at night, which is the equivalent of 5 capsules in the morning and 5 at night. Make sure you take 3 *Omax3 Professional Strength Ultra-Pure* fish oil supplements and 5 tablets of *Bioperine* by Biosource (Amazon) before taking your turmeric. The 50 mg of piperine (black-pepper extract) will significantly increase the bioavailability of your turmeric. As previously mentioned, one study showed that piperine caused a 2,000% improvement in curcumin bioavailability [17].

Resveratrol

Resveratrol, found in grapes, peanuts and pomegranates, has been found to make cancer more susceptible to radiation treatments. This is called "radiation sensitization." In a study conducted at the University of Missouri, melanoma cells became more susceptible to radiation when given resveratrol prior to treatment. When treated with resveratrol alone, 44% of the cancer cells underwent cell suicide [18]. I use a supplement called *Methylated Resveratrol Plus* made by Douglas Labs and sold on Amazon. I take one in the morning and one at night.

Other supplements that give protection to the normal cells during radiation while not affecting the end result are garlic, melatonin, selenium, alpha-lipoic acid, beta-1,3-glucan and many other flavonoids. These and others will be discussed in the chapter on targeted supplements.

For now, just realize that the prodigious amount of science irrefutably demonstrates that an antioxidant-rich, whole food, plant-based diet is an impressive protection for normal cells being exposed to radiation and is an potent inhibitor of cancer growth. Notice I used the word "inhibitor" and not the word "eradicator." From the science thus far, it appears that a whole food, plant-based diet primarily suppresses cancer's growth . . . thus causing cancer to stay in an inert state. And remember that, when cancer is in a dormant state, it cannot harm you.

SUMMARY

Most cancer patients fear their radiation treatments because of the stories they have heard from other people about extreme fatigue, nausea and vomiting, hair loss, and numerous other horrible complications. Thankfully, most of these complications can be subdued without sacrificing the effectiveness of the conventional treatments. In fact, as we have seen, nutritional supplements and a whole food, plant-based diet can actually enhance the effectiveness of the treatments, making a true cure more probable. Cancer patients I speak with who are following this kind of a regimen tell me that they feel much better after beginning their nutritional program. They have significantly more energy, little or no nausea, better endurance, improved mood, and significant improvement in their symptoms, including pain. Pain can be a horrific problem for patients with bone metastasis. This metastatic pain can improve once they are on a whole food, plant-based diet and a targeted supplement program. As we will see in the next several chapters, the fear expressed by some oncologists that nutritional supplements can interfere with the conventional treatments or even make cancers grow faster is not generally supported in the scientific literature and denies patients a powerful weapon in beating back this horrific disease called "cancer."

PART TWO

PART TWO

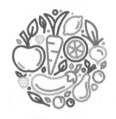

CHAPTER 4

The 5 Natural and Plant-Based Ways to Prevent, Survive and Thrive with Cancer

I n this brief chapter, I will give you an overview of the 5 scientifically proven natural ways to prevent, survive, and thrive with cancer.

In chapter 5, I will review the *Common Myths* that I frequently encounter with patients and individuals attending my lectures or reading my posts. I am certain that you have some of the same questions and concerns. Read through them, and, if you have questions about these common myths, send them to my email address at *info@naturalinsightsintocancer.com*, and I will try answer them. Also, if there are other common myths that you want me to discuss in the second edition of this book, let me know. I would love to address them.

In chapter 6, on *The Power of a Whole Food, Plant-Based Diet*, I will examine the scientific literature which points out consistently that cultures that eat a whole food, plant-strong diet, along with exercise and a robust social network live anywhere from 10 to 15 years longer that Western populations eating a standard Western diet of high meat, dairy and processed foods. They also have much lower cancer risks. For example, in an earlier mentioned Oxford University study of 60,000+ patients followed over 12 years, vegetarians had half the blood-cancer risk as compared to meat eaters. In an even larger Harvard study of 545,000+ individuals followed over 10 years, the research group reached the same result, which prompted an accompanying editorial in the AMA's *Archives of Internal Medicine* to recommend a worldwide reduction in meat consumption.

In the book *The Blue Zones*, the author, Dan Buettner, examined the 5 regions of the world that live the longest. The general theme of all 5 regions is that they eat primarily fruits, vegetables, whole grains, legumes, mushrooms, nuts and seeds, and very few animal products. The Okinawa people, for example, ingest only 2% of their diet in animal products in the form of fish. Loma Linda, another Blue Zone, is the home of the Seventh Day Adventists, who are vegetarian, exercise daily, are very religious and have strong social community. The average woman in Loma Linda lives to the age of 90. An average Western woman, on the other hand, will live to be 75–78, depending on the country. There is power in the 25,000+ phytonutrients in plants.

In chapter 7, I will discuss *The Power of Targeted Supplements*. In that chapter, I will plow through the many supplements that are available on the market such as freeze-dried plants, herbs, phytonutrients, vitamins and minerals. This is an area of much confusion. As you will see in this chapter, one of the common questions that cancer patients ask their oncologist is whether or not they can take any antioxidants. I will clear this up with a multitude of studies that show that antioxidants generally do not interfere with chemotherapeutic and radiation-therapy results but do protect the normal tissue from peripheral damage. I will go through the targeted supplements that I personally take. I take only supplements that I have thoroughly reviewed in the scientific literature. So when I make a recommendation, I am actually using that recommendation, not just throwing it out there for you to take without any intensive research.

I must warn you, I take an enormous number of supplements, which can be quite expensive. I will try to prioritize them for you so that you can buy the ones that are going to give you the most bang for your buck. *Turmeric Curcumin with Piperine*, for example, is the one supplement that all people, cancer patients or not, need to incorporate into their daily regimen. It can be purchased on Amazon very inexpensively, and this herb has thousands of studies in the scientific literature backing up its effects against cancer and a multitude of other diseases.

During chapter 8, I will review *The Power of Exercise*. This is one area that frustrates me as a physician because I know about the tremendous benefits to not only the body but to the mind. Unfortunately, I find that most people are just too lazy to do it. If its benefits came in a pill form, everyone in the world would be taking it.

As I was starting my bike ride yesterday, I noticed as I was going up the first steep hill of my ride, I was feeling very uncomfortable inside. This feeling comes when you are not getting enough oxygen. At this point in your exercise, your body converts to a fermentation type of energy production, which produces lactic acid. Once I continue my ride onto more-level surfaces, my normal energy-production pathway of oxidation phosphorylation takes over (does not produce lactic acid), making that uncomfortable feeling go away. And as I proceed through the ride, I start feeling a high, because endorphins (narcotic-like substances) begin being released from my brain, making it highly enjoyable. Unfortunately, many people don't get to the endorphin stage and remember only the uncomfortable lactic-acid stage, so they refuse to ever do it again.

You will learn that only 6 minutes of aerobic exercise can stimulate natural killer-cell activity against cancer by 50%. That is enormous! That is why every morning, I start my day with a 15-minute resistance-band routine, while thinking to myself how I am kicking myeloma's ass. Later in the day, I do a half-hour bike ride, or, if it is raining (it does it a lot in Pittsburgh), I do my elliptical while watching television.

I will go through the various studies showing you the incredible reductions in cancer-relapse rates of patients who exercise. You will get motivated to add this change to your life. On top of this, you will likely have a much-better mood. I will go through the studies that show that exercise works as well as anti-depressants in many cases. The icing on the cake is that, with all of these above-mentioned benefits, you also end up looking better. It doesn't get much better than that!

In chapter 8, I will also briefly discuss the benefits of fasting and detoxification. I personally feel that, if you are doing anything more than a daily intermittent fast, you should do it under the supervision of a physician. I personally fast for around 15–16 hours per day. I eat my last food at around 8:00 PM and do my next day smoothie between 11:00 AM and noon. I will review the research on why I do that on a daily basis and will give a recommendation of where to go if you want to do a very long water fast to jump-start your life change.

An extremely important chapter in this book is chapter 9 . . . *The Power of Stress Reduction.* Chronic stress is one of the primary instigators of chronic inflammation, which, you have already learned, is the main initiator of almost all chronic diseases and cancer. We will learn the biochemistry of how that happens and the scientific studies that have demonstrated that stress-reduction techniques equate to lower cancer and cancer-relapse rates in those who have cancer. The stress-reduction techniques that we will discuss will include meditation, deep slow breathing, exercise (there it is again), laughter, mindfulness, gentle motion, prayer, time management, guided imagery, biofeedback, self-hypnosis and a good book.

We know from the research that stress reduction can improve our immune and endocrine function, blood-vessel formation, DNA damage and repair, cancer-cell suicide, how our genes express themselves (epigenetics), cancer-treatment response, disease progression, survival and quality of life. That is why it is critical for everyone, but especially for cancer patients, to assess the stress in their lives and engage in practices that manage that stress.

We will also learn how social interaction is a key to longevity, as demonstrated so well in the Blue Zone areas of the world. This is an essential element that cancer patients need to take seriously. Being a cancer patient myself, I can tell you that it would be a very lonely and scary place without a loving wife, family and good friends that I interact with frequently. I am certain that they have all played a key role in helping me thrive with an incurable cancer.

We will also look at the power of prayer in this same chapter. When doing the research for this book, I was surprised at the amount of scientific studies looking at how prayer can positively affect disease outcomes. I will go through these studies to demonstrate that praying for yourself and people from afar has a powerful effect on treatment outcomes.

In chapter 10, entitled *The Power of Sleep* we will review why we sleep. What are all the many biochemical processes going on during that 6–8 hour period? While you are sleeping, how does the body repair damaged DNA and clean up unwanted proteins in the cells that otherwise would cause destruction? Why do people who work night shifts have much higher cancer rates? You will learn how adequate sleep keeps cancer at bay. I will go through several techniques to help you not only get to sleep, but to stay asleep.

So here we go into learning how you can naturally prevent, survive, and thrive with cancer. Enjoy and learn!

CHAPTER 5

Common Myths

Before we get into the 5 scientifically proven ways to beat back cancer naturally, I would like to address some common myths that I encounter on a continual basis as I speak and write about this topic. I debated where to place this chapter in the book, but the more I thought about it, my mind told me to knock some of these out right at the beginning . . . so here we go.

HIGH PROTEIN INTAKE IS GOOD FOR YOU

If you read the back cover for this book, you probably noticed I strongly recommend a whole food, plant-based diet to combat cancer. The question I continually get is, "Where do you get your protein?"

If you review the protein recommendations of the U.S. government, you can use the following equation to get your protein requirement:

Pounds X 4 divided by 10.

My weight is 155 pounds. Therefore 155 X 4 = 620

620 divided by 10 = 62 grams

If you use the metric system, use kilograms X 0.8.

I eat a strict whole food, plant-based diet (no animal products), and I have checked my protein intake on consecutive days for a whole week; I normally get more than 100 grams per day, which, in my view, might be a little more than my goal.

The average Westerner who eats a lot of meat and dairy products is easily getting 2–3 times the recommended about of protein, and this can be harmful to one's health—especially someone who is combatting cancer, as you will learn while you read this book. For now, let's look at some of the negatives of high meat, dairy and protein consumption.

High IGF-1

As I discussed previously, one of the concerning aspects of high animal-protein consumption is that it stimulates the liver to produce a growth-promoting hormone called Insulin-like Growth Factor-1 (IGF-1), which, at higher levels in adults, has been shown to be a major instigator of cancer initiation and growth [1,2]. This does not happen when our liver is exposed to incomplete plant proteins. Apparently, because animal protein is a complete protein, it sends a signal to the liver that growth is about to occur, so IGF-1 is manufactured. In studies, meat eaters consistently are shown to have much higher IGF-1 levels compared to vegans.

When we are young, our body needs IGF-1 for growth to allow us to become a full-grown adult. Our levels normally peak in our late teens and then gradually decline every year as we age. This gradual decline is built into our bodies to help us stay alive, because, as we age, we also accumulate thousands of DNA mutations. We do not want a stimulus for high cellular growth and replication in the setting of high levels of DNA mutations. This is a device that Nature has built in to protect us from cancer initiation, growth and metastasis. We will discuss this more at length in the chapter on "the power of a whole food, plant-based diet."

It is also important to note that, since IGF-1 can promote muscle growth, growth hormone has been promoted and prescribed by anti-aging physicians as an anti-aging hormone. However, studies are finding that restoring growth-hormone levels to youthful levels in adulthood is not beneficial; in fact, it has been found to increase death rates and diabetes, even in formerly healthy adults.

High mTOR Activation

Another promoter of cancer growth in the body that I already alluded to is the mTOR gene [3]. This gene, which is a prime regulator of cellular growth and replication (similar to IGF-1), is primarily stimulated by the amino acid leucine, which is found in high levels in all animal products and in very low levels in plants. Therefore, lowering animal products lowers leucine levels, which lowers mTOR activity. This is an effective way to decrease cancer initiation and growth. We will discuss this gene in more detail later in this book.

Kidney stress

High animal-protein intake also puts inordinate stress on the kidneys. Animal protein (but not vegetable protein) causes what is called "kidney hyper-filtration" [4]. This is an inflammatory response in the kidney caused by high levels of sulfur-containing amino acids that are present in animal proteins. When anti-inflammatory drugs are given at the time of animal protein ingestion, the hyper-filtration does not occur. This hyper-filtration also does not occur with the ingestion of vegetable protein. High animal-protein consumption is also extremely acidic, which puts additional stress on the kidney while also, in the cancer patient, creating a favorable pH for enzymes like collagenase to assist the cancer to progress and metastasize [5].

High pesticide levels

Because all animals are high on the food chain, the blood and tissue levels of pesticides and heavy metals is always much higher in meat eaters versus vegans. To help you understand this concept, if a grasshopper ate a bunch of pesticide-laden grass, it would absorb those pesticides, which would then be dissolved into its fat tissue . . . something we call "bioaccumulation." A bird then eats many grasshoppers. The bird's pesticide levels will now be greater than the grasshopper's levels. If a human eats a lot of the birds, a chicken for example, the human's levels will be higher than the chicken's. A similar situation occurs in the oceans. If you analyze mercury and PCB levels in small fish versus large fish, like tuna, the larger fish will consistently have higher mercury and PCB levels than the smaller fish.

One of many studies analyzing this bioaccumulation was published in the *British Journal of Nutrition*, and it found that PCB levels were much higher in meat eaters compared to vegans [6]. Similar studies routinely demonstrate this same result . . . the levels of pesticides and heavy metals in blood and tissue are consistently much higher in meat and dairy consumers.

Animal products also carry viruses such as bovine leukemia virus as well as bacterial endotoxins that cannot be destroyed by heat and that create much inflammation and other negative health issues in the body.

ANTIOXIDANTS CANNOT BE TAKEN DURING CHEMO AND RADIATION

This is one of the most common questions that I get asked by cancer patients. When cancer patients ask their oncologists if they can take antioxidant supplements during chemo and radiation treatments, there is almost always an international knee-jerk reaction that says "No," even though the scientific literature, in general, shows that antioxidants can be beneficial during conventional treatments and not harmful. The same goes for a whole food, plant-based diet, which has 63X the antioxidant power compared to animal-meat and dairy-based diets.

Here's the concern with taking antioxidants with chemo and radiation treatments. Both radiation therapy and many chemotherapy drugs (not all) kill cancer by producing molecules, called "free radicals," that damage the DNA of the tumor cells. Once the DNA is damaged, many of the cancer cells commit cell suicide . . . something we call "apoptosis."

Most of our normal cells have a mechanism that signals them to die when the DNA damage cannot be fixed quickly. Cancer cells, on the other hand, have a defective DNA damage-repair system, unlike normal cells. This slows down their ability to repair DNA damage, making them vulnerable to apoptosis. Because of these facts, radiation and chemo can kill many cancer cells while sparing most normal cells. Antioxidants are compounds that can neutralize the free radicals produced by radiation and chemotherapy—thus, the concerns about taking antioxidants with these treatments.

The fact is . . . the preponderance of evidence generally demonstrates that antioxidants do not negatively affect radiation therapy or chemotherapy when taken during those conventional treatments. In fact, many studies validate that they often exert a positive effect.

The only adverse effect that I could find in the scientific literature was the combination of green tea's polyphenols (which have a 1,2-benzene-diol molecular component), vitamin C, and alpha-lipoic acid reacting with the boronic-acid component of bortezomib (a protesome inhibitor used for myeloma). When the above 3 antioxidants were combined with bortezomib in animal studies, it was not as effective [7,8,9]. Other proteosome inhibitors tested that did not have the boronic component in its molecular structure were unaffected. So the bortezomib interaction seems to be peculiar to the boronic-acid moiety.

In one of the most comprehensive studies ever done on antioxidant use with chemo and radiation, Dr. Keith Block and his group systematically reviewed the entire body of scientific work evaluating the effects of concurrent use of antioxidants with chemotherapy [10]. He performed a search of literature from 1966 to 2007, using MEDLINE, Cochrane, CinAhl, AMED, AltHealthWatch and EMBASE databases. Randomized, controlled clinical trials reporting antioxidant-based lessening of chemotherapy toxicity were included in his final tally.

Only 33 of 965 articles, including 2,446 subjects, met the criteria that qualified for his high standards. The antioxidants he evaluated were: glutathione (11), melatonin (7), vitamin A (1), an antioxidant mixture (2), N-acetylcysteine (2), vitamin E (5), selenium (2), L-carnitine (1), Co-Q10 (1) and ellagic acid (1).

The majority (24 of the 33 studies) he looked at reported evidence of decreased toxicities from the concurrent use of antioxidants with chemotherapy. Nine studies reported no difference in toxicities between the 2 groups. Only one study (vitamin A) reported an increase in toxicity in the antioxidant group due to overdose. Five studies reported the antioxidant group completed more full doses of chemotherapy or had less dose reduction than control groups.

His conclusion after reviewing the entire scientific literature was that antioxidant supplementation during chemotherapy appeared to limit toxicities without affecting the results of the chemotherapy and many times improved the results.

How could the results improve? As we've already discussed, free radicals produced by many chemotherapeutic drugs cause cancer cells to "commit cell suicide," a process we described as "apoptosis." We also know that apoptosis is triggered, in part, by free-radical damage to parts of the cancer cell. We've also discussed that many oncologists recommend that their cancer patients avoid antioxidants entirely because of a theoretical fear that antioxidants might neutralize this free-radical damage and impede apoptosis. Dr. Block and his research team, however, realized that this was in direct contradiction to strong data, that is well recognized among scientists who study natural products. There are, in fact, numerous antioxidants that are well known to actually cause apoptosis in cancer cells. Curcumin, EGCG from green tea, and melatonin are just 3 of the best-known antioxidants that are widely known to cause apoptosis in a variety of types of cancer cells. But they don't cause apoptosis in normal cells. In fact, they can protect them from many kinds of carcinogenic damage.

So how is it that these well-known antioxidants can be causing apoptosis if they impede free-radical activity? When Dr. Block's research team delved into the scientific literature, they found an explanation for this phenomenon—and also for why it might occur in cancer cells, but not in normal cells. Interestingly, laboratory scientists have discovered ways to tell when a substance causes free radicals to be formed inside of cells. There are substances that are described as "molecular probes" that can test for these intracellular free radicals. Researchers can easily test any substance to see if it causes apoptosis in either cancer cells or normal cells. What researchers have discovered is that many antioxidants cause apoptosis in cancer cells when they are applied in high doses to cells grown in test tubes. The same doses, however, do not cause apoptosis in normal cells. When the molecular probes are used, scientists find that the high-dose antioxidants actually cause cancer cells to produce free radicals. This is what is most likely triggering apoptosis.

Why would this happen in cancer cells and not normal cells? It turns out that antioxidants can undergo reactions with metals. Specifically, many of the natural antioxidants that are known to trigger apoptosis in cancer cells have been found to form free radicals when they interact with copper. Cancer cells are well known to have high concentrations of copper and other metals, such as iron. Copper, in particular, plays an important role in the basic metabolic processes of the cancer cells as well as angiogenesis and metastasis. Cancer cells need copper for these processes, which are absent in normal cells. When natural antioxidants react with these extraordinarily high copper levels, they become pro-oxidants, which can then trigger cancer-cell apoptosis. This is most likely the reason that they cause apoptosis in cancer cells, but not in normal cells.

So when we give antioxidants that generate intracellular free radicals, along with chemotherapy that also creates free radicals, what happens? Do the antioxidants neutralize or interfere with the chemotherapy, or do their pro-oxidant effects dominate? In almost all of these cases, the research indicates that the antioxidants actually enhance the effect of the chemotherapy drugs. These studies have been done not only in a petri dish, but also in animals and in humans. A large review article, for instance, described many experiments in which curcumin was given with chemotherapy (or radiation) and was discovered to improve the effectiveness of the chemo. A series of clinical trials conducted in Italy found that high-dose melatonin increased the effects of chemotherapy, but reduced its toxicity to normal tissues. And, while petri-dish studies required high doses of antioxidants to obtain their pro-apoptosis effects, the studies in animals and humans used very reasonable doses. This very interesting pro-oxidant phenomenon may explain why antioxidants did not eradicate the effects of chemotherapy in the randomized trials Dr. Block's research team reviewed.

Another important gem to back up Block's findings is that the FDA approved a very potent antioxidant drug called "ethiofos" for use during radiation therapy and chemotherapy to protect sensitive tissues from the damaging effects of conventional treatments. As I mentioned in the chapter on radiation therapy, the FDA approval was based on an extensive review of the data, which found no reduction in the efficacy of radiation or chemotherapy when ethiofos was administered during treatment.

130 | BEAT BACK CANCER NATURALLY

As I emphatically stated before . . . so, on the one hand, some oncologists are telling patients not to ingest weak antioxidants like vitamin C, vitamin E, curcumin and green tea, while they are prescribing an extremely potent FDA-approved antioxidant (given through an IV) that has been found to decrease toxicity while not having a negative effect on the conventional therapeutic result.

A note of caution, however. To date, 9 randomized, controlled trials, that I already reviewed in the radiation therapy chapter, have investigated antioxidants for cancer prevention, regardless of diet. These primarily looked at synthetic-beta-carotene and synthetic-d-alpha-tocopherol (vitamin E) as single vitamins and not as they appear in nature (as one of many antioxidants in their natural mixed-carotenoid or mixed-tocopherol/tocotrienol complexes). These 9 studies have been referenced previously. Five of the studies showed no effect, 2 showed a positive effect, and 2 revealed a negative effect in smokers. Because these results are essentially neutral and the fact that fat-soluble vitamins can accumulate in the fatty tissues, I strongly advise to have your fat-soluble vitamins levels regularly checked (every 6–12 months) by your physician. I use a test from Genova Labs that measures the fat-soluble antioxidants beta-carotene, vitamin D, d-alpha tocopherol (vitamin E), vitamin K and Coenzyme Q10 levels. If your levels get above the normal range, I would highly recommend that you cut back on the strength of the supplements, because levels in excess of normal are not ideal.

In foods and herbs, the recycling of the contributed electrons of antioxidants balances out as Nature intended. To help you understand this concept . . . when an antioxidant contributes its electron to neutralize a free radical, it then becomes a pro-oxidant free radical itself, because it just lost one of its electrons. The accompanying antioxidants in foods and carotenoid and tocopherol complexes then contribute their electrons to the antioxidant that just lost one of its electrons to keep all in a neutral state. That is why, with individual vitamin supplements (especially fat-soluble vitamins), we need to be more cautious. Furthermore, when I recommend antioxidants like beta-carotene or vitamin E, they are always in their natural form. For instance, the beta-carotene supplement that I recommend is called *Full Spectrum Carotene*, which is a combination of many carotenoids. The vitamin E supplement is called *Tri-En-All 400*, which is a combination of d-alpha, beta, gamma, and delta tocopherols with 4 tocotrienols.

Ideally, a diverse whole food, plant-based diet will provide you with a hefty dose of phytonutrient antioxidants that have their contributed electrons naturally recycled by the body. The problem is, however, that only 3% of the Western population consumes the required amount of fruits, vegetables, whole grains, legumes, mushrooms, nuts and seeds to keep antioxidants at appropriate levels. I, therefore, would recommend that those individuals take, at a minimum, a high-quality multivitamin supplement with no iron. I recommend *Ultra Preventive X* made by Douglas Labs that can be purchased on Amazon. Take 4 in the morning with food.

In my chapter on "the power of targeted supplements," you will learn that most of the supplements that I recommend are herbs in a tea, capsule or freeze-dried-powder form. There are very few supplements that I recommend in a single vitamin form because of this electron recycling issue, which I do think is important. When I do recommend a single vitamin such as alpha-lipoic acid, for example, it is primarily being used as a drug to combat a specific cancer-treatment complication (e.g., peripheral neuropathy).

MODERATE ALCOHOL INTAKE IS HEALTHY

In recent years, there has been a false narrative propagated that moderate alcohol intake is healthy. This was driven by some older studies showing that people in France who eat a very high saturated-fat diet had fairly low levels of cardiovascular disease.

In a meta-analysis of the scientific data on the relationship of alcohol consumption to disease, Dr. Fillmore and his research group demonstrated that these studies were erroneously performed. In his analysis of these studies, he discovered that many individuals who described themselves as teetotalers were actually individuals who previously had severe liver disease due to alcoholism or other grave diseases [11]. They totally stopped alcohol consumption because of their life-threatening situations. Subsequent studies defining a teetotaler as someone who never drank alcohol revealed totally different results, with the no-alcohol group having much less cardiovascular disease, cancer and all-cause mortality.

Additionally, research consistently shows that drinking alcoholic beverages increases a woman's risk of hormone-receptor-positive breast cancer. Alcohol not only damages DNA, but also triggers higher levels of estrogen and other hormones linked to breast cancer. Compared to women who don't drink at all, women who have 3 alcoholic drinks per week have a 15% higher risk of breast cancer. The estimated alcohol-related breast-cancer risk increases another 10% for each additional drink women have each day according to *breastcancer.org*.

Here are more risk findings about alcohol and breast cancer:

- A large meta-analysis (reviewing many studies in one) looking at the relationship between alcohol and breast-cancer risk discovered that women who drank about 3 alcoholic drinks per week experienced a moderate increase in breast-cancer risk.
- A 2009 study found that drinking just 3–4 alcoholic beverages per week increases a women's risk of breast-cancer recurrence in women diagnosed with early-stage breast cancer.

Another very large meta-analysis of 572 studies, including 486,538 cancer cases, was recently published in the *British Journal of Cancer* [12]. That analysis concluded that even moderate alcohol intake increases the risk of cancer of the oral cavity and pharynx, esophagus, colorectum, liver, larynx and female breast. It also found evidence that alcohol drinking is associated with some other cancers, such as pancreas and prostate cancer and melanoma.

The bottom line is that regularly drinking alcohol can harm your health, even if you don't binge drink. All types of alcohol count. One drink equals 12 ounces of beer, 5 ounces of wine and 1.5 ounces of hard liquor. When you drink beverage alcohol, around 2%-8% is lost through urine, sweat or the breath. The other 92%–98% is metabolized by your body. All ethyl alcohol, which is broken down in the human body, is first converted to acetaldehyde, and then acetaldehyde is converted into an acetic-acid free radical. It is important to note that acetaldehyde is a poison that is a close relative of formaldehyde. Having this poison floating around in the blood, before moving further down the metabolic chain in the liver, is a cause of much free-radical activity that is at the core of aging, chronic diseases, and our big concern . . . cancer.

ONCE MY CANCER IS GONE FOR 5 YEARS, I AM CURED

Unfortunately, this is not the case. As I communicated in chapter 1, reports show that 70% of individuals who get into a remission from their cancer will have a relapse, and often the relapse comes back with a greater vengeance. The reality of this comes from my previous statements in chapter 1 about how the cancer stem cell is at the core of cancer development. This cell divides at a slow rate, but the daughter cells that it spurs off divide rapidly. If you remember, chemotherapy and radiation can very easily knock off these rapidly dividing daughter cells, because most of them have very rapid cell division. It is during this cell-division period that DNA strands can be easily damaged to cause the cancer cell to die. Chemo and radiation therapy, however, also have the same DNA-damaging effects to normal cells but not to the same degree, because normal cells have better DNA-repair mechanisms than cancer cells.

The bottom line is that, when you get into a complete remission, treat yourself as an individual who never had cancer before, but has been given a second chance. What would you do differently? Would you stop smoking? Would you stop drinking alcohol? Would you start eating 9 servings of fruits and vegetables per day? Would you add legumes, whole grains, mushrooms, nuts and seeds to your diet while lowering animal products or, ideally, eliminating them? I hope that, by the end of this book, you will be convinced to make many of these life-enhancing changes. It could mean many years of added longevity with a high quality of life.

NO MILK EQUALS BAD BONES

If you are on a whole food, plant-based diet, you are not eating or drinking dairy products, so you you may be wondering, "What's going to happen to my bones? Doesn't milk keep me from getting osteoporosis?" It turns out that the promised benefit of ingesting dairy products may be just another empty marketing ploy by the dairy industry. A large meta-analysis of cow's-milk intake and hip-fracture studies established no significant protection [13]. One study showed that, even if you attempt to bolster peak bone mass by drinking lots of milk during your teenage years, it won't reduce your chances of a fracture later in life [14]. One recent set of studies involving 100,000+ men and women followed for up to 20 years even suggested that milk consumption may increase bone- and hip-fracture rates [15]. These researchers also looked at the connection between milk consumption and mortality, as well as the risk of fracture in large populations of milk drinkers. In addition to dramatically having more bone and hip fractures, scientists found a higher incidence of premature death, more cardiovascular disease, and dramatically higher cancer rates for each daily glass of milk women drank. Three glasses a day was correlated with almost twice the risk of dying early. Men with higher milk consumption also had a higher rate of death, although they didn't have higher fracture rates. An editorial in the *British Medical Journal* addressing this published study underscored that, "given the rise of milk consumption around the world, the role of milk in mortality needs to be established definitively now" [16].

EGGS ARE GOOD FOR YOU

Millions of men across the world are currently living with prostate cancer. If the cancer is caught early within the prostate, the probability of it causing death within the next 5 years is almost zero. However, if the cancer spreads, your chances of surviving 5 years may be as low as 33% [17]. Hoping to identify possible inciting factors in prostate cancer's spread, researchers recruited more than 100,000 men with early-stage prostate cancer and followed them for several years. Compared with men who rarely ate eggs, men who ate even less than a single egg a day appeared to have 2X the risk of prostate cancer metastasizing into the bones. The only thing possibly worse for prostate cancer than eggs was the consumption of poultry. Men with more aggressive prostate cancer who routinely ate chicken and turkey had up to 4X the risk of prostate-cancer metastasis. The researchers hypothesized that the link between eating lots of poultry and metastasizing cancer may be due to the carcinogens, such as heterocyclic amines, that are induced by cooking. Interestingly, for some unknown reason, these carcinogens build up more when cooking chickens and turkeys than with other animals.

But what carcinogen is there in eggs? How could eating less than an egg a day double the risk of cancer metastasis? The answer may be with choline, a chemical found highly concentrated in eggs. First off, we do know that high blood levels of choline have been associated with an increased risk of developing prostate cancer [18]. This, then, logically explains the association between eggs and cancer progression [19]. But what about cancer mortality? In a well-known research paper published in the *American Journal of Clinical Nutrition*, it was demonstrated that men who consumed the most choline from food also had an increased risk of cancer death [20]. This same research group also established that men who ate 2.5 or more eggs per week had an 81% increased risk of dying from prostate cancer [21]. The choline in eggs, like the carnitine in red meat, is converted into a toxin called trimethylamine (TMA) [22] by the bacteria that exist in the guts of those who eat meat [23]. And TMA, once oxidized to trimethylamine oxide (TMAO) in the liver, appears to increase the risk of heart attack, stroke and premature death [24].

Ironically, the presence of choline in eggs is something the egg industry brags about [25] while completely ignoring the cancer connection. In fact, Dr. Michael Greger's research group, through the Freedom of Information Act, was able to get their hands on an e-mail from the executive director of the Egg Nutrition Board directed to another egg-industry executive that discussed the Harvard study suggesting that choline is a culprit in promoting cancer progression. "Certainly worth keeping in mind," he wrote, "as we continue to promote choline as another good reason to consume eggs." [26].

Eggs also have an enormous amount of cholesterol, and we have already learned how higher cholesterol levels are correlated with higher cancer rates and cardiovascular disease.

WHITE MEAT IS BETTER THAN DARK MEAT

There is a common belief that those watching their cholesterol should opt for chicken. A recent study, however, found that consuming high quantities of meat—red or white—can equally raise cholesterol and threaten heart health [27]. Scientists recently monitored a group of 113 healthy men and women as they cycled through 3 different types of diets: a diet that contained white meat, a diet that contained red meat, and a diet that contained plant-based protein and no meat. The participants spent 4 weeks eating each diet. As an add-on test, researchers split the participants into 2 groups, one that ate higher-saturated fat versions of all 3 diets and one that ate lower-saturated fat versions, to evaluate the impact on heart health. Researchers took samples of blood at the start and end of each diet cycle and counseled the participants on the importance of adherence to each diet. After a cycle would be completed, the participants returned to their regular diet for 2 weeks before moving to the next diet.

The results totally disproved the common myth that white meat, such as chicken and turkey, is better for cholesterol than red meat, such as beef and pork. In fact, the scientists discovered no difference in the way both meat types raised blood-cholesterol levels. Furthermore, total cholesterol increases were similar whether the participants ate a diet high or low in saturated fats; however, eating more saturated fat led to a greater rise in LDL (bad cholesterol).

The final overall result from the study was that a plant-based diet was found to be healthiest for blood cholesterol. Researchers concluded that these findings support growing evidence of plant-based diets being much more healthy for the cardiovascular system compared to diets heavy in meat. Remember that cholesterol is only present in animal products and not at all in plants. We also know from the scientific evidence that a plant-strong diet is also the best diet in the fight against cancer.

SOY CAUSES BREAST CANCER

Soybeans naturally contain a class of phytoestrogens called isoflavones. People hear the word "phytoestrogens" and immediately deduce that means soy acts like estrogen. Phytoestrogens do lodge onto the same receptors as your true, innate estrogen but have a very weak protective effect, in that they can block the powerful effects of your innate estrogen.

Let me explain. There are 2 kinds of estrogen receptors in the body . . . alpha and beta. When estrogen binds to alpha-receptors, that is a trigger for growth and pro-estrogenic activity. When an estrogen binds to a beta-receptor, there is an anti-growth protective effect. There are 3 basic types of estrogen in a woman's body . . . estriol, estradiol, and estrone. Estriol is the weakest of the 3 and has a high affinity for the protective beta-receptor. Women in Japan have much higher estriol levels than American women and also a much lower incidence of breast cancer. Estriol is also the estrogen of pregnancy and reaches very high levels during the pregnancy process. Studies have shown that those with the highest estriol levels during pregnancy, followed over a long period of time, have lower cancer rates. Estrone, on the other hand, binds almost exclusively to the pro-growth alpha-receptor. This is typically the hormone that remains when women enter menopause. Estradiol, our last estrogen for discussion, binds ⅔ to the alpha-receptor and ⅓ to the beta-receptor . . . so it has an effect on cellular replication, but not to the degree of estrone.

As I stated, estrone and estradiol prefer the alpha-receptors, while estriol and the phytoestrogens in soy have an affinity for the beta-receptors. The effect of soy phytoestrogens on different tissues, therefore, depends on the ratio of alpha to beta-receptors. Therefore, your native estrogen has positive effects in some tissues and possible negative effects in other tissues. For example, high levels of estrone and estradiol can be positive for your bones, but can also increase the probability of developing breast cancer. Ideally, what you want is a "selective estrogen-receptor modulator" that would have pro-estrogenic effects in certain tissues and anti-estrogenic effects in others. Well, for heaven's sake . . . these are the exact characteristics that phytoestrogens possess [28]. Soy seems to lower breast-cancer risk [29] (an anti-estrogenic effect) but can also help reduce menopausal hot-flash symptoms [30] (a pro-estrogenic effect). So, by eating soy, you get the best of both worlds.

So what about women with breast-cancer eating soy? There have been 5 really good studies on breast cancer survivors and soy consumption. Researchers, in general, have discovered that women diagnosed with breast cancer who ate the most soy lived much longer and had a dramatically lower risk of breast-cancer relapse than those who ate less soy [31]. Another study found that just a single cup of soy milk daily may reduce the risk of breast-cancer recurrence by a whopping 25% [32]. Surprisingly, the increase in survival rate for those soy-food eaters was shown to be evident in both women whose tumors were responsive to estrogen (estrogen-receptor-positive breast cancer) and those whose tumors were not (estrogen-receptor-negative breast cancer). This effect was also found to be equally true in both young and older women. In one study, for instance, 90% of the breast-cancer patients who ate the most soy after their breast-cancer diagnosis were still alive 5 years later, while 50% of those who ate little to no soy succumbed [33].

Other than binding onto the protective beta-receptors, another way that soy may decrease cancer risk and improve survival is by reactivating the BRCA genes [34]. BRCA1 and BRCA2 are 2 of the 100+ cancer-suppressing genes in our bodies responsible for DNA repair. Mutations in this specific repair gene can cause a rare form of hereditary breast cancer. As I mentioned before, Angelina Jolie decided to undergo a preventative double mastectomy because of a detected mutation in her BRCA genes. Hereditary breast cancer happens in only 2.5% of breast-cancer cases, however.

Interestingly, the BRCA gene can be involved in breast-cancer spread once the cancer gets started. The tumor can actually turn off the DNA-repair power of the BRCA gene through a methylation process. Even though the gene is still operational, the cancer has a way of turning off or diminishing its expression [35]. This is where soy comes into play, in that it seems to have an ability to prevent this methylation process from occurring, allowing the BRCA genes to do their DNA-repair activities unimpeded [36]. The bottom line is that women should eat a lot of soy products whether they have breast cancer or not because of their clearly demonstrated breast-cancer-protective effects.

Even though we know that soy can be extremely good for your body, there are certain caveats. It must always be organic. It must always be non-GMO, because GMO soy is loaded with the pesticide Roundup. So always buy soy with the labels USDA ORGANIC and non-GMO. If you do that, you are on solid ground.

The 2 primary isoflavones in soy, genistein and daidzein, also have significant health benefits other than its cancer-protective effects.These 2 phytonutrients have been found in many studies to decrease bad LDL cholesterol and increase the good HDL cholesterol. These isoflavones also have powerful antioxidant properties that protect LDL cholesterol from oxidation, which would have progressed to atherosclerosis. It also increases the flexibility of the blood vesels, which has been found to lower blood pressure.

Other very health-promoting properties are that soy is loaded with fiber; has quite a bit of healthy plant protein; is cholesterol free and low in saturated fat; has has high amounts of vitamin K2, which helps bring calcium into the bones, enhancing bone strength while simultaneously removing calcium from the blood vessels, thus preventing atherosclerosis.

VEGANS MUST PLANT COMBINE TO GET ALL OF THEIR AMINO ACIDS

All nutrients come from the sun or the soil. Vitamin D, the "sunshine vitamin," is created when skin is exposed to sunlight. All the other nutrients come from the surface or sea ground. Minerals come from the Earth's soil, and vitamins come from the plants and micro-organisms that grow from the soil. Remember, the calcium in cow's milk came from all the plants she ate . . . plants that derived their calcium from the soil. Shouldn't we be able to cut out the cow and get our calcium directly from the plants?

Protein contains what are called "essential amino acids," conditionally essential amino acids, and non-essential amino acids. There are:

- 9 essential amino acids (leucine, methionine, histidine, isoleucine, lysine, phenylalanine, threonine, tryptophan and valine)
- 6 conditionally essential amino acids (arginine, cysteine, glutamine, glycine, proline and tyrosine)
- 6 non-essential amino acids (alanine, aspartic acid, asparagine, serine, selenocysteine and pyrrolysine)

Our bodies cannot manufacture the 9 essential amino acids, so we must get them from our diets. The other conditionally essential and non-essential amino acids can be manufactured by the body and stored for 3–4 days if needed for future activities.

Remember, other animals don't make their essential amino acids, either. All essential amino acids originate from plants and microbes, and eating a variety of plants easily provides you with all of the essential amino acids. Studies have shown that those eating a whole food, plant-based diet eat about twice the U.S. government's average daily protein requirement. My wife and I regularly calculate our protein requirement for the day, and our protein intake is always at least 1.5X the recommended amount. As Dr. Michael Greger always says, "Those who don't know where to get protein on a plant-based diet don't know beans!"

So far we have been talking about protein quantity. How about protein quality? The concept that plant protein is inferior to animal protein arose from studies performed on rodents more than a century ago. Scientists discovered that infant rats didn't grow as well on plants. However, they also found that infant rats don't grow as well on human breast milk, either. Does that mean we shouldn't breastfeed our babies? That is absurd! They're rats, and rat milk has 10X more protein than human milk, because rats grow about 10X faster than human infants.

It is true that some plant proteins are comparatively low in some essential amino acids. So, about 40 years ago, the myth of "protein combining" came into vogue. The concept was that we needed to eat so-called complementary proteins together (for example, rice and beans) to make up for their relative shortfalls. However, this falsehood was totally debunked many years ago. The myths that plant proteins are incomplete, aren't as good as animal proteins, or need to be combined with other proteins at meals have all been dismissed by the nutrition community a long time ago. But many in conventional medicine didn't get the message.

Finally, Dr. John McDougall called out the American Heart Association for a 2001 publication that questioned the completeness of plant proteins. Thankfully, they've changed that publication, which now states that *"plant proteins can provide enough of the essential and non-essential amino acids" and that we "don't need to consciously combine . . . complementary proteins . . ."* Thank God for John McDougall for his courage and energy to combat this formerly widely held fallacy.

It turns out that our body is not stupid. Our body maintains pools of free essential, non-essential, and conditionally essential amino acids that can be used to do all of the complementing for us. And that is not to forget about our body's massive protein-recycling program. Some 90 grams of protein are dumped into the digestive tract every day from our own body to get broken back down and reassembled, so our body can mix and match amino acids to whatever proportions we need, regardless of what we eat, making it almost impossible to even create a diet of plant foods that has enough calories but not enough protein. Thus, plant-based eaters do not need to be concerned a single iota about amino-acid imbalances.

ALL OILS ARE BAD FOR YOU

This is a big debate in the whole food, plant-based community. Many say that you should consume no oil whatsoever. My personal feeling from much research is that the only oil that should ever be used with cooking or over salads is a very minimal amount of FIRST COLD PRESSED EXTRA VIRGIN OLIVE OIL. The reason I have capitalized FCPEVOO is because there is a big difference between "first cold pressed extra virgin olive oil," "extra virgin olive oil," and "olive oil"—don't even consider buying "light olive oil." First cold pressed is the first pressing go around without any chemicals or refinement and contains the highest levels of phytonutrients, as well as the best taste. The main problem with recommending olive oil and why I believe many whole food, plant-based doctors steer away from recommending it, is that most people do not use a teaspoon (40 calories, which I use) on their salads but use several tablespoons (120 calories per tablespoon). I believe that high amounts routinely can lead to weight gain, which creates a whole series of health problems. In regard to its naysayers saying that it has a negative effect on the endothelium (a measure of blood-vessel behavior and blood flow), there are isolated studies that demonstrate this to be the case. This was likely because of the dose of the oil administered, the nature of the oil used, or both. In general, FCPEVOO intake has been associated with improved endothelial function. To put such opposing findings into context, exercise is also routinely correlated with improved endothelial function and better cardiovascular health . . . but isolated studies have shown endothelial dysfunction, comparably related to the intensity and timing of the exercise.

My opinion is that a diet does not require FCPEVOO to be optimal; I am equally convinced that an optimal diet certainly allows for FCPEVOO and may benefit from it.

Some whole food, plant-based doctors state that olive oil has no nutrient value, but I know that this is categorically wrong. Fifteen olives are required to make one teaspoon of olive oil. One olive has 5 calories, so 15 olives equals 65 calories. One teaspoon of olive oil has 40 calories. Although some of the water-soluble phytonutrients are squeezed out during the pressing process, there are very many remaining fat-soluble phytonutrients that have powerful antioxidant, anti-tumor and anti-cancer activity. And remember, olive oil is placed on high-fiber vegetables . . . not on meat. Many "absolutely no olive oil" proponents seem to forget that we don't ingest olive oil in a vacuum. We are placing it on high-phytonutrient, high-fiber vegetables that will help slow the absorption of calories. The other point that needs to be emphasized is that placing a small amount of olive oil on a salad allows the fat-soluble vitamins, such as vitamin E, vitamin A, vitamin K, and the many fat-soluble phytonutrients, such as the carotenoids, to be absorbed. Without some healthy fat on that salad, none of these vital nutrients will be absorbed into the bloodstream.

Some of the olive oil's phytonutrients are oleuropein, hydroxytyrosol, tyrosol, oleocanthal, and oleic acid, which have been shown to enhance your immune system plus have potent anti-inflammatory, antioxidant and anti-angiogenic properties. One study wanted to see if substituting butter, corn oil and soybean oil for FCPEVOO would enhance a person's immune response. The researchers picked 41 overweight volunteers, all older than 65 [37]. The subjects ate a typical Western diet, which was high in saturated fat and low in dietary fiber. The scientists gave all of the subjects a bottle of oil and spread. One group received FCPEVOO from Spain. The other group was given a mix of corn and soybean oil and a butter spread. For 3 months, the subjects continued to eat a standard Western diet, but used only their authorized oil and spread. Both groups used approximately 3 tablespoons of oil per day. After 3 months, blood-lab assay revealed that the immune T-cells in the olive-oil group increased their capability to become activated and multiply in number by 53%. The same immune cells in the group eating corn-soy oil and butter had no change in immune activity.

FCPEVOO also has been found to diminish the body's reaction to allergens. The phytonutrient hydroxytyrosol, found in extra virgin olive oil, aids immune cells in manufacturing interleukin-10, which allays inflammation [38]. These combined effects show that substituting FCPEEVO for other cooking oils used in a standard Western diet can have both immune-boosting and anti-inflammatory health benefits. It is important to note that not all olive oils contain the same concentration of hydroxytyrosol. In Dr. William Li's excellent book *Eat to Beat Disease*, he points out a study from the Instituto de la Grasa in Spain that compared the polyphenols found in 4 types of Spanish extra virgin olive oils made from olive monovarietals (Arbequina, Hojiblanca, Manzanilla, Picual) [39]. The highest levels of hydroxytyrosol were present in the oil made from Picual olives.

FCPEVOO also contains a class of phytonutrients known as secoiridoids, which represent up to 46% of the total polyphenols present in olive oil. These phytonutrients can be detected in the blood plasma and in urine after ingestion, proving their bioavailability in the body [40]. Scientists validated that olive oil secoiridoids could dramatically diminish the growth of breast-cancer stem cells [41]. When mice were injected with breast-cancer stem cells that were given secoiridoids, 20% of the mice did not get cancer. In the 80% that did develop cancer, the tumors were 15X smaller and grew at a much slower rate than the breast-cancer cells not exposed to the secoiridoids. This result demonstrates undoubtedly that secoiridoids repress breast-cancer stem cells. The power of the olive-oil secoiridoids on cancer stem cells was also found to demonstrate effectiveness at the genetic level. After the breast-cancer stem cells were exposed to the secoiridoids, its phytonutrient power changed the expression of 160 genes involved with the regulation of cancer-stem-cell activity. As we already learned, this is called "epigenetics". . . the ability of phytonutrients to change the way genes act. So even if you have bad genes, your lifestyle can make bad genes act in a more positive way. In this secoiridoid study, one gene was curtailed in its activity 4-fold, while the activity of another gene that counteracts cancer stem cells was increased 13-fold. We, therefore, now know for certain the powerful activity of FCPEVOO against formidable cancer stem cells.

In Dr. Li's book, he pointed me to a fascinating study conducted in Milan that examined 27,000 subjects in Italy for their use of FCPEVOO, butter, margarine, and seed oils [42]. Their usage was correlated to different types of cancer. They found that 3–4 tablespoons per day of FCPEVOO was associated with a diminished risk of esophageal cancer by 70%, laryngeal cancer by 60%, oral and pharyngeal cancer by 60%, ovarian cancer by 32%, colorectal cancer by 17%, and breast cancer by 11%. These benefits were not seen with any of the other types of oils or fats. Butter, in fact, was correlated with an increased risk of esophageal, oral, and pharyngeal cancer by 2-fold. There was no cancer-risk-reducing benefit seen with any seed oils. As I have reiterated before, make sure you buy "first cold pressed extra virgin olive oil." To find the oil with the highest levels of health-generating polyphenols, look carefully at the label, and see if the type of olive used is identified. Dr. William Li feels the best olives for good health are Koroneiki (from Greece), Moraiolo (from Italy), and Picual (from Spain). The oils from these olives have wonderful flavors and work well for cooking, on salad dressings, or bread dipping.

COCONUT OIL IS GOOD FOR YOU

Over the past decade, there has been a message sent throughout the media that coconut oil is good for you. But is it really? If you have never seen what coconut oil looks like in a glass container, go to your nearest Whole Foods or Trader Joe's and take a look. It is a solid. And the reason it is solid at room temperature (similar to lard) is that coconut oil is 94% saturated fat.

As most of us know, high saturated-fat intake is correlated with many chronic diseases such as atherosclerosis as demonstrated in thousands of studies over 40 years. Why people began to believe that coconut oil might be good for them is the fact that coconut oil contains some MCTs (medium chain triglycerides). Some studies have shown that these MCTs can help in the process of excess-calorie burning, thus helping in weight loss [43]. MCTs have also been observed to cause increased fat oxidation and reduced food intake [44], and some in the bodybuilding and endurance-athlete community have touted MCTs as having performance benefits [45]. While some health benefits from MCTs may occur, a link to improved exercise performance is not very strong [46]. Additionally, there are studies that back the use of MCT oil as a weight-loss supplement, but these claims are also very inconclusive [43].

The other important fact is that MCTs make up only 5% of coconut oil. I, therefore, strongly advise against its regular use because of its incredibly high saturated-fat content and extremely low MCT content.

FRUIT JUICES ARE GOOD FOR YOU

In July of 2019, the *British Medical Journal* published a study that focused on investigating whether drinking sugary drinks could increase cancer risk. The objective of the study was to "assess the associations between the consumption of sugary drinks (such as sugar-sweetened beverages and 100% fruit juices), artificially sweetened beverages, and the risk of cancer." The study, which included 101,257 healthy French adults used data for 97 sugary drinks and 12 artificially sweetened drinks. The sugary-drink group consisted of all sugar-sweetened beverages containing more than 5% of simple carbohydrates, as well as 100% fruit juices (with no added sugar). This includes soft drinks (carbonated or not), syrups, 100% juice, fruit drinks, sugar-sweetened hot beverages, milk-based sugar-sweetened beverages, sport drinks and energy drinks. Artificially sweetened beverages included all beverages containing non-nutritive sweeteners, such as diet soda, sugar-free syrups and diet milk-based beverages. The mean intake of sugary drinks and artificially sweetened beverages in the study was ½ cup. Results from the study revealed that a 3.5-ounces-per-day increase in the consumption of sugary drinks is correlated with an 18% increase in overall cancer risk and a 22% increased risk of breast cancer [47]. In general, the study made evident that the drinking of sugary beverages was conclusively related with the risk of overall cancer and breast cancer.

The partaking of artificially sweetened beverages, however, was not associated with the risk of cancer. This is a finding that came as a surprise to the researchers. Even the consumption of 100% fruit juice was inescapably correlated with increased cancer risk. These findings suggest that "sugary drinks, which are widely consumed in Western countries, might represent a modifiable risk factor for cancer prevention."

How might sugary drinks increase cancer risk? It's believed that there are innumerable negative effects of sugary drinks. There is a mountain of evidence that consuming sweetened beverages is associated with an increased risk of obesity, which in turn, is recognized as a strong risk factor for many cancers. Studies show that excess weight is a potent risk factor for mouth, pharynx, larynx, esophageal, stomach, pancreatic, gallbladder, liver, colorectal, breast, ovarian, endometrial, prostate and kidney cancers. Sugary drinks also appear to create increases in deep abdominal fat, exclusive of body weight. And scientists know that high amounts of visceral fat is linked to the growth of tumors through transformation of cell-signaling pathways.

Aside from contributing to weight gain/obesity, we know that cancer cells need an enormous amount of sugar just to survive because of its crude use of Warburg's anaerobic glycolysis for energy production. For example, one sugar molecule produces 2 ATP energy molecules in a cancer cell versus one sugar molecule producing 36 ATP energy molecules in our normal cells. Therefore, when you drink sugary artificial drinks or fruit juices, you are feeding the monster.

Additionally, there are certain chemicals in sugary drinks, such as 4-methylimidazole, which give the caramel colorings, that may also cause cancer, a finding based on research by the International Agency for Research on Cancer.

So, what should we drink? Purified plain water is the single best way to stay hydrated, since water contains zero calories or sugar and is essential for overall health for many reasons. I personally drink purified, alkalinized water with lime and lemon juice to alkalinize my pH throughout the day. I use organic stevia as a sweetener in my morning caf and decaf anti-cancer concoctions that I will discuss later in this book. In the evening before retiring, I drink a tea medley with lemon and lime juice, which I will also discuss later in this book.

Since the above study did not show that artificially sweetened beverages were correlated with cancer risk, should we consume them? The answer is "No." Even though there is no increased cancer risk, there are many studies that link artificially sweetened beverages to a higher rate of hypertension, obesity, type 2 diabetes and impaired glucose intolerance, negative changes in gut microbiota, and potentially more cravings, headaches and other symptoms.

The only sweeteners that I recommend are very small amounts of natural sweeteners like the herb stevia, molasses, maple syrup, date sugar and guava nectar.

VEGANS DO NOT GET ENOUGH IRON

Compared with people who eat meat, vegetarians tend to consume more iron (as well as more of most nutrients), but the iron in plant foods is not absorbed as efficiently as the heme iron in meat. While this is advantageous in preventing iron overload with its iron free-radical excess, 3% of women in the United States lose more iron than they take in, which can lead to anemia. Studies reveal that women who eat plant-based diets do not appear to have higher rates of iron-deficiency anemia compared to women who eat a lot of meat [48], but all women of childbearing age need to make sure they consume enough iron. Those diagnosed with iron deficiency should first try to improve iron levels with diet, as iron supplements have been shown to increase free-radical activity in the body. The healthiest and best sources of iron are whole grains, legumes, nuts, seeds, dried fruits, and green, leafy vegetables. You should also abstain from drinking tea with meals, as tea has been established to inhibit iron absorption. One way to boost iron levels is to eat vitamin C-rich foods, as it has been revealed in studies to improve the absorption of iron from the GI tract.

Should we even be thinking about increasing our iron levels through consuming more heme iron present in meat? Two extremely large studies (50,000+ [49] and 500,000+ [50]) determined that people with high meat intake (processed and unprocessed) had a much higher frequency of cancer, heart disease, diabetes and all-cause mortality. One theory is that the increased consumption of heme iron creates high levels of iron-based free radicals. And as we learned in chapter 1 . . . free radicals cause innumerable DNA mutations that lead to cancer and a multitude of other diseases.

YOU ARE STRICTLY A PRODUCT OF YOUR GENES

In the next chapter, we will look deeply into a previously mentioned study that Dr. Dean Ornish carried through on 93 men with early prostate cancer which revealed that those who ate a whole food, plant-based diet, along with lifestyle changes, had a reversal of their cancer progression. The Standard American Diet group, on the other hand, had significant progression of their disease.

With that same group of individuals, Dr. Ornish and Nobel Prize-winner Dr. Elizabeth Blackburn decided to study how each group's genes would be expressed utilizing heat-map technology. To their surprise, after only 3 months on a whole food, plant-based diet, combined with lifestyle changes, more than 500 genes were found to act in a more positive fashion, demonstrating that you can actually change the way your bad genes act by making good lifestyle choices [51]. Earlier in this chapter, we also were exposed to a similar study that established that first cold pressed extra virgin olive oil made 160 genes act in a more positive way. This ability of our bodies to change gene expression is called "epigenetics" and is an exciting, rapidly evolving area of scientific study.

COFFEE IS BAD FOR YOU

Most people equate coffee with being a bad health habit, but most don't realize that the typical Western diet provides more antioxidants from coffee than from fruits and vegetables combined [52,53].

Because of the high antioxidant content of coffee, coffee drinkers have been found in many studies to have a lower risk of diabetes, Parkinson's disease, Alzheimer's, liver disease and depression. Coffee drinkers also appear to live longer. Long-term research involving 402,260 individuals aged 50–71 found that coffee drinkers had a much lower risk of dying over the 12- to 13-year study period [54].

You will notice later in my daily regimen that I start off every day with a cup of organic coffee with a number of added anti-cancer freeze-dried powders followed by a cup of organic decaf coffee with the same powders. I also must inform you that I always add ⅛ teaspoon of baking soda to neutralize the acidity of the coffee. You will learn later in this book how cancer tends to spread more easily in an acidic extracellular environment. So keeping a slightly alkaline pH is extremely important.

SUMMARY

These are just a few of the many myths propagated over the years about health, nutrition and a whole food, plant-based diet. If you have any other myths that you would like me to address in the second edition of this book, please send them to my email address *info@naturalinsightsintocancer.com.*

CHAPTER 6

The Power of a Whole Food, Plant-Based Diet

Every year, Americans lose more than 5 million years of life that could have been prevented [1]. Most experts in the field of preventive medicine think that only a small percentage of all cancers are due to purely genetic factors. The rest involve what we do on a day-to-day basis . . . with diet being one of the main determining factors [2].

We also know that The National Cancer Institute recommends 9 servings of fruits and vegetables for the prevention of cancer. The reason that recommendation was made was because the preponderance of the scientific studies show that fruits and vegetables have some kind of magical effect against cancer. We will go through the evidence with various cancers to sort out the facts.

PLANTS AGAINST BLOOD CANCERS

One of the largest prospective studies ever done on diet investigated the correlation between vegetarians' and meat eaters' cancer occurrence [3]. This study, that we briefly reviewed before, was performed at Oxford University and looked at 61,566 British men and women, comprising 32,403 meat eaters, 8,562 fish eaters, and 20,601 vegetarians. After an average follow-up of 12.2 years, the results were collated for various cancers occurring during that follow-up period.

In general, this study revealed that those who ate a plant-based diet had the lowest cancer rates, but the decreased rates were extraordinary for blood cancers. The incidence of leukemia, lymphoma and multiple myeloma (the cancer that I have) among vegetarians was nearly half of those eating meat. But how did this happen?

As most of us know by now, chemotherapy can wipe out rapidly dividing daughter cells very effectively, but in the process, a great number of normal cells are either destroyed or severely mutated in the process. Phytonutrients in plants, on the other hand, have been shown to have anti-cancer activity, using some of the same mechanisms as conventional therapeutic drugs, but with zero damage to normal cells.

For example, sulforaphane, considered one of the potent phytonutrients in cruciferous vegetables, kills leukemia cells very effectively in a petri dish without harming any of the normal cells at all [4]. Cruciferous vegetables include broccoli, cauliflower, brussel sprouts, bok choy, watercress, kale, collard greens, kohlrabi, rutabaga, turnips, arugula, radish, horseradish, wasabi and cabbage. These vegetables should be included in your diet every day if you are trying to prevent cancer and certainly in high volumes if you have cancer or had it and are trying to prevent a relapse.

We know that dripping cruciferous-vegetable extracts on cancer cells will kill the cancer, but what happens to people who already have cancer who go on a whole food, plant-based diet? Yale researchers wanted to find out the answer, so they did an 8-year study following more than 500 women being treated for non-Hodgkin's lymphoma. Those who started out consuming 3 or more servings of vegetables per day had a 42%-improved survival rate compared to individuals who ate less. In this study, green, leafy vegetables and citrus fruits appeared most protective [5].

The researchers were not sure whether the improved survival was due to the vegetables' phytonutrients keeping the cancer in check or to the patients' better ability to tolerate the chemotherapy and radiation due to the antioxidant-protective effects of the plants. An accompanying editorial in the *Journal of Leukemia and Lymphoma* suggested that a "lymphoma diagnosis may be an important teachable moment to improve diet" [6].

Additionally, "The Iowa Women's Health Study," published in the *International Journal of Cancer*, followed more than 35,000 women for decades and found that higher cruciferous-vegetable intake correlated with a lower risk of getting non-Hodgkin's lymphoma in the first place [7].

Another study published in the *Journal of Agricultural Chemistry* looked at the effect of açaí berries on leukemia cells [8]. During this study, the researchers dripped an extract of açaí berries on leukemia cells removed from a leukemia patient. When the extract was applied to the cancerous cells in a petri dish, 86% of the cells were destroyed. Also, when açaí was applied to macrophages (cancer, bacteria, and virus-fighting immune cells), the macrophages were able to destroy 40% more bacteria than the control [9].

PLANTS AGAINST PROSTATE CANCER

Prostate cancer is the most common cancer in men. In fact, autopsy studies show that about 50% of men older than 80 have prostate cancer

[10], and most men die with prostate cancer without ever knowing they had it. That is why PSA screenings can be a problem due to the fact that the detected prostate cancers may never have caused a problem if they went undiscovered [11]. Regrettably, many men are not so fortunate, because approximately 28,000 men die each year from prostate cancer.

As I alluded to in the chapter on common myths, one factor that has been correlated with prostate cancer is dairy consumption. Since the U.S. National Dairy Board was first established by the Dairy and Tobacco Adjustment Act of 1983, it has spent more than $1 billion on pushing their product. We are probably all familiar with their slogan "Milk Is Natural." But is drinking another species' milk natural? Aside from drinking another species' milk, humans are the only species that drinks milk after weaning. Then on top of that, we drink milk from a species (cows) that grows 40X faster than us. And that 40X faster means more cancer-causing proteins like casein and growth hormones. One point that many proponents of high-meat diets forget is that all animal foods have their own innate sex and growth hormones, even if sex and growth hormones are not added by the farmers.

When it comes to cancer, however, growth hormone is the hormone that is of the gravest concern [12]. As I previously communicated, cow's milk is designed to make a calf grow 40X faster than an infant . . . putting on a few hundred pounds within a few months. Being exposed to these powerful growth hormones and factors in milk may help explain the correlation found between dairy consumption and certain cancers [13]. Leading experts in the field of nutrition have communicated grave concern that the growth hormones and growth factors in dairy products could propagate the growth of hormone-sensitive tumors [14]. The scientific literature also points to the correlation of dairy products with precancerous lesions being converted into invasive cancers [15]. One of the growth hormones of gravest concern to scientists is our next topic of discussion . . . Insulin-like Growth Factor-1 (IGF-1).

IGF-1 (Insulin-like growth factor-1)

One fact that has been noticed from the scientific literature over the years is that, as we age, our risk of developing and dying from cancer grows every year—until we hit 85–90, when, interestingly, our cancer risk starts to drop [16]. What accounts for this resistance to cancer when we start nearing the age of 100? The science is showing more and more that it may have to do with a cancer-promoting growth hormone called "Insulin-like Growth Factor-1" (IGF-1) [17].

As we discussed before, when we are born, we need growth hormone to cause our cells to divide at an appropriate speed so that we can become a full-grown adult. To cause that to happen, the pituitary gland secretes human growth hormone (HGH), which then signals the liver to manufacture Insulin-like Growth Factor-1 (IGF-1). This hormone will then promote and guide the heightened cellular proliferation that is required to reach adulthood. The level of this hormone will steadily increase into our teenage years, at which time the levels start declining gradually each year with age.

Remember in chapter 1 how we discussed the fact that, as we age, we also develop DNA mutations that accumulate. When these mutations hit a critical level is when a precancerous cell can turn cancerous. Mother Nature designed us so that, as we age, with these increased mutations, our IGF-1 levels simultaneously decline, which protects us from precancerous cells converting to a full-blown cancer. If your levels of IGF-1 remain too high once you reach adulthood, your cells will continually receive a message to grow and divide. Not surprisingly, the more IGF-1 you have in your bloodstream as an adult, the higher your risk for developing cancers, such as prostate cancer [18].

Another interesting fact (that we've already learned) that adds to the evidence that high IGF-1 levels lead to cancer has to do with a rare form of dwarfism called "Laron Syndrome," which is caused by their genetic incapability to produce IGF-1. Affected individuals grow to be only a few feet tall, but, as you may remember, there has never been a reported case of an individual with "Laron Syndrome" ever acquiring cancer [19]. Because of these findings, scientists started to wonder how they could down-regulate IGF-1 so that cancer incidence would decline with advancing age instead of increasing. What they found was that you can do it through a simple dietary change . . . a whole food, plant-based diet.

The release of IGF-1 appears to be triggered by the consumption of animal protein [20], and, by reducing our animal-protein intake, we reduce our IGF-1 levels [21]. This, however, does not happen with plant protein. As I explained before, the theory is that when the liver is exposed to a complete protein, which is found in animal products, this complete protein sends a signal to the liver that growth is about to take place, which then causes the liver to start manufacturing IGF-1. In one aforementioned study where they looked at the IGF-1 levels in vegans versus meat eaters, the vegans consistently had significantly lower IGF-1 levels. The vegan group had an average IGF-1 level of 139 pmol/L, with meat eaters coming in at 201 pmol/L. This should not worry anyone, however, because a drop in IGF-1 can occur very rapidly after adopting a whole food, plant-based diet. In fact, in one study, it was demonstrated that in just 11 days after adopting a whole food, plant-based diet, the IGF-1 levels dropped by 20% and the levels of IGF-1 binding protein (holds onto the IGF-1, which keeps it inactive) jumped by 50% [22].

The Landmark Dean Ornish Studies

Many of you know that atherosclerotic heart disease is the number-one killer in the United States and even worldwide. This process of atherosclerosis starts at a very young age in countries like the United States. I was first exposed to this fact about 35 years ago, when I first read some of the writings of Nathan Pritikin. He referred to a study of U.S. soldiers killed in the Korean War who had autopsies of their coronary arteries [23]. In that study, the average age was 22 years and the incidence of atherosclerosis was 70%. Another study of Vietnam soldiers killed in action revealed that 45% had coronary atherosclerosis and that 55% already had gross evidence of severe coronary atherosclerosis [24]. These were detected by post-mortem angiograms and dissections. Still another study looked at the coronary arteries of American children 10–14 years old who had been killed in motorcycle accidents and found that 50% of them already had evidence of early atherosclerosis [25].

Dr. Dean Ornish decided to study this significant health problem and see if he could demonstrate definitively, with coronary angiograms, cardiac PET scans, cholesterols, triglycerides, blood pressure and symptom follow-up, if a whole food, plant-based diet, along with stress management and exercise, could actually reverse this atherosclerotic process [26].

He had 48 patients randomized into a whole food, plant-based group and a Standard American Diet (SAD) group; after 5 years, the results were astounding. The individuals in the plant-based group had an amazing 7.9% average improvement in their stenosis, while the SAD group had a resounding 27.7% continuing closure of their coronary arteries. Subsequent to this landmark study, Dr. Caldwell Esselstyn and others have been able to duplicate this work, with the clear conclusion that individuals can reverse advanced atherosclerosis with a whole food, plant-based diet. And this was all proven with advanced diagnostic technology like angiograms and very sensitive cardiac PET scans.

Because of these dramatic results with heart disease , Dr. Ornish decided to perform a similar experiment with prostate cancer. In this study, he recruited 93 men diagnosed with early prostate cancer. They were divided similarly, as with the heart study, into a whole food, plant-based-with-lifestyle-changes group and a Standard American Diet (SAD) group. Their PSAs (biomarker for prostate cancer) ranged between 4 and 9ng/ml [27].

The results of this study were fascinating. Even though the whole food, plant-based diet did not totally obliterate the cancer, it reversed it and, at the very least, held it in check over a one-year period without any conventional therapy. The PSA levels (biomarker for prostate cancer) in the plant group came down by 4% and went up 9% in the SAD group. Another amazing finding was that, when the blood of each group was placed onto petri dishes growing LNCaP prostate cancer cells, the blood of the plant group killed the cancer cells 8X more effectively than the blood of the SAD group . . . 70% obliteration of the cancer cells versus 9% for the control!

So, for those of you who have cancer, this should be great evidence that a whole food, plant-based diet with stress-management techniques and exercise will be an excellent adjunct to your conventional therapy . . . one that should not only help you beat the cancer, but keep you from relapsing once you get into remission. And for you lucky ones who have not had cancer, this is a wonderful way to help yourself from ever getting it in the first place.

While Dr. Ornish had this group of prostate-cancer-patient participants available to him, he decided to do another study with Nobel Prize-winner Dr. Elizabeth Blackburn to see what a whole food, plant-based diet with lifestyle modifications would do to genetic expression . . . something we call "epigenetics" in the medical community. RNA samples were taken from the prostates of both groups before the aforementioned prostate cancer study ever began, and, at 3 months after the food and lifestyle interventions. The genetic expression was then analyzed at a 3-month time interval using heat-map technology. What was found was extremely interesting and exciting . . . the whole food, plant-based-diet-with-lifestyle-changes group up-regulated 48 good genes and down-regulated 453 bad genes. Therefore, 501 genes had their gene activity modified in a positive way simply through a change in diet and lifestyle to make the genes behave in a health-improving way. [28]. This is exciting news . . . you are not always a victim of your genes.

Another study that Drs. Ornish and Blackburn did while having this same group of prostate-cancer patients available to them was to analyze what happens to the telomere length of individuals on a whole food, plant-based diet with exercise and stress-management techniques [29]. For those of you unfamiliar with telomeres, they are the DNA caps on the end of our chromosomes that protect the DNA helix structure from totally unraveling. Think of them as the plastic ends of your shoelaces. As we age, the length of those telomeres shorten, and that is why all animals have a definitive lifespan. Normally, however, the speed at which these telomeres shorten has been thought (but never studied) to be affected by our lifestyle. With this study, as with the other Ornish/Blackburn study, the results were quite conclusive. After 5 years, the whole food, plant-based diet group had actually increased telomere length while the SAD control group had significant shortening. This is some impressive, concrete, scientifically based information for you to know that lifespan can be significantly altered by a whole food, plant-based diet along with exercise and stress-management techniques.

PLANTS AGAINST BREAST CANCER

Breast cancer is the second-most-common cancer among American women after skin cancer. Approximately 230,000 cases are diagnosed each year, and about 40,000 women die from it [30]. One thing that most people don't understand is that a breast-cancer lump is not something that started overnight. Cancers typically take 20–40 years to develop to the point that you can palpate them [31]. So what your doctor is calling an "early detection" is actually the detection of a tumor that has been acquiring thousands and thousands of new mutations over the course of many years. What is scary is that many women have breast-cancer cells growing in their breasts and have no clue that they are there. One research paper in the *British Journal of Cancer* revealed that as many as 20% of women aged 20–44 who died from accidents had hidden breast cancers growing inside of them revealed by autopsy [32].

The good news is that even if you have an occult cancer growing in your body, a plant-strong diet along with lifestyle changes can keep that cancer from ever becoming deadly. As long as your body can keep it to the size of the tip of a ballpoint pen, or smaller, you can exist perfectly normally without it having any effect on your overall health. I will show you the power of certain plant foods to help you achieve that goal.

Cutting Risk Factors

The American Institute for Cancer Research (AICR), the world's leading authority on diet and cancer, came up with 10 recommendations for cancer prevention based on a thorough review of all the scientific literature available to them. Their drive-home message was: "Diets that center around whole-plant foods—vegetables, whole grains, fruits and beans—cut the risk of many cancers, and other diseases as well"[33]. Also, many of us know that The National Cancer Institute recommends 9 servings of fruits and vegetables for the prevention of cancer. As I stated before, this recommendation was not made out of thin air, but was based on a high volume of scientific evidence that shows that those individuals and cultures that eat more fruits and vegetables have much lower cancer rates. To illustrate just how significantly lifestyle choices can impact breast-cancer risk, researchers followed a group of about 30,000 postmenopausal women with no history of breast cancer over a 7-year period. They found that women who accomplished just 3 of the 10 AICR recommendations (limiting alcohol, eating mostly plant foods, and maintaining a normal body weight) had a 62% lower risk of breast cancer [34].

Another very interesting study validated that simply eating a plant-based diet, along with walking every day, could improve your cancer defenses within just 2 weeks. Scientists applied the blood of women before and after 14 days of plant-strong eating onto breast-cancer cells growing in petri dishes. The blood taken after they started eating healthier suppressed cancer growth significantly better and killed 20%-30% more cancer cells than the blood taken from the same women just 2 weeks before [35]. The researchers attributed this positive effect to a decrease in levels of a cancer-promoting growth hormone called "IGF-1," likely due to the reduced intake of animal protein. As Dr. Michael Greger often asks in many of his *nutritionfacts.org* videos, "What kind of blood do you want flowing through every nook and cranny of your body? Blood that rolls over at the sight of cancer or blood that is in constant battle mode?"

The Alcohol Question

We've already discussed this in the common-myths chapter, but I want to touch on some additional critical points because we, as a culture, have become so blasé about alcohol use. Nowadays, many seem to view it like drinking water. However, in 2010, the official World Health Organization formally raised its classification of alcohol as an absolute human-breast carcinogen. In 2014, they were even more intense in their position, stating that, regarding breast cancer, no amount of alcohol is safe. But what about so-called "responsible drinking"? In 2013, researchers did a meta-analysis of more than 100 studies looking at the correlation between breast cancer and light drinking (up to one alcoholic beverage a day). The scientists discovered a modest but statistically significant rise in breast-cancer risk even among women who had at most one drink per day. They estimated that, every year around the world, nearly 5,000 breast-cancer deaths may be attributable to light drinking [38]. Scientists believe that the cancer-causing chemical isn't the alcohol itself. The offender is actually the toxic enzymatic metabolic byproduct of alcohol called "acetaldehyde," which is a relative of formaldehyde. Red wine may be slightly better than white wine and other alcoholic beverages, but "The Harvard Nurses' Health Study" found that even a little less than one drink of red wine per day day is correlated with some elevation in breast-cancer risk [37].

In regard to specific plant foods that have anti-breast-cancer action, we will discuss those at the end of this chapter and in the chapter on "the power of targeted supplements." I will also teach you about the amazing power of exercise against breast cancer in the chapter on "the power of exercise."

PLANTS AGAINST COLORECTAL CANCERS

Cancers of the digestive tract kill 100,000+ Americans every year. Colorectal (colon and rectal) cancer, which kills 50,000+ lives per year, is one of the most frequently diagnosed of all cancers. The good news is that it is one of the most treatable if caught early enough. Conversely, pancreatic cancer is pretty much a death sentence for the 46,000+ individuals who contract it every year. Very few of these people will live beyond one year after they are diagnosed, which means prevention is the key. Esophageal cancer is another digestive cancer that is also usually a death sentence for its 18,000+ annual victims. The foods that create acid reflux can directly affect esophageal-cancer risk by causing a constant irritation to the esophageal lining.

The average person has about a 5% chance of contracting colorectal cancer over the course of his or her lifetime and it is the second-leading cause of cancer-related deaths in the United States. Fortunately, it is among the most treatable cancers, as regular screening has enabled doctors to detect and remove the cancer before it spreads. There are more than one million colorectal cancer survivors in the United States alone, and, among those diagnosed before the cancer has spread beyond the colon, the 5-year survival rate is about 90% [38].

As we've already stated, colorectal cancer is the second-leading cause of cancer-related death in the United States, yet in some parts of the world, it is almost non-existent. America has one of the highest colon-cancer rates in the world, yet many African countries have virtually no colon cancer at all

[39]. It most likely is the fact that many Africans eat primarily a whole food, plant-based diet [40]. However, in some countries, where people eat more fiber than other countries, the colon-cancer rates are slightly higher [41].

The Power of Phytates

So what is happening with this unexpected correlation? Ensuing research is demonstrating that dietary prevention of cancer may involve not only fiber but also natural compounds called "phytates," which are found in the seeds of plants—that means in all whole grains, beans, nuts, and seeds. One of the ways that phytates may have this positive anti-cancer effect is that they have been shown to detoxify excess iron in the body. And excess iron can generate a very harmful type of free radical called an "hydroxyl radical," and, if you remember from the first chapter . . . free-radical formation is at the root of almost all cancers. The Standard American Diet, therefore, has some major problems when it comes to colorectal cancer. Americans consume a lot of meat, and meat contains the type of heme iron that is highly correlated with colorectal cancer [42]. The other problem with meat and refined foods is that they also lack phytates that get rid of these iron-induced free radicals.

Of all the wonderful nutrients in beans, whole grains, nuts and seeds, why do we credit the phytates with reduced cancer risk? Petri-dish studies have demonstrated that phytates constrain the growth of just about every human cancer investigated . . . including cancers of the colon, breast, cervix, prostate, liver, pancreas, and skin . . . while not affecting normal cells at all [43]. What we are finding is that, when you consume phytates, your body rapidly absorbs them into the bloodstream and they are very quickly absorbed by cancer cells. In fact, you can do a radioactive phytate scan, similar to a PET scan (uses radioactive glucose), and it will show where the cancer is present in the body [44]. How do phytates fight cancer? Besides having known powerful antioxidant and anti-inflammatory effects, phytates have been found to significantly increase the activity of natural killer cells, which are white blood cells that form your initial defense against cancer cells [45]. Phytates can also prevent tumors from getting enough blood supply. There are many phytonutrients in many plant foods, including phytates, that have this very important anti-angiogenesis effect [46].

THE MCLELLAND TRIANGLE

I would highly recommend reading a book by Jane McLelland called *How to Starve Cancer*. In this is highly researched book, Jane McLelland describes the 3 pathways that cancer cells utilize for energy production. The first one is the glucose pathway that we discussed in chapter 1. This is Warburg's anaerobic glycolysis, which is essentially a fermentation process that creates 2 ATP energy molecules per one glucose molecule. To reiterate how inefficient this process is . . . our normal metabolic process creates 36 ATP molecules from one glucose molecule.

If cancer cells are not presented with enough glucose, they can convert to a cholesterol- or glutamine- (an amino acid) fermentation pathway for their energy production. Her research, in fact, shows that some cancers, like breast, prostate, and colon cancer, may actually prefer the cholesterol pathway over the glucose pathway.

For this reason, I feel that a whole food, plant-based diet is the best diet to starve the cancer stem cell at all 3 levels. If you are eating an extremely high-fiber, whole-plant-based diet (no refined carbs), the blood-sugar levels should never get into an abnormal range. I told you before that, if I drink my smoothie one hour before my monthly blood work, my blood-sugar level never goes above 85 mg/dl. A fasting blood-sugar level of more than 100 md/dl is considered abnormal, and a level of 140 mg/dl, even after 4 hours of eating, is considered a normal blood sugar. Remember . . . my blood-sugar level before my monthly blood work is not a fasting blood-sugar level.

Besides keeping the blood sugar low, an individual eating a whole food, plant-based diet is eating about 10% fat/cholesterol and 10% protein. All of these levels are such that the normal cells are getting excellent nutrition with a huge anti-cancer phytonutrient payload, while the cancer cells (dividing at an extremely fast rate), which need an enormous amount of fuel, are starving.

PLANTS AGAINST ANGIOGENESIS

Another book that I previously recommended is Dr. William Li's book called *Eat to Beat Disease*. I also told you about Dr. Li's amazing TED Talk, *Can We Eat to Starve Cancer?* that you can view on YouTube, dealing with the science establishing that certain plant foods have an amazing ability to inhibit the formation of new blood vessels to cancers (angiogenesis).

As we have formerly discussed, a cancer cannot grow beyond the size of the tip of a ballpoint pen if it does not have enough blood supply. As the tumor rapidly grows, it relies on the creation of new blood vessels to make certain it has enough fuel to feed the growing mass of tumor cells. Through intensive research, Dr. Li points out the foods that have been shown to have the greatest anti-angiogenesis effect. They are, from strongest to weakest . . . soy extract, artichoke, parsley, berries, soy, garlic, red grapes, cruciferous vegetables, citrus fruits, green tea, turmeric, black tea and vitamin E.

FOODS THAT ARE STRONGLY ANTI-CANCER

Broccoli and the Cruciferous Vegetables
Broccoli contains sulforaphane, a plant compound found in cruciferous vegetables that may have potent anti-cancer properties. One petri-dish study validated that sulforaphane reduced the size and number of breast-cancer cells by up to 75% [47]. Similarly, an animal study found that

treating mice with sulforaphane helped kill off prostate-cancer cells and reduced tumor volume by more than 50% [48]. Some studies have also found that a higher intake of cruciferous vegetables such as broccoli may be linked to a lower risk of colorectal cancer. One meta-analysis of 35 studies showed that eating more cruciferous vegetables was associated with a lower risk of colorectal and colon cancer [49].

Carrots and High Beta-Carotene Foods

Several studies have found that eating more carrots is linked to a decreased risk of certain types of cancer. For example, an analysis looked at the results of 5 studies and concluded that eating carrots may diminish the risk of stomach cancer by up to 26% [50]. Another scientific inquiry discovered that a higher intake of carrots was correlated with an 18% lower chance of contracting prostate cancer [51]. One study analyzed the diets of 1,266 participants with and without lung cancer. It found that current smokers who did not eat carrots were 3X more likely to fall victim to lung cancer, compared to those who ate carrots more than once per week [52]. Because of these and many other important studies verifying the above findings, you should try to incorporate carrots and other high beta-carotene foods into your diet as a healthy snack or tasty side dish every day to increase your intake and reduce your risk of cancer. Other high beta-carotene foods are mangos, sweet potatoes, cantaloupes, kale, spinach, romaine and parsley.

Beans

Beans, as I have already shown, help to protect against colorectal cancer [53]. One study followed 1,905 people with a history of colorectal tumors and ascertained that those who consumed more cooked, dried beans had a decreased risk of tumor recurrence [54]. An animal study also found that feeding rats black beans or navy beans and then inducing colon cancer blocked the creation of cancer cells by up to 75% [55].

According to these results, eating a few servings of beans each week may increase your fiber intake and help lower the risk of developing cancer. I actually recommend 2 servings per day, and Dr. Greger, in his *Daily Dozen App*, recommends 3 servings per day. Remember from earlier in this chapter . . . phytates, along with the high content of fiber in the beans, are the main players in cancer prevention.

Berries
Berries are high in anthocyanins, plant pigments that have antioxidant properties and are linked with a reduced risk of cancer. In one human study, 25 people with colorectal cancer were treated with bilberry extract for 7 days, which was established to reduce the growth of cancer cells by 7% [56]. Another small investigation gave freeze-dried black raspberries to patients with oral cancer and showed that it decreased levels of certain biomarkers identified with cancer progression [57]. One animal study observed that feeding rats freeze-dried black raspberries diminished esophageal tumor rates by up to 54% and decreased the number of tumors by up to 62% [58]. Similarly, another rodent research project made evident that fueling rats with a berry extract decreased several cancer biomarkers [59]. Based on these findings, you should try to include a couple of berry servings into your diet each day, which will decrease your chances of coming down with cancer. I personally use a Trader Joe's prepackaged ***Organic Blueberry, Blackberry, Raspberry and Strawberry Fancy Berry Medley*** in my smoothie every morning.

Cinnamon
Cinnamon is well known for its health benefits, including its capability to reduce blood-sugar levels and calm inflammation [60]. Furthermore, some petri-dish and rodent studies have brought to light that cinnamon may help arrest the spread of cancer cells. One petri-dish study demonstrated nicely that cinnamon extract had the ability to decrease the

proliferation of cancer cells and induce their death [61]. Another research project validated that cinnamon's essential oil restrained the growth of head- and neck-cancer cells and also dramatically reduced tumor size [62]. Still another study determined that cinnamon extract triggered cell suicide in tumor cells and also decreased the effectiveness of the tumor's ability to grow and spread [63]. Because of these and many other studies verifying cinnamon' anti-cancer effects, I would highly recommend adding ½–1 teaspoon of cinnamon to your diet per day. Not only will it reduce your chances of getting cancer, but it will also reduce your blood-sugar levels and decrease inflammation. Personally, I give 10 shakes of *Organic Ceylon Cinnamon* by Frontier Co-Op (Amazon) into my morning caf and decaf coffee. I also use a teaspoon on my sweet potatoes with a pinch of clove. Tastes great and gives an incredibly high antioxidant boost.

Nuts

Research has recognized that eating nuts is linked to a lower risk of certain kinds of cancer. For instance, one observational analysis investigated the diets of 19,386 people and discovered that those eating a greater amount of nuts had a decreased risk of dying from cancer [64]. Another research project that followed 30,708 participants for up to 30 years validated that eating nuts regularly equated with a decreased risk of colorectal, pancreatic and endometrial cancers [65]. Other studies have brought to light that certain types of nuts may be linked to a decreased cancer risk. For example, Brazil nuts, which are high in selenium, may safeguard against lung cancer in those with a low selenium levels [66]. Furthermore, an interesting rodent study indicated that feeding mice walnuts decreased the growth rate of breast-cancer cells by 80% and slashed the amount of tumors by 60% [67]. These results suggest that adding a serving of nuts to your diet each day may reduce your risk of developing cancer in the future. I personally eat nuts before I take my supplements to ensure that the fat-soluble vitamins are absorbed. I eat 2 organic almonds, 2 organic walnuts, 2 organic pecans, 2 organic cashews, an organic Brazil nut, a few organic raw peanuts, a few organic pistachios and a few pumpkin seeds. Remember that variety is the key to health and cancer prevention. Eating a full handful of walnuts is not as cancer protective as eating a small amount of several types of nuts each day.

First Cold Pressed Extra Virgin Olive Oil

As I discussed in the "common myths" chapter, first cold pressed extra virgin olive oil (FCPEVOO) is loaded with health benefits. As I stated in that chapter, several studies have found that a higher intake of FCPEVOO helps protect against cancer. One massive review, made up of 19 studies, established that people who regularly consume the highest amount of FCPEVOO have a lower risk of getting breast and digestive cancers when compared to those with the lowest intake [68]. Another scientific fact-finding mission looked at the cancer rates in 28 countries around the world and discovered that the regions with a greater intake of FCPEVOO had decreased rates of colorectal cancer [69].

There are some doctors in the whole food, plant-based community who tell people to eat no olive oil because they feel that all oils negatively affect the cardiovascular system. I, however, have done a very thorough search of the entire scientific literature and have found that it is very difficult to find studies showing a negative effect on the cardiovascular system. They are largely positive. I do feel very strongly, however, that you should use only FIRST COLD PRESSED EXTRA VIRGIN OLIVE OIL. It has the highest polyphenol and vitamin E levels and has consistently been found to be the most health promoting. Also, don't use it extravagantly! I use only about a teaspoon on my salads. Remember, one tablespoon of any oil is 120 calories. The basic breakdown of FCPEVOO is 70% healthy monounsaturated fat, 15% saturated fat, and 15% polyunsaturated fat. About 2% is made up of the health-promoting polyphenols and vitamin E. A typical tablespoon of FCPEVOO, therefore, has 2 grams of saturated fat. If you add 3 tablespoons to your salad . . . now you are adding 6 grams of saturated fat and 360 calories, which could start changing the risk-to-benefit ratio. I think this is the fear of some plant-based doctors who are treating patients with severe atherosclerosis. Also, I would limit or, ideally, not use olive oil for cooking. The polyphenols get destroyed as you near the smoking point of 350°F, and toxic chemicals are produced at the smoking point and above. I would encourage you to learn to cook with organic-vegetable broth. Chef AJ has some very good videos on YouTube on how to do this easily and effectively.

Turmeric/Curcumin

Turmeric is a spice well known for its health-promoting properties. Curcumin, its most active ingredient, is a phytonutrient with potent anti-inflammatory, antioxidant and anti-cancer effects. There are literally thousands of peer-reviewed papers in the scientific literature verifying curcumin's anti-cancer activity. One study investigated how curcumin would affect 44 patients with precancerous lesions of the colon. The results were amazing. In just one month, 4 grams of curcumin daily reduced the number of lesions by a whopping 40% [70]!

In a different analysis, curcumin was also discovered to decrease the advancement of colon cancer by zeroing in on an essential enzyme required for cancer metastasis [71]. Still another study demonstrated that curcumin could eradicate head- and neck-cancer cells [72]. Other investigations reveal that curcumin can decelerate the growth of lung-, breast-, and prostate-cancer cells [73].

In the chapter on "the power of targeted supplements" we will discuss curcumin in further depth because of its importance in the battle against cancer. In fact, if you are going to take one supplement, this is the one I would recommend.

For use on your food, I would aim for at least ½–3 teaspoons of ground turmeric per day. Use it as a ground spice to add flavor to foods, and pair it with black pepper to help boost its absorption. As a supplement for cancer patients, I recommend supplement made by aSquared Nutrition called *Turmeric Curcumin with Piperine* that you can purchase on Amazon. Take 5 capsules in the morning and 5 at night. For the prevention of cancer, I recommend 2 in the morning and 2 at night. I always eat nuts and take 3 *Omax3 Professional Strength Ultra-Pure* fish oil capsules before taking turmeric, because it requires fat for proper absorption.

Citrus Fruits

Eating citrus fruits such as lemons, limes, grapefruits and oranges has been correlated with a lower risk of cancer in several analyses. One large study found that participants who ate a larger volume of citrus fruits had a lower risk of contracting digestive- and upper-respiratory-tract cancers [74]. A meta-analysis of 9 studies also ascertained that a greater consumption of citrus fruits was coupled to a reduced risk of pancreatic cancer [75]. Finally, another meta-analysis of 14 studies validated that an intake of at least 3 servings of citrus fruit per week decreased the risk of stomach cancer by 28% [76]. These studies and many other in the scientific literature strongly indicate that including a few servings of citrus fruits in your diet each day is an effective way to lower your risk of contracting certain types of cancer. I personally always include lemon and lime juice in my drinking water. I eat one orange every night, put a lemon wedge in my smoothies, and add a lemon and lime wedge to my nightly tea concoction, which we will discuss in the chapter on "the power of targeted supplements."

Flaxseeds/Chia seeds

Flax and chia seeds are high in fiber as well as the health-promoting, anti-inflammatory omega-3 fatty acid—alpha linolenic acid. In fact, several scientific studies have demonstrated that omega-3 fatty acids can literally kill cancer cells. In one interesting study, more than 30 women with breast cancer were given either a flaxseed muffin or a placebo each day for 30+ days. When each group's cancer biomarkers (tumor-growth and cancer-cell-death measurements) were assessed at the end of the study, the flaxseed group had significantly better results when compared to the control [77]. In another experiment, the researchers looked at 500+ men with prostate cancer who were fed ground flaxseeds on a daily basis. The results revealed that the flaxseed group had a lower rate of cancer progression [78]. Possibly because flaxseeds are so high in fiber, some studies have revealed it to be protective against colorectal cancer [79].

Try adding at least one tablespoon of ground flaxseed into your diet each day by adding it to smoothies, sprinkling it over cereal and yogurt, or adding it to your favorite baked goods. Chia seeds also have similar cancer-fighting and anti-inflammatory benefits. I place 1 tablespoon of organic ground flaxseeds and chia seeds into my daily morning smoothie.

I will discuss these seeds in further detail in the chapter on "the power of targeted supplements."

Tomatoes

Lycopene is the phytonutrient found in tomatoes that confers its beautiful red color. It is also linked to its anti-cancer properties. Several studies have indicated that consuming more lycopene gives rise to a reduced risk of prostate cancer. A meta-analysis of 17 studies illustrated that a higher consumption of raw tomatoes, cooked tomatoes and lycopene were all correlated with a lessened probability of getting prostate cancer [80]. Another study of more than 47,000 people determined that a higher consumption of tomato sauce, in particular, equated to a lower probability of succumbing to prostate cancer [81]. So try to get a tomato into your diet each day by adding it to sandwiches, salads, sauces, or pasta dishes. Being an Italian American and loving whole-wheat pasta with garlic-infused marinara sauce, I get cooked tomatoes into my diet every single day.

Garlic, Onions, Leeks and Shallots

One of the most active anti-cancer components in garlic is allicin, a compound that has been illustrated to kill off cancer cells in multiple experimental studies [82]. Several studies have established a link between garlic intake and a lower risk of several types of cancer. One study of 543,220 participants discovered that those individuals who consumed a lot of *Allium sativum* vegetables, such as garlic, onions, leeks and shallots, had a lower chance of acquiring stomach cancer compared to those who rarely ate them [83]. Another interesting analysis of more than 450 men indicated that a greater regular consumption of garlic was linked with a diminished probability of acquiring prostate cancer [84]. Still another research project demonstrated that the men who ate lots of garlic, as well as fruit, deep-yellow vegetables, dark-green vegetables, and onions were less likely to become afflicted with colorectal cancer. This study, however, did not uncouple the positive effects of garlic from the other consumed vegetables [85]. Based on the vast amount of science, it is a great idea to include a fresh clove of garlic in your diet on a daily basis. As I stated before, I eat lots of garlic-infused tomato sauce on my whole-wheat pasta, but to make sure I get a daily dose, I do take a garlic supplement called **Garlic** by Douglas Labs that you can purchase on Amazon. I take 2 tablets in the morning and 2 at night.

Fatty Fish

This is the only time I will diverge from recommending a solely whole food, plant-based diet, but there is some scientific literature demonstrating that fatty fish may have some cancer-fighting activity. One large study demonstrated that a greater consumption of fatty fish corresponded with a lower probability of coming down with digestive-tract cancer [86]. Another study that tracked 478,040 adults discovered that ingesting more fatty fish decreased the chance of contracting colorectal cancer, while red and processed meats actually inflated the probability [87]. In particular, it is the fatty fish such as salmon, mackerel, and anchovies that have critical nutrients such as vitamin D and omega-3 fatty acids, which have been associated with a lower cancer risk. Several scientific reviews have indicated that having adequate levels of vitamin D most likely protects us against cancer [88]. Furthermore, omega-3 fatty acids, through their powerful anti-inflammatory effects, deter the initiation of chronic disease and cancer [89]. If you are not strictly vegan like me, aim for one serving of fatty fish per week or every other week to get a dose of omega-3 fatty acids and vitamin D, and to maximize the potential health benefits of these nutrients. Just remember that nowadays most fish are highly contaminated with PCBs, mercury, microplastics and prescription drugs. I personally take a fish-oil supplement called ***Omax3 Professional Strength Ultra-Pure***. I take 3 in the morning and 3 in the evening before taking my other supplements.

PHYTONUTRIENT ACTIVITY IN A NUTSHELL

As I have reiterated over and over again, plant foods contain over 25,000 phytonutrients. These are their amazing cancer-killing activities in a nutshell:

- Increase natural killer T-cell activity
- Block cancer-cell-blood-vessel growth (anti-angiogenesis)
- Cause cancer-cell suicide (apoptosis)
- Disrupt cancer gap-junction cell signaling
- Inhibit cancer proteosomes (allows contaminated cancer proteins to accumulate killing the cancer cell)
- Fragment cancer DNA
- Make tumor-suppressor genes suppress more
- Make cancer cell apoptosis genes cause more apoptosis (cancer cell suicide)
- Help prevent chemotherapy resistance

- Stop cancer cell division at various phases of division
- Stop the methylation process that inactivates BRCA-DNA-repair genes
- Become cancer-killing pro-oxidants in the presence of cancer's high copper and iron levels
- Protect from further mutations to normal and cancer cells
- Significantly reduces inflammation (cancer thrives on inflammation)

CONCLUSION

As new research continues to emerge, it is becoming more and more clear that your diet has a major impact on your risk of cancer. Although there are many foods that have potential to reduce the spread and growth of cancer cells, current research is limited to a petri dish, animal and observational studies. As time goes on more and more studies will clarify how these incredibly powerful foods directly counter cancer initiation in humans. In the meantime, it's a safe bet that a diet rich in whole plant foods paired with a healthy lifestyle, will help you in your battle against cancer while improving many other aspects of your health.

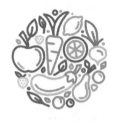

CHAPTER 7

The Power of Targeted Supplements

When I give lectures on cancer, the one fact that I drive home continually is that fruits, vegetables, whole grains, legumes, nuts, seeds, mushrooms, herbs, and spices have more than 25,000 phytonutrients that have powerful antioxidant, anti-inflammatory and anti-tumor effects. Many of these phytonutrients scientists do not even know what they do, but when they do start performing experimentation on the ones that they do discover, they find that Nature put them there for a specific purpose, and that purpose is to protect us from disease. So what I will do in this chapter is go through some of my favorite phytonutrients that are present in foods and herbs that have been shown to have anti-cancer activity. I will also let you know how I personally incorporate them into my daily routine. Every single supplement that I take has been scientifically validated to have anti-cancer properties. I am not going to waste my hard-earned money on a phytonutrient or herbal supplement that has not been shown in multiple scientific studies to have an anti-cancer effect. Sometimes these supplements will be a freeze-dried powder, a tea or a capsule that I can usually purchase on Amazon.

I must emphasize at the start that a whole food, plant-based diet is the absolute best, most effective way to get the 25,000+ phytonutrients that fight cancer. Additionally, the phytonutrients in these plant foods are in the perfect balance that Nature intended. The sad fact, however, is that only 3% of the Western population follow this type of diet and are not getting nearly the amount of nutrients necessary to fend off a formidable enemy like cancer. And even if you are eating a whole food, plant-based diet, the level of nutrient concentration needed to fight an incredibly formidable enemy like cancer cannot be obtained through 3 meals a day.

As you will notice, I take a lot of supplements . . . more than 30. I don't expect many of you to do what I do. I, however, have asterisked the ones that I do think are the most important. Go through each one that I describe; do some of your own research, and decide which ones work best for your budget, your lifestyle and the type of cancer that you are fighting.

NUTS FIRST

As you will see in chapter 12 describing my daily-maintenance program, before I take my supplements, I start off with eating 2 organic walnuts, 2 organic pecans, 2 organic almonds, 2 organic cashews, a few raw organic peanuts, a Brazil nut for selenium, a few organic pumpkin seeds, and a few organic pistachio nuts. I do this not only to ensure that I am getting the important varied phytonutrients in those nuts and seeds but also to get some healthy fats into my system to be able to absorb any fat-soluble vitamins or phytonutrients in the supplements that I will be taking. If those supplements are taken with no fat, there will be no absorption. That is one reason why I always put a teaspoon of first cold pressed extra virgin olive oil on my salads. Below are all of the supplements that I take daily. So let's begin.

INDOLE-3-CARBINOL

This is one of the better-known phytonutrients found in cruciferous vegetables like broccoli, cabbage, brussel sprouts, collard greens and kale. Most of the scientific studies on I-3-C have focused on its ability to alter estrogen metabolism and other effects on the cell. These results show that its anti-cancer effects are most likely due to its ability not to allow toxins to bind to DNA. The first evidence of anti-cancer activity by I-3-C in humans was claimed by the Dashwood group in 1989 [1].

I-3-C and its metabolite 3,3'-diindoylmethane (DIM) have also been demonstrated to target multiple aspects of cancer-cell-cycle regulation and survival, which include better BRCA gene activity (a DNA-repair gene), inducing cancer-cell suicide, positively affecting estrogen metabolism and estrogen-cell-receptor signaling, and lowering inflammation [2].

There are innumerable other, well-done scientific studies demonstrating remarkable anti-cancer activity. Go to *pubmed.gov* and type in "indole-3-carbinol against cancer," and you will be impressed. Because of the science backing its anti-cancer effects, I personally take an Indole-3-Carbinol supplement made by Douglas Labs and purchased on Amazon. It is called **Ultra I-3-C** and is in a capsule form. It has 200 mg of I-3-C and a proprietary blend of broccoli extract (sprouts), cauliflower (entire plant), and brussel sprouts (entire plant). I take one in the morning and one at night. I would strongly recommend this for breast-cancer patients.

*RESVERATROL

Resveratrol is another phytonutrient that has received lots of attention in the media due to its anti-cancer and anti-atherosclerosis effects. It is found in many plant species such as grapes, raw cacao, pomegranate, peanuts and berries, and it is produced by these plants in response to mechanical injury, fungal infection and UV radiation [3].

It belongs to a family of compounds known as "polyphenols," which are known to combat damaging free radicals. Research shows that resveratrol has the ability to penetrate deeply into the center of the cell's nucleus, allowing our DNA to be protected from free-radical damage, which, you know by now, if not protected, leads to cancerous growth. Furthermore, resveratrol has potent anti-inflammatory activity, which helps prevent certain enzymes from triggering tumor development.

Besides helping to prevent cancer, resveratrol can be very helpful to those receiving conventional cancer therapy and acts as a:

- Chemo-sensitizer—a substance that can help you overcome resistance to chemotherapy drugs.
- Radiation-sensitizer—making cancer more susceptible to radiation treatments.

Radiation sensitization was shown in a study conducted at the University of Missouri, where melanoma cells became more susceptible to radiation when given resveratrol prior to radiation. When treated with resveratrol alone, 44% of the cancer cells underwent cell suicide [4].|

I personally take resveratrol in a vegetarian-capsule form twice daily. It is called **Methylated Resveratrol Plus** made by Douglas Labs and can be purchased on Amazon. One capsule contains Vitamin D3 1,000 IU, MERIVA® curcumin phytosome 250 mg, resveratrol 100 mg, pterostilbene (methylated resveratrol) 50 mg, proprietary cruciferous

150 mg and a vegetable-and-fruit blend of Wasabia japonica, broccoli powder, and organic pomegranate powder.

CHINESE RED YEAST

Because Chinese Red Yeast is sometimes called "Red Yeast Rice," I will use the abbreviation RYR in this section. So what is RYR? It is created by fermenting a type of yeast called *Monascus purpureus* with rice. When the rice is added to the fermenting yeast, the result is RYR, with its reddish-purple color. The interesting thing about RYR is that it has naturally occurring chemicals in it called "monacolins," which block the production of cholesterol . . . similar to statin drugs.

In fact, the first statin drug made by Merck, called "lovastatin," had the exact same chemical structure as monacolin K, found in RYR. This fact actually turned into a lawsuit when the first RYR supplement, called "Cholestin," was brought to market. Merck sued over it but fortunately lost the lawsuit, which has allowed a safer way to lower cholesterol with many fewer side effects.

Experts aren't clear on whether RYR successfully lowers cholesterol solely because of the monacolins or because of the additional phytonutrients present in RYR. It is very likely due to a combination and is why I prefer it over taking a statin drug.

So why do we want to lower cholesterol? A multitude of studies in the scientific literature show that, when looking at large groups of individuals taking statins or RYR, they have lower rates of cancer [5]. I previously described how there are 3 pathways that cancer can use for energy . . . a sugar, cholesterol, or glutamine pathway. In some cancers, like prostate cancer, it has been shown by several researchers to actually have a predilection for the cholesterol pathway. Therefore, I think it is prudent to lower the amount presented to each pathway. What is the best way to do this? I strongly think that a whole food, plant-based diet is by far the best way to accomplish this task. But to get additional help with the cholesterol-mevolanate pathway, I think taking RYR, without the major side effects of statin drugs, is a prudent choice. In fact, you can ask your doctor if he or she would be willing to add an old generic blood thinner called "dipyridamole." A few studies have demonstrated a powerful synergistic anti-cancer effect when a statin and dipyridamole are combined [6]

I personally take a supplement by Douglas Labs called **Beni Koji RYR** which can be purchased on Amazon. Each capsule contains 500 mg of organic red yeast rice. I take 2 in the morning and 2 at night. It is important that, when you take RYR, you also take coenzyme Q10, which is the next topic of discussion. If you have breast, prostate, or colon cancer, I fully recommend this supplement. Also, if you are a cancer patient with a total cholesterol greater than 150 mg/dl, I would strongly recommend taking RYR, because many studies show that heart attacks, strokes and blood clots kill a high number of cancer patients due to the side effects of the chemo drugs, lack of exercise and poor dietary habits.

COENZYME Q10

Coenzyme Q10 is a natural antioxidant made by the body, found in many foods and available as a supplement. There are 2 basic forms: ubiquinol (the active antioxidant form) and ubiquinone (the oxidized form), which partially converts to ubiquinol. Many of the CoQ10 supplements contain both forms of this antioxidant.

CoQ10's primary function is as a vital participant in the chain of metabolic reactions that generate energy within the cells. This antioxidant is found in every single cell in the body, but is found in the highest concentrations in organs that have very high energy requirements such as the heart, kidneys and liver.

This antioxidant is especially beneficial for heart health. It helps maintain the normal oxidative state of the bad LDL cholesterol (preventing atherosclerosis) and supports optimal functioning of the heart muscle. The reason you should make sure you take CoQ10 if you are taking a statin or RYR is that they can deplete CoQ10 levels in the tissues. So, it is very prudent to make sure you are taking CoQ10 with a statin or RYR.

An interesting study, dealing strictly with cancer, looked at the prognosis of melanoma-skin-cancer patients' long-term survival in correlation to their CoQ10 levels. Researchers prospectively followed 117 early-stage (none with metastatic disease) melanoma and 125 healthy volunteers (control group). The first thing to note is that the CoQ10 levels were significantly lower in the cancer patients when compared to the control group. Secondly, those with a CoQ10 level less than 0.6 mg/L (low) had a 790% increased risk of developing metastatic disease compared with those who had higher CoQ10 levels . . . and the time to develop metastasis was nearly double in patients with CoQ10 levels of 0.6 or less.

Among the 82 melanoma patients with a CoQ10 level less than 0.6 mg/L (low), 17 of them died during the study period, with none of the higher level CoQ10 patients dying [7].

I personally take a capsule supplement from Douglas Labs called *Ubiquinol-QH* that can be purchased on Amazon. I prefer *Ubiquinol-QH* because it is the active antioxidant form. I take 2 capsules in the AM and 2 in the PM for a total of 400 mg per day. Because this is a fat-soluble antioxidant, you must take it with some nuts and/or fish-oil capsules for excellent absorption.

*OMEGA-3 FAT SUPPLEMENTS

We have previously discussed the critical importance of chronic inflammation for not only cancer's initiation, but also for its maintenance and progression. We also discussed the importance of the essential fats and getting the proper balance to keep inflammation at bay. We learned that omega-6

184 | BEAT BACK CANCER NATURALLY

fats are very inflammatory, omega-3 fats are very anti-inflammatory, and that the current Western diet is balanced heavily in favor of omega-6 fats, because we eat so many processed foods and because livestock is now fed grain instead of grass. The ideal omega-6 to omega-3 ratio is around 2:1. The average Western ratio is 20:1 up to 40:1 in various studies [8].

The best way to increase the amount of omega-3 fats is through plant-based sources, which are walnuts, edamame, flaxseeds, chia seeds, kidney beans, black beans, and winter squash. If you are a meat eater, fatty fish is your best way; this would include wild caught salmon, tuna, mackerel, sardines, herring, and anchovies. Their fillets contain up to 30% oil, although this figure varies among species.

The problem with getting your omega-3 fats from fatty fish is that, as you go up the food chain, fat-soluble pesticides and heavy metals such as mercury begin to accumulate in the fatty tissues. This is called "bioaccumulation" and is one of the major reasons, among others, that I am not a proponent of animal products. In fact, in one study in the *International Journal of Environmental Pollution* found 81 different drugs, including illegal narcotics, stimulants, anti-depressants, and other classes of drugs in the fillets of wild caught salmon outside of Seattle. Fish also have the highest PCB and microplastic contamination of any animals on earth.

I, therefore, personally eat as many plant-based sources as possible of omega-3 fat, including a tablespoon of ground flax and chia seeds, in my morning smoothie. I also think it is critical to take an omega-3 supplement to get your omega-6 to omega-3 ratio around 2:1. I use ***Omax 3 Ultra-Pure Professional Strength*** capsules. I take 3 in the AM and 3 in the PM right before taking my supplements. Again, the reason that I take these (and my nuts) right before my other supplements is to make sure the fat-soluble vitamins and phytonutrients are properly absorbed. As I previously alluded to, without healthy fat being present, fat-soluble nutrients will just pass through the gut without absorbing the needed nutrition to fight disease.

Three capsules of **Omax3 Ultra Pure Professional Strength** give me 2,265mg of EPA and 564mg of DHA. Therefore, in one day, 6 capsules will provide 5,658mg of omega-3 fats. When I had my omega-6 to omega-3 ratio checked with an inexpensive lab test by Quest Laboratories, my ratio was 2.6:1, and my DHA was a little on the lower side. I, therefore, added 2 capsules of **Omax Cognitive**, which adds 200 mg of EPA and 800 mg of DHA. I, therefore, upped my total omega-3s to 6,658mg per day, and, when I rechecked my omega-6 to omega-3 ratio it was 1.9:1, with the EPA and DHA levels in perfect balance.

In regard to DHA, it is very important to make sure that this level is ideal because several studies demonstrate a strong anti-cancer effect with this form of omega-3 fat. It incorporates into the cellular membrane of the cancer cell and has been shown to cause cancer-cell suicide and reduce proliferation in in-vitro and in-vivo studies [9].

By the way, **Omax3 Ultra-Pure Professional Strength** is the only fish-oil supplement that I would recommend. I have researched many of these fish-oil supplements, and this one is totally clear of extraneous toxins. In fact, a little test that you can do at home is to place an **Omax 3** supplement and a CVS or other fish-oil supplement in the freezer overnight. The **Omax 3** will be crystal clear the next morning, and the other fish-oil supplement, I guarantee you, will be cloudy.

If you are totally opposed to anything animal based, there are several algae-based omega-3 supplements that can be purchased on Amazon. The only problem with these supplements is that they typically have very little EPA and a lot of DHA—so the proper balance between EPA and DHA is not ideal.

MANGOSTEEN

Mangosteen (*Garcinia mangostana*), also known as the purple mangosteen, is a tropical evergreen with edible fruit grown in Southeast Asia, southwest India, Colombia, Puerto Rico, and Florida. The fruit of the mangosteen is sweet and tangy, and, because of the taste, it is sometimes called the "queen of fruits." It has an inedible, deep-purplish-colored rind (pericarp) when ripe. The pericarp is actually where most of the the anti-cancer nutrients are present. The interest in the mangosteen's pericarp phytonutrients, called "xanthones," has greatly increased in recent years, demonstrated by the dramatic increase in scientific reports. A search of available literature in Pubmed, Science Direct, Google Scholar, and Scirius showed 158 reports from 1980 to 2008. By contrast, there were 454 published articles from 2008 through March 2013.

Sixty-eight of these xanthones have been discovered in the pericarp, but the most-studied xanthone is alpha-mangostin, for which strong anti-cancer and anti-inflammatory effects have been demonstrated [10]. After reviewing a large segment of the articles published between 2008 and 2019, I decided to incorporate mangosteen into my daily regimen. I personally take a mangosteen capsule (morning and evening) by Solaray "*Mangosteen*," that can be purchased on Amazon. Each capsule has 475mg of the whole fruit. I also add one teaspoon of *Mangosteen Fruit Powder* by Terrasoul (Amazon) to each of my morning organic coffees (one caf and one decaf). This powder is made solely from the pericarp, where the xanthones are concentrated.

*TURMERIC

Turmeric (*Curcuma longa*) is really the king of anti-cancer herbs. Of all of the herbs, phytonutrients and supplements that I am recommending in this book, turmeric is the one everyone should take . . . cancer patient or not. It is the primary spice in curry, and it is agreed upon by many to be the most powerful herb on the planet for fighting and reversing disease.

At the time of this writing, there are more than 12,500 peer-reviewed scientific articles that prove turmeric's powerful benefits. In regard to cancer, the anti-tumor activities have been shown to include the inhibition of tumor proliferation, the inhibition of angiogenesis (new-cancer-blood-vessel growth), the ability to push back against cancer invasion and metastasis, the induction of tumor apoptosis (cancer-cell suicide), the increase of chemotherapy sensitivity, and the ruining of the cell cycle in the cancer stem cell . . . indicating that turmeric works by modulating innumerable aspects of cancer progression.

In regard to my cancer, multiple myeloma, there is a lab value that monitors the activity of plasma-cell-tumor proliferation. The cancerous plasma cells release a paraprotein that can be measured in the bloodstream, and this lab value is called the "M-spike."

With myeloma, the individual progresses from MGUS (monoclonal gammopathy of underdetermined significance) to smoldering myeloma, to a full-blown multiple myeloma. This progression is actually an excellent way to view how cancer progresses from "under control by the immune system" to a "full-blown cancer." In an article published in *Nature*, famous genomic myeloma researcher Dr Nikhil Munshi, wrote that, at the time of diagnosis of myeloma, the cancer cell has approximately 5,000 mutations. Then, when the disease relapses, there are approximately 12,000 mutations. Therefore, it is my projection that, to get to MGUS, an individual probably requires approximately 2,000 mutations, and, to get to smoldering myeloma, around 3,500 mutations. The developing cancer then needs another 1,500 mutations (total of 5,000) to get you to a full-blown myeloma.

In 2 very-well-done scientific studies, turmeric was put to the test on MGUS to see if it had an effect on the progression of the M-spike [11,12]. In both studies, about half of the patients had a 33% drop in the level of the M-spike. In the larger study by Golombick's group [13], there were also improvements in other biomarkers of multiple myeloma, such as free monoclonal light chains and uDPYD, a biomarker of bone resorption.

In regard to how to add it to your diet, I would recommend incorporating turmeric into as many recipes as possible. Dr. Greger recommends a quarter-teaspoon per day in his *Daily Dozen App*. When battling cancer, I personally recommend 4–8 grams per day . . . 8 grams preferably. If you are on blood thinners, consult with your oncologist.

I personally use a turmeric product made by aSquared Nutrition called **Turmeric Curcumin with Piperine** and take 5 capsules in the morning and 5 in the evening. One attractive aspect about this product is that every 1600 mg has 2.5mg of piperine (black-pepper extract) included in each capsule. Studies show that 20mg/kg of piperine increases the bioavailability of curcumin by 2000% [14]. This is accomplished through better absorption and decreased breakdown in the intestinal wall and liver.

Since an average male weighs 70 kg, that means a person should intake about 1,400 mg of piperine, which is an extraordinarily high amount. Ten capsules of **Turmeric Curcumin with Piperine** by aSquared Nutrition gives you 25 mg of piperine. I, therefore, take a separate piperine supplement called **Bioperine** by Source Naturals, which provides 10 mg per tablet. I take 5 tablets with the 5 turmeric capsules in the morning and the night. Even though I am not even close to the 1,400 mg that was used in the above study, I believe it still enhances the bioavailability of the turmeric. Another important point about bioavailability . . . make sure you always ingest fat before taking turmeric supplements . . . a point I have emphasized over and over again in this book.

One other reason that I use the **Turmeric Curcumin with Piperine** supplement by aSquared Nutrition is because it is primarily the whole turmeric root rather than being standardized to 95% curcumin, like most turmeric supplements. Studies over the past decade have indicated that curcumin-free turmeric (CFT) components possess numerous anticancer activities that surpass using curcumin in isolation [14]. Some of the individual components of turmeric are phytonutrients such as turmerin, turmerone, elemene, furanodiene, curdione, bisacurone, cyclocurcumin, calebin A, and germacrone. As I continue to preach in this book, the combination of many phytonutrients in plants is usually much more effective than isolating one component of the whole.

*GINGER ROOT

When you were a little kid, your mom may have given you ginger ale to fix your upset stomach. For ages, ginger has been well known as an effective treatment for nausea, but in recent years, it has been seriously researched as a treatment for cancer.

Ginger (*Zingiber officinale*) is a tropical plant that has green-purple flowers and an underground stem called a rhizome. In the rhizome, there is a mixture of various compounds, including gingerol, paradol, zingiberene and shogoal. Such compounds have been found to have anti-inflammatory and anti-tumor activity. These phytonutrients have proven roles in cancer management through their anti-inflammatory activity, making tumor-suppressor genes suppress cancer more effectively, muddling the cancer-cell cycle, inducing apoptosis (cancer-cell suicide), confusing cancer's transcription factors (coordinate cell division), preventing angiogenesis (cancer-blood-vessel growth), and interfering with cancer-cell-signaling pathways [15].

Additionally, because ginger also has anti-nausea effects, its combination with chemotherapeutic agents may offer the advantage of being efficacious at helping to defeat the cancer while helping to reduce toxicity [16].

I personally take a supplement made by Douglas Labs called **Ginger Root Max-V**, which which can be purchased on Amazon. Each capsule has 350mg of ginger root standardized to 5% gingerols. I take one capsule in the morning and one in the evening.

*MILK THISTLE

Milk thistle (*Silybum marianum*) is an annual or biennial plant that has reddish-purple flowers that can be found throughout the world.

Traditional milk-thistle extract is made from the seeds, which contain approximately 4–6% silymarin. Silymarin is a complex mixture of polyphenolic molecules, including 7 closely related flavonolignans (silybin A, silybin B, isosilybin A, isosilybin B, silychristin, isosilychristin, silydianin) and one flavonoid (taxifolin).

Lab and animal studies are showing that these phytochemicals in milk thistle may, indeed, fight cancer. If you go back to the first chapter on how cancer starts and progresses, you might remember that STAT3 (signal transducer and activator of transcription 3) has a prominent role in the initiation of cancer. What scientists are finding is that STAT3 is also playing a critical role in starting the resistance to conventional chemo-/radio-therapies and modern targeted drugs.

Silibinin, one of the components of the above silymarin phytochemical complex, is being discovered to significantly lower STAT3 activity, and it is, therefore, a viable player not only in fighting cancer but also in helping to fight the liver toxicity so common with many cancer chemotherapeutic regimens [17].

Because of the abundant studies showing that milk thistle has antitumor activity and the fact that I am on 2 medications that can cause liver toxicity, I choose to include milk thistle in my daily regimen. I use *Milk Thistle Max-V* from Douglas Labs that can be purchased on Amazon. This product consists of 250 mg of milk-thistle extract standardized to provide 200 mg of silymarin flavonoids and 100 mg of milk-thistle seed, which is non-standardized.

ASTRAGALUS

Astragalus gummifer is an herb used in Traditional Chinese Medicine, as well as by herbalists and alternative health practitioners in the West. The biologically active ingredients in *Astragalus* include polysaccharides, beta-sitosterol, saponins and flavonoids. Astragaloside is a saponin and is reported to be the primary phytonutrient in the herb that has anti-cancer effects. But as I have repeated over and over again in this book, it is the synergy of many phytonutrients (some discovered and some not) that give herbs their phytonutrient punch. The phytonutrient cocktail in *Astragalus* stimulates the growth of bone-marrow stem cells, promotes the maturation of stem cells into white blood cells, and activates white blood cells' natural killer cells to knock out cancer cells.

Another usage of *Astragalus* with cancer treatment is in the area of resistance to chemotherapy. This is a significant obstacle encountered in cancer treatment and is frequently associated with what is called multi-drug resistance (MDR). Many recent screenings have shown the success of *Astragalus* saponins, flavonoids and polysaccharides in decreasing or eliminating tumors in this scenario. Also, according to a study published in the *Journal of Pharmacy and Pharmacology* [18] investigating chemo-resistance when treating liver cancer, *Astragalus* demonstrated potential in reversing multi-drug resistance. A review of 34 randomized scientific studies, which involved 2,815 patients receiving *Astragalus* with chemo-therapy, found that 30 of the 34 studies demonstrated improvement in response to treatment [19].

I personally take an *Astragalus* product made by Douglas Labs called **Astragalus Max-V** that can be purchased on Amazon. I take one capsule in the morning and one at night. It can also be taken in the form of a tea decoction or an extract, but I chose a capsule for convenience. If you are having difficulty keeping your white-blood-cell count in normal range, I would strongly suggest taking *Astragalus*.

CHLOROPHYLL IN GREEN FOODS

Several studies have shown that chorophyll binds to carcinogens and inhibits the way that they are absorbed into the body. This prevents them from entering your bloodstream, which could then generate DNA mutations in predisposed organs.

Researchers have investigated the effect of chlorophyll and chloro-phyllin (the synthetic form in some supplements) on cancer. One animal study found that chlorophyll reduced the incidence of liver tumors by 29%–64% and stomach tumors by 24%–45% [20].

It has only been of late that there have been some human experiments. A very small study of 4 human volunteers found that chlorophyll may limit the absorption of ingested aflatoxin—a compound known to cause cancer and found primarily in corn, corn products, peanuts, tree nuts and milk. This trial was based on the findings from an old study [21] where chlorophyllin (synthetic form) consumption led to a 55% decrease in aflatoxin biomarkers.

This older study, done by the Linus Pauling Institute, demonstrated that chlorophyllin was very efficient at inhibiting the gastrointestinal absorption of aflatoxin-B1 in humans, which then lowered the biomarkers of aflatoxin-caused DNA mutations. Results from several other scientific peer-reviewed studies on both animals and humans validate that binding the aflatoxin helps lower the risk of cancers of the liver and colon. It has been found to decrease the risk for cancer not only by affecting aflatoxin absorption, but also by interfering with the metabolism of several other toxic carcinogens that the liver must first metabolize for there to be DNA damage.

Diets that are high in red meat and low in green vegetables have long been correlated with a higher risk of colon cancer. A lot of this increased risk is due to the toxins that are released when cooking meat, such as heme iron (found only in meat and not in plants) and heterocycline amines. Both of these are well known to increase colon-cell toxicity and cancer-cell multiplication. This is why in 2005, the Wageningen Centre for Food Sciences in the Netherlands initiated a study to see if green vegetables could hinder the toxic effects of heme iron inside the

the colon [22]. Rats were fed either a control diet with high amounts of heme iron or an identical diet supplemented with chlorophyll for 14 days. The results established that the rats eating the control high heme iron with no chlorophyll experienced about 8X the amount of cell toxicity compared to the start of the study.

The rats given the chorophyll supplements with the high-heme-iron diet were dramatically protected from the formation of the cell-toxic heme metabolites. This made the researchers come to the conclusion that green vegetables diminish the risk of colon cancer, because the chorophyll prevents the cell-toxic and cell-multiplication effects of dietary toxins such as heme. Therefore, if you do decide to go to Ruth Chris Steakhouse, make sure that, when you eat the red meat (which I advise against), to add some of those green veggies!

To get an adequate amount of chlorophyll, I always add kale to my smoothies and eat lots of greens like spinach, collard greens, romaine lettuce, arugula and mixed greens. I take a supplement called **G.F.S.-2000** by Douglas Labs every morning. This can be purchased on Amazon. I take 4 capsules only in the morning, because there is green-tea extract included in the supplement, which has caffeine and might prevent a good night's sleep. Some of the many ingredients in this supplement include wheat grass, barley grass, alfalfa, spirulina, spinach and blue green algae.

*BERBERINE

Berberine is a compound that can be elicited from several different plants, including a group of shrubs called *Berberis*. It belongs to a class of compounds called "alkaloids." Berberine has been used in traditional Chinese medicine for many years, where it has been used to treat many different health conditions. Now with modern technology and advanced research techniques, researchers have shown conclusively that it has many significant benefits for several health problems [23].

In recent years, berberine is the rage in the scientific community, with hundreds of studies demonstrating that it has compelling effects on many different organ systems and has been shown to destroy cancer cells in a variety of ways [24].

Once berberine enters your cells, it binds to a variety of biologic-receptor sites, which then changes the activity of the cell [25]. One of the most important things that berberine does is to activate an enzyme inside the cell called "AMP-activated protein kinase" (AMPK) [26], which is called the "metabolic master switch" by many scientists [27]. This master conductor of metabolism [28] is present in almost every cell in our body and has been found to affect the way our cells' genes are expressed (epigenetics) [29].

Besides activating AMPK to help us fight cancer, it also affects cancer through its blood-sugar control. If you remember from chapter 1, we talked about how cancer uses a very crude method of energy production called "Warburg's anaerobic glycolysis." This fermentation process requires huge amounts of sugar to keep the cancer growing and progressing. Many studies have demonstrated that berberine can effectively lower blood-sugar levels in people with type 2 diabetes [30]. In fact, its blood-sugar-lowering ability has been validated to compete with the in-vogue diabetes drug metformin [31]. It appears to work by making the blood-sugar-lowering insulin more efficient; supporting the body to metabolize sugars inside cells; diminishing the amount of manufactured sugar in the liver; abating the metabolism of carbohydrates in the gastrointestinal tract; and increasing the number of good probiotic bacteria in the gut [29]. In addition to these impressive effects, berberine has also exhibited anti-proliferative effects and direct toxicity against cancer cells [32,33].

I, therefore, take a supplement called **Berberine 1200** mg made by Naturulse, which can be purchased on Amazon. I take one capsule in the morning and one in the evening. If you are having trouble with blood-sugar control, I would also take one in the mid-afternoon. If you are on blood-sugar-lowering drugs, make sure you consult with your physician.

NONI FRUIT

Noni fruit (*Morinda citrifolia*) is a lumpy, mango-sized fruit that is yellow in color, is very bitter tasting, and has a smell like stinky cheese. Polynesians have used it in traditional folk medicine for thousands of years and is commonly used to treat health issues like constipation, infections, pain, and arthritis [34]. In recent years, Noni fruit has been investigated for its anti-cancer effects. It has been shown to activate cancer-cell suicide and reduce cancer-cell multiplication and progression in certain kinds of cancers [35]; in one study, it actually shrunk tumors by an amazing 50% [36]. Other ways that it has been ascertained to help in the battle against cancer is through its well-studied anti-inflammatory and antioxidant effects [37].

I, therefore, take a noni-fruit supplement by Doctor's Best called **Noni Concentrate** that can be purchased on Amazon. I take one in the morning and one at night. Each capsule contains 650 mg of noni concentrate (morinda citrifolia). I also add one teaspoon of freeze-dried **Organic Noni Fruit Powder** made by Naturevibe Botanicals (Amazon) in my morning smoothie.

SOURSOP (GRAVIOLA)

Soursop, also known as graviola, is the fruit of the *Annona muricata* tree, which is indigenous to tropical areas of the Americas. This green fruit with little horns has a buttery consistency, with a pineapple or strawberry flavor. Most people eat soursop by cutting it in half and then scooping out the fruit.

In regard to cancer, most of the scientific studies have been performed on a petri dish or in a test tube. The ones that have been carried

196 | BEAT BACK CANCER NATURALLY

through show that soursop has a strong capability to kill cancer cells. One of these scientific studies applied treatment to breast-cancer cells with soursop extract. It revealed that the soursop extract diminished the tumor's size and weight, abated cancer spread and progression, and generated cancer-cell suicide. Furthermore, it decreased the level of nitric oxide inside the tumors (decreases blood flow) while it also increased the blood concentrations of cancer-destroying white blood cells, T-cells, and natural killer cells [38]. Another study investigated how soursop would affect leukemia cells, and it also validated that it generated leukemia-cell suicide and hampered the leukemia cells' ability to proliferate [39].

The other ways that soursop may work to fight cancer is through its antioxidant, anti-inflammatory effects and its capability to lower blood sugar. One experiment scrutinized the antioxidant properties of soursop and discovered that it had the ability to strongly neutralize free-radical activity [40]. Another study that used rats investigated soursop's anti-inflammatory effects, and it was discovered that it lowered several inflammatory biomarkers in arthritic rats [41]. In regard to its ability to keep blood-sugar levels down, another rodent study indicated a striking difference between the blood-glucose concentrations of treated and untreated high-blood-sugar groups [42]. As we know . . . cancer craves sugar. So, the better we can control blood-sugar levels, the better we control cancer growth.

I personally take a supplement made by Horbaach called **Graviola 2000 mg** that can be purchased on Amazon. Each capsule is a blend of the soursop (graviola) leaf and fruit, and has 1,000 mg per capsule. I take one in the morning and one in the evening.

*MUSHROOMS (BETA-1,3-GLUCAN)

While almost all of the nutritional supplements in this chapter will protect the cells from the damaging effects of radiation and chemotherapy, there are some that work especially well in this regard. One that stands out is beta-1,3-glucan, a polysaccharide extract from mushrooms and found in the outer wall of baker's yeast. Beta-1,3-glucan has been shown to induce impressive protection against the destructive effects of radiation, especially for the immune cells of the spleen, bone marrow, and lymph nodes. Besides these protective effects, beta-1,3-glucan is also a powerful stimulator of the immune cells that are at the forefront in the battle against cancer. One of the more critical cells in this battle is the macrophage, which has the ability not only to fight cancer directly but also to recruit T-lymphocytes from the bone marrow to join in the battle.

In one study, mice administered high doses of whole-body radiation had strikingly higher survival rates if they were first treated with beta-1,3-glucan [43]. Not only is beta-1,3-glucan protective of the bone-marrow cells, but it also impedes the development of infections that so commonly occur following extensive radiation exposure. The best attribute of this supplement is that it does all of this protection while also decimating cancer cells.

In another important study, it was established that beta-1,3-glucan not only diminishes cancer-cell survivability but also reduces its migration, progression and spread. These attributes resulted in decreases in tumor burden and the incidence of metastasis [44].

I personally have 2 ways to get my beta-1,3-glucans. In the morning I use ¼ of a teaspoon of a freeze-dried mushroom powder called *Thrive 6* in my morning caf and decaf coffees. This powder includes chaga, cordyceps, turkey tail, reishi, lion's mane, and maitake mushrooms. *Thrive 6* can be purchased on Amazon.

I also take a capsule called *Myoceutics* by Douglas Labs that can also be purchased on Amazon. One capsule contains 1,200 mg of an organic-mushroom combination of cordyceps, reishi, maitake, shiitake, coriolus, polyporus, wood ear, tremella, poria and hericium. I take one in the morning and one in the evening. Most importantly, make sure you eat a lot of cooked mushrooms on a daily basis. This is the absolute best way to get your beta-1,3 glucan protection. Also, use nutritional yeast as a flavoring on popcorn and other foods, as it has a high concentration of beta-1,3 glucan.

MORINGA

Moringa oleifera is a plant that is native to the sub-Himalayan areas of India, Pakistan, Bangladesh, and Afghanistan. It is also grown in the tropics. The leaves, bark, flowers, fruit, seeds, and root are used to treat a number of diseases, including cancer.

In a study published in the *Journal of Medicinal Food*, South African researchers looked into the ability of *Moringa oleifera* to inhibit the proliferation of esophageal-cancer cells, which is very common in South Africa. The researchers found that *Moringa* has an anti-proliferative effect on esophageal-cancer cells, thanks to its ability to break the cancer-cell DNA into fragments as well as induce cancer-cell suicide [45].

In another study looking at the effects of *Moringa* against breast and colorectal cancer, the plant was found to have remarkable anti-cancer activity [46]. Cancer-cell survival was very low in both the breast- and colorectal-cancer-cell lines when treatment was applied with *Moringa* leaves and bark extracts. There was also noted a 7-fold increase in cancer-cell suicide with *Moringa* treatment when compared to the control. Some of the phytonutrients in *Moringa* thought to be playing a role in this anti-cancer activity are eugenol, isopropyl isothiocynate, D-allose, and hexadeconoic acid ethyl ester.

Because of these 2 studies and many others that I found in the scientific literature, I take a *Moringa* capsule called **Pure Premium Moringa** made by Fresh Healthcare that can be purchased on Amazon. Each capsule contains 500 mg of organic *Moringa* powder. I take one capsule in the morning and one in the evening.

ASHWAGANDHA

Ashwagandha (*Withania somnifera*) is a medicinal plant that has been utilized in traditional medicine in many parts of South Asia for millennia. In recent years, scientific research is discovering its anti-cancer properties.

In a study coming out of the University of Pittsburgh (my home town), it was shown that ashwagandha had impressive activity against breast-cancer cells [47]. It was found to incite cancer-cell suicide, fragment the DNA of the cancer cell, and also negatively affect its ability of to repair its induced-damaged DNA.

Another way that ashwagandha appears to work against cancer is by combating new-blood-vessel growth to the expanding cancer (anti-angiogenesis). In a study analyzing this previously known effect of this herb, it was found to exert potent anti-angiogenic activity in vivo at concentrations that were 500-fold lower than those revealed in previous peer-reviewed scientific studies [48].

An additional study coming out of India discovered that ashwagandha not only shielded mice exposed to high-dose radiation but also boosted the number of blood-forming cells in the mice's bone marrow [49]. With bone-marrow depression being a common and major problem in cancer patients treated with radiation or chemotherapy agents, ashwagandha may be very useful for keeping the number of immune cells in the normal range. My medication, lenalidomide, is well known to cause this problem, and I have found that ashwagandha has consistently helped me keep my blood counts in the normal range.

Because of the above-mentioned and other studies confirming its anti-cancer activity, radiation, and chemo-protective effects and blood-cell-boosting properties, I take *Ayur-Ashwagandha* capsules by Douglas Labs that can be purchased on Amazon. I take one in the morning and one in the evening. Each capsule contains 300 mg of ashwagandha root extract. Ashwagandha does increase energy levels, so if you have trouble sleeping at night, eliminate the evening dose.

ALPHA LIPOIC ACID (PERIPHERAL NEUROPATHY PREVENTION)

Alpha-lipoic acid is a fat- and water-soluble antioxidant that the body can actually manufacture. Good plant sources are yeast, spinach, broccoli, and potatoes. It can also be made in the laboratory for use as a medicine. Alpha-lipoic acid is most commonly taken by mouth for diabetes and its accompanying peripheral neuropathy. This latter problem can cause significant burning, pain, and numbness in the legs and arms. Besides being taken by mouth, alpha-lipoic acid can also be given as an injection into the vein (by IV). High doses of alpha-lipoic acid are actually approved in Germany for the treatment of these nerve-related problems.

As we discussed in the chapter on chemotherapy, the vast majority of cancer drugs cause chemotherapy-induced peripheral neuropathy (CIPN), which can be quite debilitating to the cancer patient and negatively affect their quality of life.

In a very recent 2018 study done at the National Cancer Institute in Rome, 18 patients being treated with the protesome inhibitor bortezomib, were given alpha-lipoic acid (600 mg) along with DHA (400 mg), vitamin C (60 mg) and vitamin E (10mg) twice daily. By the way, bortezomib is known to be one of the greatest inducer of painful peripheral neuropathy and is the treatment that I rejected at the beginning of my cancer journey. The results of this study were rather remarkable in that 17 of the 18 patients receiving this preventive formula had no peripheral nerve pain [50].

It is important to note, however, that there is one published petri-dish study in the journal *Blood* that showed that alpha-lipoic acid may negatively affect bortezomib's anti-myeloma activity [51], so I would first consult with your doctor before taking alpha-lipoic acid with bortezomib. Since bortezomib is typically administered 2 days per week, you may want to forgo taking alpha-lipoic acid on your bortezomib days. Other proteosome inhibitors exposed to alpha-lipoic acid were not affected. It is thought that the alpha-lipoic-acid molecule interacts with the boronic-acid component of the bortezomib molecule in a way that makes it ineffective.

I personally do not take alpha-lipoic acid because of the aforementioned study [51], which also demonstrated that alpha-lipoic acid may cause myeloma cells to become more viable. Therefore, I would have a serious discussion with your oncologist before taking this supplement. If you are going to try it, I would recommend *Super R-Lipoic Acid 240 mg* by Life Extension available on Amazon. Take one in the morning and one in the evening.

VITAMIN E (MIXED TOCOPHEROLS AND TOCOTRIENOLS)

Vitamin E is an extremely well-known fat-soluble vitamin that is naturally found primarily in nuts, seeds, avocados, spinach, butter nut squash, kiwi fruit, broccoli and olive oil.

I take vitamin E primarily for the prevention of neuropathy, but it has also been found in several studies to be advantageous in the fight against cancer [52].

In one study evaluating its anti-peripheral-neuropathy effects, 30 patients participated. Fourteen received 600 mg of vitamin E per day and 16 patients received a placebo. These results were impressive in that the group taking the vitamin E supplementation had a much lower incidence and severity of cisplatin-induced peripheral neuropathy [53].

Because of its antioxidant, anti-cancer and peripheral-neuropathy-preventive effects, I include a vitamin E that has a variety of tocopherols and tocotrienols. Most cheap vitamin E supplements have only d-alpha tocopherol, but the the other tocopherols and the tocotrienols have been shown to possess superior antioxidant and anti-inflammatory properties over d-alpha tocopherol alone. I, therefore, take a vitamin E supplement called *Tri-En-All 400* made by Douglas Labs and available on Amazon. It contains d-alpha, beta, gamma, and delta tocopherols, along with a variety of tocotrienols from palm. I take one in the morning. I also get my vitamin-E level, along with my beta-carotene, vitamin-D, vitamin-K, and Coenzyme-Q10 levels checked every 6–12 months with a test from Genova Labs, because they are all fat-soluble vitamins that can accumulate in the fat tissues and get abnormally high if taken at inappropriate doses.

*GARLIC

Garlic (*Allium sativum*) has been used for centuries as a therapeutic and preventive medicine because of its many known effects against infections, atherosclerosis, hypertension and cancer. When garlic is chopped or crushed, the allinase enzyme is activated and produces allicin from alliin (present in intact garlic). Allicin is one of the primary medicinal phytochemicals found in garlic, but it has been determined through considerable research to possess an impressive number of other powerful bioactive compounds with anti-cancer properties, mainly allysulfides (sulfur derivatives). These sulfur compounds have been found to counter cancer in many different ways. These include not allowing carcinogens to attach themselves to DNA; the neutralization of free radicals; the protection against mutation formation; the blockage of cancer-cell multiplication; and the impedance of cancer angiogenesis (new-blood-vessel production).

The growth rate of cancer cells is reduced by garlic and occurs by blocking what is called the "G2/M phase of cell division." Apoptosis (cancer-cell suicide) is also triggered by garlic. Activation of of this cell suicide has been related to garlic's inactivation of the cancer cell's AKT pathway, which is the most important pathway regulating cell growth and cell division. In an interesting rodent study, rats with induced prostate cancer had a reduction in the serum concentration of prostate-specific antigen (a prostate-cancer biomarker) when given high doses of garlic [54]. In addition to inhibiting primary cancer, garlic's sulfur compounds also inhibited metastasis in this study. The water-soluble *Allium* derivative, *S*-allyllmercaptocysteine, inhibited metastases to the lung and adrenal gland by a remarkable 90%. Furthermore, garlic is what is called a "seleniferous plant," which means that it accumulates selenium from the soil against a concentration gradient. Selenium has many anti-cancer actions, particularly in the expression of genes involved in cancer initiation. That is one reason that I eat a Brazil nut (has high selenium content), among other nuts, before I take my morning supplements.

Because the scientific literature is replete with articles showing the anti-cancer properties of garlic, I try to incorporate garlic into as many dishes as possible. I also take a garlic supplement called **Garlic** made by Douglas Labs and available on Amazon. I take 2 tablets in the morning and 2 in the evening.

*QUERCETIN

Quercetin is one of the most common bioflavonoids consumed by most Westerners and has been shown in more and more scientific papers to have proven anti-cancer activity. The foods with the highest quercetin levels are capers, red onions, berries, kale, apples, spinach, red grapes, and plums. In my research, I found that even The Sloan Kettering Cancer Center, a renowned cancer center, has it on their web page as having anti-cancer properties.

If you do a *pubmed.gov* search on "quercetin against cancer," you will find a slew of scientific studies demonstrating how quercetin fights cancer. In one study, it was determined to have anti-proliferative and enhanced cancer-cell-suicide effects against prostate cancer [55].

In an excellent meta-analysis article looking at the scientific literature as a whole, it was made evident that there are a number of mechanisms that make it a potent anti-cancer agent. These include damaging the cell-division cycle of cancer cells, interaction with type II estrogen-receptor sites, and the hinderance of tyrosine kinase-signaling pathways [56]. This last method of cancer fighting comprises the blocking of tyrosine kinase inside the cancer cell but not in normal cells. These tyrosine kinase-directed signaling pathways are normally involved with keeping normal cells from dividing abnormally and causing cell death when the normal cell's life-sustaining mechanism goes haywire. These signaling pathways are often genetically modified somehow in cancer cells, which gives significant superiority to the cancer cell. Quercetin appears to inhibit tyrosine kinase, which, as we have seen, is profoundly embroiled with this abnormal signaling.

The great thing is that quercetin appears to have little toxicity when administered orally or intravenously. As I previously alluded to, there is much in-vitro and animal and human data indicating that quercetin inhibits tumor growth. More research is, however, needed to clarify the oral doses we should be taking and the magnitude of its anti-cancer effects.

Because of the enormity of the data, I take a supplement called **Querciplex** made by Douglas Labs and available on Amazon. Each capsule has Quercetin dihydrate 333 mg and Bromelain 100 mg. Bromelain has been shown to increase the absorption of quercetin. I take one capsule in the morning and one in the evening.

*GYMNEMA SYLVESTRE

In chapter 1, we discussed how cancer cells have a ravenous desire for sugar because it uses a fermentation method called "Warburg's anaerobic glycolysis" for its energy production. One sugar molecule in a normal cell produces 36 ATP energy molecules versus only 2 ATP molecules by one sugar molecule in the cancer cell. Therefore, cancer needs a lot of sugar just to survive. One of the ways to starve the cancer cell is by eating a whole food, plant-based diet, which not only starves the sugar pathway but also the glutamine- and cholesterol-feeding pathways. In order to help keep the blood-sugar levels as low as possible, I personally take a *Gymnema sylvestre* supplement because of its known anti-diabetic properties.

Gymnema sylvestre is a woody, climbing plant that grows in the tropical forests of Central and Southern India and in parts of Asia. As a supplement, it has been used in combination with other diabetes medications to lower blood-sugar levels. In Hindi it is called gurmar—"destroyer of sugar." One of the ways that *Gymnema sylvestre* lowers blood sugar is to block receptors in your intestines and thus, sugar absorption, which then causes a lowering of your post-meal blood-sugar levels.

Studies have established that consuming 200–400 mg of gymnemic acid (a primary component of *Gymnema sylvestre*) decreases the intestinal absorption of the sugar glucose [57]. In another study, *Gymnema sylvestre* was validated to improve blood-sugar control in individuals with type 2 diabetes. The study deduced that *Gymnema's* ability to reduce blood-sugar levels after a meal could diminish long-term complications of diabetes if taken on a regular basis [58]. For people with a chronically high blood sugar or a high HbA1c blood level, *Gymnema sylvestre* has the potential to keep those levels in check.

Besides helping to keep your blood-sugar levels low, *Gymnema sylvestre* has cancer-fighting properties in its own right. In a study where they isolated 5 polysaccharides from the *Gymnema* plant and put them to the test, they were able to establish immunological and anti-tumor activities of these polysaccharides. All of the polysaccharides exhibited anti-tumor activity in a dose-dependent manner (the higher the strength—the stronger the anti-tumor effect). These polysaccharides displayed impressive cancer-inhibitory rates of 78.6% and 83.8%, respectively [59].

Because of these studies and other important scientific data, I take a supplement called **Gymnema Sylvestre 400 mg** made by Now Foods and available on Amazon. As with berberine, if you are taking blood-sugar-lowering medications, make sure you first consult with your doctor.

BLACK SEED OIL

Black seeds, also known as "black cumin," "nigella," or by its scientific name *Nigella sativa*, belongs to the buttercup family of flowering plants. The oil is the focus of a lot of anti-cancer research primarily because it has a very high concentration of a well-studied anti-tumor ingredient, thymoquinone.

Thymoquinone (TQ) has exhibited anti-cancer activities in a variety of tumors by homing in on several cancer pathways. One of these many activities is to affect the epigenetic code of cancer cells. As we have discussed previously in this book, epigenetics is the science of how nutrients and lifestyle choices affect the way genes act. A good dietary choice, for example, can make a gene that is causing cancer to grow, to stop acting in that negative way.

In an extremely interesting study on thymoquinone's effects on T-cell acute lymphoblastic leukemia cell lines, scientists found that thymoquinone affects many key epigenetic players [60]. I don't want to bore you with science, but I thought this paragraph was so detailed and interesting about the epigenetic findings. This is directly from the abstract:

"Interestingly, several tumor-suppressor genes, such as *DLC1, PPARG, ST7, FOXO6, TET2, CYP1B1, SALL4*, and *DDIT3*, known to be epigenetically silenced in various tumors, including acute leukemia, were up-regulated, along with the up-regulation of several downstream pro-apoptotic genes, such as *RASL11B, RASD1, GNG3, BAD*, and *BIK*."

What this is saying is that, in cases where cancer starts, tumor-suppressor genes (genes that normally suppress out-of-control cell division) lose their ability to suppress the growth of cancer cells. The thymoquinone made tumor-suppressor genes start to suppress tumor growth again. The same thing happened to pro-apoptotic (pro-cell-suicide) genes. Pro-apoptotic genes make normal cells commit cell suicide when the inner machinery of the cell is mutated or functioning improperly, as it is with cancer. When cancer is growing out of control, these genes are not instructing the cancer cell to kill itself like they should. The thymoquinone apparently reverses this gene's malfunctioning by making it start to instruct the cancer cell to commit suicide again.

Because of this study and the multitude of other good studies that I found in the scientific literature, I include black-seed oil in my daily regimen. I take liquid capsules of **Black Seed Oil** by Healths Harmony that can be purchased on Amazon. Each capsule contains 500 mg of black-cumin-seed oil. I take one in the morning and one in the evening.

POMEGRANATE POWDER

During my daily scientific research, one food that continually pops up because of its anti-cancer activity is the fruit pomegranate (*Punica granatum*). I love the fruit, but I must tell you that it is almost impossible for me to quickly and accurately remove all of the seeds. And when I buy the seeds already removed in the grocery store, if I don't eat them immediately, they seem to ferment very quickly. I, therefore, use a freeze-dried powder.

The scientific data on the effectiveness of pomegranate against cancer is prodigious, but the one study that popped out at me was one concerning its effects against multiple myeloma, since that is the cancer that I have. In a study coming out of Italy, the researchers found that the pomegranate affected a part of the cancer-cell-division cycle called G0/

G1, which caused the myeloma not to be able to proliferate [61]. They also investigated the effect of pomegranate on angiogenesis (new-blood-vessel growth) and myeloma-cell migration/invasion. Interestingly, they observed an inhibitory effect on microvessel outgrowth and decreased cancer-cell migration and invasion. Analysis of angiogenic gene expression in endothelial cells lining the inside of the blood vessels verified the anti-angiogenic activity of pomegranate. Interestingly, a sequential combination of bortezomib (a chemotherapy drug used to treat myeloma) with pomegranate enhanced bortezomib's cancer-killing effect.

Because of this article and the many other peer-reviewed scientific studies establishing pomegranate's anti-tumor effects, I place a teaspoon of a freeze-dried *Organic Pomegranate Powder* made by Navitas Organics (Amazon) in my morning caf and decaf coffees. Freeze-dried powders, by the way, maintain all of the nutrients found originally in the fruit.

GOJI BERRY POWDER

Another freeze-dried powder that I use in my morning coffees is goji-berry powder. The goji berry (*Lycium barbarum*) is a traditional Chinese berry widely used in Asian countries and has been validated in scientific studies to be protective against several chronic diseases and to have potent anti-cancer properties.

Goji berries are famous for having an exceptionally high antioxidant concentration, which is most likely one of the central factors behind its anti-tumor activity. In one study evaluating goji-berry carotenoids against colon cancer, it was established to have robust epigenetic activity, which acted similar to black-seed oil's thymoquinone—made tumor-suppressor genes suppress more, and made cell-suicide genes cause more cancer-cell suicide [62]. A comparable epigenetic effect was discovered against breast-cancer cells [63]. When goji-berry nanoparticles were added to the chemotherapeutic drug doxorubicin, this blend was much more deadly to liver-cancer cells when compared to using the doxorubicin alone [64].

Because of the prodigious amount of science behind using goji berries against cancer and because of its extraordinary antioxidant potency, I use *Organic Goji Powder* made by Navitas that can be purchased on Amazon. I place one teaspoon in my caf and decaf coffees in the morning.

AÇAÍ BERRY POWDER

Another freeze-dried powder that I use in my morning coffees is açaí-berry powder. Açaí (*Euterpe oleracea*) is lavishly found in South and Central America and is helpful to our health due to its elevated levels of phytochemicals, including lignans and polyphenols. While reviewing the scientific literature, I came across a good meta-analysis review of all the studies done to date on açaí against cancer [65]. In all, 60 publications were found in the databases. Interestingly, anti-cancer activities of açaí were observed in all the experimental models of cancer, and it was found to reduce the incidence of cancer and diminish tumor-cell proliferation, multiplicity, and size of the tumors due to its anti-inflammatory, anti-proliferative and pro-cancer-cell-suicide properties.

Because of these significant anti-cancer properties and because I can't buy açaí berries locally, I use a freeze-dried powder called *Organic Açaí Powder* made by Whole Foods Market that can be purchased on Amazon or at Whole Foods. I place one teaspoon in my morning caf and decaf coffees.

CINNAMON

Another herb that I place in my morning coffees is cinnamon (*Cinnamomum verum*). Cinnamon is probably one of the most commonly used herbs in the world. From childhood, I have frequently used it on my oatmeal and sometimes in my coffee for its amazing flavor. After my cancer diagnosis, when I started investigating natural ways that I could enhance my results, cinnamon kept popping up as an anti-cancer herb. One of the primary ways that cinnamon seems to battle cancer is through its ability to increase cancer-cell suicide, demonstrated in a good Iranian study [66].

Low oxygen levels in the cancer microenvironment is positively correlated with tumor aggressiveness and hence is a negative prognostic factor in cancer. In response to low oxygen, a master gene regulator called "HIF-1-α" (hypoxia-inducing factor-1-α) has been found to activate new-blood-vessel growth to the cancer and increase its metastasis. In a study that looked at how cinnamaldehydes in cinnamon affect cancer, it was found that it decreased the amount of HIF-1-α production, which then negatively affected the mTOR-cell-growth pathway [67]. Remember mTOR from chapter 1? Remember that animal products activate mTOR? Remember that the more mTOR activity in adulthood—the more cancer?

Cinnamon is also well known as a blood-sugar regulator [68]. Therefore, because cancer needs an enormous amount of glucose for its very survival, cinnamon's ability to help keep blood-sugar levels low may be one of the additional ways that it combats cancer.

Because of its blood-sugar-lowering and anti-cancer effects, I give 10 shakes of **Organic Ceylon Cinnamon** made by Frontier Co-Op that I buy from Amazon in my morning coffees.

CACAO POWDER

Flavanols in fruits and vegetables have attracted a great deal of attention due to their cancer-preventive effects with no toxicity. Cacao (*Theobroma cacao*) has the highest concentration of flavonols out of all foods per weight. Experimental studies on cacao and its many phyto-nutrients have established that they have potent antioxidant effects, protect cells from free-radical damage, combat inflammation, constrain cancer-cell growth, prevent new-blood-vessel growth to cancer, cancer-cell suicide, and impede metastasis [69,70]. Animal studies using a cacao-rich diet or cacao extracts have demonstrated its effectiveness against breast, pancreatic, prostate, liver and colon cancer, as well as leukemia [71].

Because of this evidence and also because cacao powder has intense mood-elevation effects [72] and also tastes so delicious, I place a whole tablespoon of freeze-dried cacao powder in my morning coffees. I use *Organic Cacao Powder* by Navitas that can be purchased on Amazon.

*MY MORNING COFFEE REGIMEN

So far in this chapter, I have covered all of the ingredients that I place in my morning caf and decaf coffees. Here they are in a nutshell. One tablespoon of *Organic Cacao Powder*; one teaspoon of *Organic Mangosteen Fruit Powder*; one teaspoon of *Organic Pomegranate Powder*; one teaspoon of *Organic Goji Powder*; one teaspoon of *Organic Açaí Powder*, ¼ teaspoon of *Thrive 6* mushroom powder, 10 shakes of *Organic Ceylon Cinnamon*, ⅛ teaspoon of baking soda to alkalinize the coffee acidity, and *Organic Stevia* made by Wholesome Mindfully Delicious to adjust the sweetness to my liking.

AMLA POWDER

AMLA powder is made from the ground-up leaves of the Indian gooseberry (*Phyllanthus emblica*). It has been used in Ayurvedic medicine for centuries to treat everything from diarrhea to jaundice. It is also known to have the highest concentration of antioxidants than any food on the face of the Earth. Experimental studies have shown that AMLA and some of its phytochemicals such as gallic acid, ellagic acid, pyrogallol, norsesqui-terpenoids, corilagin, geraniin, elaeocarpusin, and prodelphinidins B1 and B2 also possess anti-cancer effects [73]. AMLA is also reported to possess radiation- and chemotherapy-protective effects, along with potent antioxidant, anti-inflammatory, anti-mutation [74], and immune-enhancing activities—properties that are efficacious in the treatment and prevention of cancer.

Because mutations are at the root of cancer formation and progression and AMLA has been shown to have the ability to prevent mutations through its very powerful antioxidant activity, I make sure I include AMLA powder in my morning smoothie every day. I use *Organic AMLA Powder* made by Terrasoul that is available on Amazon. I place one teaspoon in my morning smoothie.

DRAGON FRUIT POWDER

Another powder that I place in my morning smoothie is dragon fruit (*Hylocereus cactaceae*) powder. Although I can purchase the actual dragon fruit in the summer from Whole Foods, it is available for only a very short period, so I use it as a freeze-dried powder all year round.

Dragon fruit is very high in vitamin C, betalains, and carotenoids—all of which have been found to promote anti-cancer activity. For example, observational studies have found correlations between vitamin-C intake and cancer risk. One investigational study involving 120,852 participants correlated more-elevated intakes of vitamin C with reduced rates of head and neck cancer [75]. Another study established that betalains high in dragon fruit can combat oxidative stress and suppress cancer cells [76]. Beta-carotene and lycopene are the plant pigments that give dragon fruit its extremely vibrant, reddish-pink color. Diets rich in carotenoids have been linked to a reduced risk of cancer and heart disease [77]. And as I mentioned in the chapter on radiation, they also give protection to normal cells exposed to cancer radiation therapy.

I use *Freeze Dried Dragon Fruit Powder* made by Wilderness Poets that can be purchased on Amazon. I place one teaspoon in my morning smoothie.

CAMU CAMU POWDER

An additional powder that I put in my smoothie is camu camu (*Myrciaria dubia*) powder. It is found in the Amazon rainforest and has gained popularity worldwide in recent years due to its many purported health benefits. Fresh camu camu berries are extremely tart in flavor, which is why they're commonly found in supplement form as powders and capsules.

As with dragon fruit, camu camu has extremely high vitamin-C content. It may have the highest vitamin-C content of any food on the face of the Earth. According to product nutritional labels, camu camu powder can deliver up to 750% of the Reference Daily Intake (RDI) of vitamin C per teaspoon. As we saw in the review of dragon fruit, higher vitamin-C intake results in lower cancer rates [75].

Other than its extremely high vitamin-C content, camu camu has impressive amounts of many other powerful flavonoid antioxidants like anthocyanins and ellagic acid, which have shown to help prevent cancer [78].

I use **Camu Camu Powder** made by Terrasoul that is available on Amazon. I place one teaspoon in my morning smoothie.

GUAVA/MATCHA POWDER

Guavas (*Psidium guajava*) are tropical trees that grow primarily in Central America. Their fruits are light green in color and contain edible seeds. What is used as a supplement are the guava leaves which can be made into an herbal tea or a leaf extract. The leaf extract has been shown to have a powerful anti-cancer effect. In fact, animal studies demonstrate that guava extract can effectively block cancer-cell proliferation [79,80]. This is likely due to its elevated levels of powerful antioxidants that prevent free radicals from damaging cells, one of the main causes of cancer and genetic mutations. Another study found that guava-leaf oil was 4X more efficacious at combating cancer-cell growth than the cancer-chemotherapeutic drug vincristine [81].

Another component of the powder that I use is matcha tea. Matcha comes from the same plant as green tea—the *Camellia sinensis* plant. However, it is grown differently, which gives it a different nutrient profile when compared to green tea. The way that matcha is made is that 20–30 days before the *Camellia sinensis* plants' harvest, they are covered so that they get no direct sunlight. This increases chlorophyll production in the plant, which gives it a darker-green tint and increases its nutritive value. In fact, one study established that the number of certain potent antioxidant catechins in matcha was up to 137X greater than the amount found in other types of green tea [82].

Matcha is especially high in epigallocatechin-3-gallate (EGCG), a type of catechin that has been shown in several studies to have impressive anti-cancer activity. One experimental study established that the EGCG in matcha could destroy prostate-cancer cells [83]. Other studies have validated that EGCG has powerful cancer-fighting activity against skin, lung, and liver cancers [84].

I, therefore, use a supplement called ***Guava/Matcha Powdered Green Tea*** made by Yavari that is available on Amazon. I place one teaspoon in my morning smoothie. Because caffeine affects my sleep . . . if I drink my smoothie after noon time, I do not add it. Matcha has much higher caffeine content compared to green and black teas.

*MY MORNING SMOOTHIE MIXTURE

At this point, you know all of the powders that I add to my morning smoothie. They are ***AMLA Powder***, ***Dragon Fruit Powder***, ***Camu Camu Powder***, ***Noni Fruit Powder***, and ***Guava/Matcha Powdered Green Tea***. I also add one tablespoon of ***Organic Ground Flaxseeds*** by 365 (Amazon) and ***Organic Ground Chia Seeds*** by Spectrum Essentials (Amazon) for their omega-3 fatty acid anti-inflammatory effects. The fruits that I use are *Trader Joe's Frozen Fancy Berry Medley* (organic strawberries, raspberries, blackberries, blueberries), frozen organic mangoes, frozen organic cranberries, frozen organic grapes, an organic apple, and an organic banana. I also add a cup of organic kale because of its known anti-cancer effects. I add one cup of organic soy milk and one cup of purified alkalinized water and use my Vitamix at high speed for 2 minutes. My wife and I share this smoothie every morning. I also use this smoothie as my drink for my morning supplements. This smoothie provides me with about 1,500 ORAC units (oxygen-radical-absorbance capacity). To put this into perspective . . . most standard American breakfasts provide about 22–40 ORAC units.

BONE HEALTH SUPPLEMENTS (VITAMIN D3, VITAMIN K2, CALCIUM/MAGNESIUM, STRONTIUM)

It is well understood that many cancer treatments for women with early-stage breast cancer can have detrimental effects on bone and may result in dramatic bone loss within the first few years of therapy. In premenopausal women, chemotherapy can cause premature menopause by causing repression of the ovaries and, in all women, accelerated bone loss [85]. Likewise, the aromatase-inhibitor therapy that is often utilized against breast cancer is correlated with profound bone loss and an increased incidence of fracture risk in postmenopausal women compared with women who received tamoxifen [86].

At diagnosis, women with breast cancer may already have several additional risk factors, unrelated to bone loss from breast-cancer therapies, which add to their fracture risk. These baseline risk factors may include age (>65 years), a history of fragility fracture after the age of 50, body mass index <20 kg/m2, family history of osteoporosis, current or history of smoking, and oral corticosteroid use >6 months [87]. Each of these risk factors has been demonstrated to elevate a woman's fracture risk independent of bone density and is critical in determining her overall fracture risk. The bone health of women with breast cancer (and other cancers) and men with prostate cancer (and other cancers) are often under attack from many different avenues; it is, therefore, of extreme importance to proactively address these risks through a combination of diet, supplements and lifestyle changes, as well as through conventional drugs when required. We will now discuss some of the supplements you can take to strengthen your bones.

Calcium

Calcium is one of the most important supplements you should take when you have osteoporosis. Taking calcium is recommended by the Endocrine Society for most women undergoing osteoporosis treatment. Ideally, you'll get enough in your diet. If you don't, however, supplements can help. While there are many calcium supplements available, your body doesn't absorb all calcium supplements the same way. For example, chelated calcium (calcium citrate, calcium lactate, or calcium gluconate) is easier for your body to absorb. "Chelated" means compounds are added to a supplement to improve its absorption. Calcium carbonate is usually the most inexpensive and contains 40% of the elemental calcium. Your body isn't physically able to absorb more than 500 mg of calcium at a time. Therefore, you should break up your supplement intake over the course of a day. Taking the supplements with food can also enhance their absorption.

I personally use a supplement called **Cal/Mag 2001** made by Douglas Labs and available on Amazon. Two tablets provide 500 mg of calcium citrate/carbonate/ascorbate complex, 250 mg of magnesium, vitamin C 100 mg, vitamin D3 50 IU, boron 3mg and glutamic acid. I take 2 tablets only in the morning. I take strontium citrate in the evening. Calcium and strontium (we will discuss later) should be taken at separate times since they compete for the same binding sites.

*Vitamin D3

As with calcium, it's important you get enough vitamin D3 if you have osteoporosis. This is because vitamin D is essential for helping your body absorb calcium and build strong bones. In addition to calcium, taking vitamin D is recommended by the Endocrine Society for most women undergoing osteoporosis treatment. However, it's not naturally present in many foods. Sun exposure causes your body to make vitamin D, but sometimes the seasons don't permit your body to make enough. To combat this issue, I use a *Sperti Sunlamp* that you can purchase on Amazon. During the winter months, I apply it to my back for 10 minutes each day while I work on my computer. Adults older than age 50 should take between 800 and 1,000 international units of vitamin D3 per day. Some studies recommend 35 IU per pound of body weight. I personally use *Liquid Vitamin D-3* made by Douglas Labs and which you can buy on Amazon. I add 1 cc to my morning smoothie, which is 10,000 IU. That high amount is what my body requires to keep my vitamin-D levels between 80 and 100 ng/ml, which is my goal for bone health and improved immunity. You should ask your doctor to regularly check your vitamin-D levels to keep them within ideal range.

Magnesium

Magnesium is a mineral naturally found in foods like whole-grain breads, dark-green vegetables and nuts. Magnesium and calcium work together closely to maintain strong bones. The recommended daily amount of magnesium is 300 to 500 mg. However, if you eat a lot of processed foods, you likely don't get enough magnesium in your daily diet. Magnesium is often incorporated into a daily multivitamin. An ideal balance is two parts calcium to one part magnesium. If your multivitamin has 1,000 mg of calcium, it should have 500 mg of magnesium. Watch for signs of excess magnesium, such as stomach upset and diarrhea. These symptoms indicate you should cut back on magnesium.

I personally use the aforementioned supplement called "*Cal/Mag 2001*" made by Douglas Labs and available on Amazon. Two tablets provide 500 mg of calcium citrate/carbonate/ascorbate complex, 250 mg of magnesium, vitamin C 100 mg, vitamin D3 50 IU, boron 3mg and glutamic acid. I take 2 tablets only in the morning.

Vitamins K1 and K2

Vitamin K activates proteins that play a role in blood clotting, calcium metabolism and heart health. One of its most important functions is to regulate calcium deposition. In other words, it promotes the calcification of bones and prevents the calcification of blood vessels and kidneys. Some scientists have suggested that the roles of vitamins K1 and K2 are quite different, and many feel that they should be classified as separate nutrients altogether. This idea is supported by an animal study showing that vitamin K2 reduced blood-vessel calcification whereas vitamin K1 did not [88]. Controlled studies in people also observe that vitamin K2 supplements generally improve bone and heart health, while vitamin K1 has no significant bone or heart benefits [89].

I, therefore, take a supplement called **K2-D3** made by Douglas Labs that can be purchased at Amazon. Each capsule contains vitamin K-2 (as menaquinone-7), vitamin D-3 (cholecalciferol), and astaxanthin 2 mg. I take one in the morning and one in the evening.

Strontium Citrate

Strontium citrate is the last piece of the puzzle for me regaining my bone strength. As I have mentioned previously, multiple myeloma releases chemicals that cause the osteoblasts (bone-building cells) to slow down while causing the bone-breaking cells (osteoclasts) to speed up.

Strontium is in row IIa of the periodic table, just below calcium. Like calcium, strontium has 2 positive charges in its ionic form. Because of its chemical similarity to calcium, strontium can replace calcium to some extent in various biochemical processes in the body, including replacing a small proportion of the calcium in hydroxyapatite crystals of calcified tissues such as bones and teeth. Strontium in these crystals imparts added strength to these tissues. Strontium also seems to pull extra calcium into bones. When rats or guinea pigs are fed increased amounts of strontium, their bones and teeth became thicker and stronger.

Although you may have never heard of strontium before, it has been safely used as a therapeutic agent for more than 100 years. It was first catalogued in *Squire's Companion to the British Pharma-copoiea* in 1884. After that, strontium was used as a medicine in the United States and Europe. As late as 1955, strontium was still tabulated in the *Dispensatory of the United States of America*. For decades in the early 1900s, strontium salts were prescribed by doctors in doses between 200 and 400 mg/day without toxic effects being reported.

In 1985, Dr. Stanley C. Skoryna of McGill University in Montreal brought strontium back into prominence by conducting a small research study that ended up demonstrating the potential for using strontium for the improvement of osteoporosis [90]. Three men and three women with osteoporosis were each prescribed 600–700 mg/day of strontium in the form of strontium carbonate. Hip-bone biopsies were then performed on each patient before and after 6 months of treatment with strontium. Biopsies disclosed an amazing 172% increase in the rate of bone production after strontium therapy, with no change in bone resorption. The patients receiving the strontium remarked that the pains in their bones had decreased and that their movability had improved.

A much larger research study included 1,649 osteoporotic postmenopausal women. These participants received 2 gm per day of strontium ranelate (providing 680 mg strontium) or placebo for 3 years [91]. Calcium and vitamin-D supplements were also taken by both groups during the study. The results were remarkable in that the patients in the strontium group had a reduced fracture risk of 49% in the first year and 41% reduced risk during the 3-year study period. Participants in the strontium group improved lumbar bone mineral density (BMD) by an average of 14.4% and femoral-neck BMD by an average of 8.3%. The authors came to the conclusion that "treatment of postmenopausal osteoporosis with strontium ranelate leads to early and sustained reductions in the risk of vertebral fractures."

Strontium for Cancer Metastasis

Dr. Skoryna also analyzed the strontium's response in patients with breast or prostate cancer that had metastasized to the bones [92]. Metastatic bone cancer is a horrific condition with an extremely poor prognosis, in which the cancer cells are multiplying exponentially and gradually eating away the bone tissue. In addition to causing agonizing pain, metastatic bone cancer can make bones so brittle that they break with the slightest of trauma or just collapse under the body's weight. Disfiguring and debilitating fractures end up with loss of mobility and tormenting pain. Metastatic cancer is exceptionally difficult to treat and generally becomes progressively worse, albeit successful treatment of the cancer will, in some cases, cause the bone lesions to recede.

In spite of this bleak prognosis, Dr. Skoryna prescribed to these metastatic-cancer patients strontium (in the form of strontium gluconate) for at least 3 months. The dosage of strontium that he used was only 274 mg/day—much lower than the 600–700 mg/day he used in his osteoporosis study. Nevertheless, since strontium gluconate is absorbed more efficiently than strontium carbonate, less strontium was needed to achieve the same blood level. In many cases, the results were indisputable and quite remarkable. X-rays taken before and after strontium treatment disclosed brand-new mineral deposition in areas of bone that had been deteriorated by the cancer. In one patient, a vertebra that was on the brink of collapse exhibited extensive remineralization. Although much of this newly deposited mineral was composed of calcium crystals, the presence of strontium was unmistakably distinguishable by its very characteristic presentation on the X-rays. Furthermore, these strontium deposits were still able to be viewed on X-rays taken several months after strontium therapy had been discontinued. Many of these cancer patients also reported feeling much better, and some actually gained weight during the strontium treatment.

Strontium citrate in doses up to 1.7 g/day has been validated to offer a safe, efficaceous, and inexpensive approach to preventing and reversing osteoporosis and may benefit patients with bone metastasis, as well as possibly helping to prevent dental cavities. Doses of 680 mg/day seem to be optimum, although lower doses are clinically efficacious. In the extensive number of scientific studies that I have reviewed, I have found zero side effects with strontium citrate even with treatment beyond 3 years.

In Europe it was actually approved by the European FDA as strontium ranelate, which is an inorganic totally synthetic form of strontium. There were some questions about it possibly increasing the chances of stroke or heart attack, so the company that manufactured it pulled it from the market. The organic form "strontium citrate," which I use, is highly effective, side-effect free, very inexpensive, and can be purchased from home on Amazon. Almost too good to be true. In fact, many people I inform about strontium don't use it because it does seem too good to be true. My oncologist knows that I am using it and has been quite amazed by my bone-density results. He has been supplied with a multitude of scientific articles by me. This is how complementary treatments gradually start becoming more mainstream.

I started taking strontium citrate after I decided to stop my zoledronic acid infusions (remember in the introduction) because I was having severe side effects and because it is highly kidney toxic; takes 55 years to be totally eliminated by the body; 4% of people get destruction of the jawbone; and 2% get a weird oblique fracture of the hip bone that does not occur in nature. There is a huge difference between getting an hour, intravenous zoledronic acid infusion every month with major side effects and a natural element found in seafood and root vegetables with no side effects that you take at home and can order from your computer.

The product that I use is **Strontium** by Douglas Labs that can be purchased on Amazon. I take three 200 mg strontium citrate capsules (600 mg total) in the evening before bed. After taking it for only 8 months, my DexaSCAN improved from osteoporosis to osteopenia. My bone mineral density (BMD) improved 8% in only 8 months. To put that into perspective, a average person older than 40 years of age loses about 0.5% of their bone density per year. My 8% increase in 8 months reversed 16 years of erosion!

ALKASELTZER GOLD

Cancer thrives in a microenvironment of high acidity and low oxygen. In fact, an acidic environment around cancer cells is necessary for spread and metastasis. This acidic pH activates metalloproteinases like collagenase and cathepsin B, both important matrix-remodeling proteases that eat away at the connective tissue surrounding the cancer cells to allow them to move freely and spread.

To keep my pH as alkaline as possible, I utilize an **Acid/Base Food Chart**, which is at the end of this book. Foods are broken down into most alkaline, less alkaline, least akaline, least acidic, less acidic and most acidic. This chart indicates the effect that these foods have on the pH after they have been utilized and metabolized by the body. For instance, a lemon is acidic if you place a pH strip on it, but after being metabolized by the body, it has an alkalinizing effect in the blood. When you review this chart, you will immediately notice that fruits and vegetables are primarily on the alkaline side and animal products on the acidic side. There are, however, some plant foods, such as beans, corn, and carrots that are on the acidic side.

I buy **Hydrion pH 5.5-8.0 Strips** made by Microessential Labs from Amazon and check my urine pH about 4 times throughout the day. I try to keep it between 6.5 and 7.5, which is correlated with a color code on the front of the plastic container. The vast majority of people I check have a urine pH between 5.5 to 6.5. That is because most people I am checking are eating a Standard American Diet, which is extremely acidic. Also, as you age, you tend to get more acidic from your kidneys deteriorating and having pockets of chronic inflammation throughout the body.

When initiating this, start with 70% alkaline/30% acidic foods, and then adjust accordingly. It took me about a month to have my pH consistently between 6.5 and 7.5. As you eat more alkaline, you will store many of the minerals present in alkaline foods.

Occasionally, when I get an acidic reading, I use an *Alkaseltzer Gold* tablet in a cup of water, which immediately gets my pH into my goal range. *Alkaseltzer Gold* contains 344 mg of potassium bicarbonate, 1050 and 1050 mg of sodium bicarbonate, and 1000 mg of anhydrous citric acid. I use this maybe once per month when I get an occasional acidic reading. You can purchase this product on Amazon.

If you remember with my coffee regimen, I add ⅛ teaspoon of baking soda to my coffee. When you look at the *Acid/Base Food Chart*, you will see that coffee is very acidic. I have checked with a pH strip, and baking soda completely neutralizes this acidic pH.

In one important study, investigators demonstrated that oral bicarbonate selectively increased the pH of tumors and reduced the formation of spontaneous metastasis in mouse models of metastatic breast cancer [93].

FERMENTED WHEAT GERM EXTRACT

Fermented-wheat-germ extract is a natural compound derived from industrial fermentation of wheat germ. In recent years, its anti-cancer properties have been investigated. A 2018 meta-analysis looked at 16 well-done studies on the topic. Various types of cancer cells treated with FWGE were analyzed, which demonstrated cancer-cell toxic effects, alteration of the cancer-cell cycle, anti-proliferative effects, and induction of cancer-cell suicide.

Strong anti-cancer effects were seen with leukemia [94], lymphoma [95], gastric cancer [96], ovarian cancer [97], breast cancer [98], colon cancer [99], and liver cancer [100]. Other types of cell lines investigated were prostate-cancer cells, endocervical adenocarcinoma, cervical-epidermoid-carcinoma cells, testicular-cancer cell lines, head and neck cancer, thyroid- and pancreatic-cancer cells, melanoma, hepatoma, glioblastoma, neuroblastoma, and oral squamous-carcinoma cells. In all cases, the effects of FWGE treatment provided similar strong anti-cancer activity.

I personally use a product called *Metatrol-Fermented Wheat Germ Extract* made by American Biosciences that can be purchased on Amazon. I take one capsule every morning. It is quite expensive, but I think the science is so good on FWGE that you should include it in your program if you can afford it.

*IODINE

Unfortunately, up to a third of people worldwide are at risk of an iodine deficiency [101]. Those at highest risk are those who are pregnant, and people who live in countries where there is very little iodine in the soil. This includes South Asia, Southeast Asia, New Zealand and European countries. People who don't use iodized salt and people who follow a vegetarian or vegan diet are also at risk.

Because I advise a whole food, plant-based diet and because much of the iodine that people intake comes from seafood, I recommend using iodized salt when using salt and also taking a kelp supplement. I personally take *Kelp* made by Nature's Way, available on Amazon. I take one capsule in the morning only. I also put a drop of nascent iodine into my morning smoothie. I use *Iodine Edge* made by Go Nutrients, also available on Amazon. In addition, I think it is a good idea to ask your physician for an iodine blood level. When I first had mine checked, it was low, and I have been able to keep it consistently in a normal range with the nascent iodine and the kelp supplement.

*VITAMIN B12

Vitamin B12 is an important water-soluble vitamin. It plays a critical role in the production of our red blood cells and DNA, and helps our nervous system function properly. For people taking chemotherapy, it is especially important to keep your B12 levels in normal range because of chemo's negative effect on red-blood-cell production and its toxic effect on nerves. This vitamin is naturally found in animal foods such as meats, fish, poultry, eggs and dairy. However, it can also be found in B12-fortified food products such as some varieties of breads and plant milks. Unfortunately, B12 deficiency is quite common, especially in the elderly, because we tend to lose our ability to absorb B12 as we age. Vegans are also at risk because they don't intake animal products.

Because I do promote a whole food, plant-based diet for the battle against cancer, I strongly recommend taking a B12 supplement. I personally take *Methyl B12 Plus* made by Douglas Labs that can be purchased on Amazon. This supplement contains 400 mcg of folate and 1,000 mcg of methylcobalamin. I place it under my tongue daily. If you choose, you can use this supplement once per week and still maintain good levels because it is stored in the liver. There is no risk for toxicity.

*MODIFIED CITRUS PECTIN

First off, what is the difference between natural pectin and "modified" pectin? Natural pectin is a fiber found in ripe berries, stone fruits and most citrus fruits. As we have learned in a previous chapter, fiber cannot be absorbed by the body. Modified citrus pectin (MCP), on the other hand, is processed to make the fiber molecules smaller so that it can be absorbed into your bloodstream. That means your body can benefit from more than just pectin's fibrous properties.

In regard to its anti-cancer effects, MCP has been investigated quite a bit in the scientific literature. In one study, intake of soluble pectin fragments inhibited the growth and metastasis of transplanted tumors in mice [102], and it has been shown that MCP inhibits the growth of colon cancer and liver metastasis [103]. With my cancer, multiple myeloma, it was found to act in several different ways to destroy the myeloma cells [104].

Because of these studies and several others establishing anti-cancer effects, I use a product called **Pectasol** made by Douglas Labs that can be purchased on Amazon. I take one capsule in the morning and one at night.

*MY NIGHT TEA CONCOCTION

Before I retire for the night, I take my lenalidomide capsule and my evening supplements. I use a concoction of 4 teas as the way to get the supplements down while getting some anti-cancer activity from the teas. In Dr. Li's book *Eat to Beat Disease*, he discusses how combining teas creates a synergistic effect. For instance . . . 2 + 2 does not equal 4. It equals 7. These are the 4 teas that I use:

Hibiscus Tea

Hibiscus (*Hibiscus amottianus*) is widely used in folk medicine due to its well-established antioxidant and anti-inflammatory effects, as well as its ability to prevent toxicity from chemotherapy. During my daily perusal of the scientific literature, I came across a good study demonstrating that *Hibiscus* has anti-cancer activity against my cancer . . . multiple myeloma [105]. In another study on breast cancer, *Hibiscus* extract was able to selectively cause cancer-cell suicide in both triple-negative and estrogen-receptor positive breast-cancer cells in a dosage-dependent manner (the higher the dose, the greater the cancer-killing effect). Most importantly, the addition of *Hibiscus* extract was found to enhance the cancer-cell-suicide effect of the chemotherapy treatments (taxol and cisplatin) in triple-negative breast-cancer cells when compared to taxol and cisplatin treatment alone [106].

Dandelion Tea

I came across a video on *nutritionfacts.org* that reviewed the literature as to what tea had the highest antioxidant activity. The winner was dandelion (*Taraxacum officinale*) tea. That prompted me to do a search of the scientific literature, and, to my delight, there was quite a bit of data establishing that it also had anti-cancer properties. One study that investigated its effects against gastric cancer demonstrated that it kept the cancer from proliferating and migrating [107]. In another study looking at dandelion extract's effects against colorectal cancer, it was discovered to instigate cancer-cell suicide in > 95% of colon-cancer cells [108].

In the previous chapter on chemotherapy, we also discussed dandelion's scientifically proven protective effects on the kidney.

Chamomile Tea

Most of us are familiar with the fact that chamomile (*Matricaria chamomilla*) tea creates a relaxant effect that can help us enter sleep more quickly. But many of you are probably not aware that chamomile is loaded with a well-known anti-cancer phytochemical called "apigenin." Apigenin and the other antioxidants found in chamomile tea have been linked with a lower incidence of certain types of cancer. In several studies, apigenin has been shown to combat cancer cells, especially those of the breast, digestive tract, skin, prostate and uterus [109,110]. Furthermore, another study of more than 500 people discerned that those who drank chamomile tea 2–6 times per week were much less likely to contract thyroid cancer compared to those who did not drink chamomile tea [111].

Decaf Green Tea

Green tea (*Camellia sinensis*) is loaded with antioxidants, which would suggest that it might have forceful effects against cancer, and that's exactly what the science shows. In one meta-analysis, reviewing several scientific studies, it was found that women who drank the most green tea had a 20–30% lower risk of getting breast cancer, the most common cancer in women [112]. Another good study validated that men drinking green tea had a 48% lower risk of developing prostate cancer, which is the most common cancer in men [113]. Still another meta-analysis looking at a total of 29 studies demonstrated that those drinking green tea were 42% less likely to develop colorectal cancer [114].

All Four Teas

Because of the magnitude of scientific evidence and the fact that multiple teas work synergistically, I place all 4 tea bags in a tea cup, add a wedge of a lemon and a lime, add hot water; then I sip it as I take my supplements. I use all-organic teas that I purchase at Whole Foods, which you can also find on Amazon.

*ZINC LOZENGES

Zinc is essential for a well-functioning immune system. Zinc supplements have been shown to stimulate the immune system and reduce oxidative stress. In a meta-analysis of 7 studies, it was demonstrated that 80–92 mg per day of zinc decreased the length of the common cold by up to 33% [115]. Zinc supplements were also shown to dramatically diminish the risk of infections and increase the immune activity in the elderly [116].

Because of these immune-enhancing effects, I eat a few high-zinc-containing pumpkin seeds before I take my morning supplements and take *Zinc Lozenges* made by Douglas Labs that can be purchased on Amazon. I suck on one as the grand finale of my morning supplements.

SUMMARY

I have included every efficacious targeted supplement that I could find in the scientific literature to help you in your fight against cancer. I have asterisked the ones that I think are the most important. I would encourage you to do your own *pubmed.gov* scientific-literature search to determine which supplement is worth taking for your individual cancer and situation.

There is also the matter of expense, in that some of these supplements, such as *Metatrol*, for example, are quite expensive. If money is no issue for you, and you are in a significant battle against cancer, I would recommend taking as many of the targeted supplements that I have described because there is a synergy when taking multiple phytonutrients simultaneously.

Most importantly, however, you should eat a whole food, plant-based diet. If you are eating a Standard American Diet and expect the supplements to counter your bad eating habits, then you will definitely be disappointed. This is a battle against a powerful and horrific enemy that wants to kill you, and you need to pull out every single weapon in your armamentarium. That means conventional treatment, a whole food, plant-based diet, targeted supplements, daily exercise, intermittent fasting, adequate sleep and stress reduction.

You can do it. It takes a desire to live, discipline and motivation. It has worked for me, and I know it can work for you.

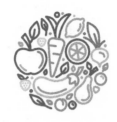

CHAPTER 8

The Power of Exercise

We always hear that people who exercise have fewer and milder colds. Exercise enthusiasts tend to boast that they hardly ever get sick when compared to sedentary folks.

Before scientists decided to start studying this, no one really knew for sure if this was true. To get to the bottom of this question, one research group collected data on more than 1,000 people from the ages of 18 to 85. Over 12 weeks, during the winter months, they tracked the number of upper-respiratory infections that these individuals acquired. The individuals were quizzed on all the variables that could affect the results. They were asked how much aerobic activity they did on a weekly basis, and each of the participants had their fitness rated on a 10-point system.

The results were stunning . . . the frequency of colds in individuals who exercised 5 or more days per week was 46% less than those who were primarily sedentary. Additionally, when these exercisers did get an illness, it was not as severe, and the number of days with the illness was 41% lower!

Other studies show that exercise not only helps our immune system fight off bacterial and viral infections but also decreases our chance of developing cancer. And if you had cancer and are in a remission, it can significantly lower your chance of developing a recurrence [1].

Several studies show that even just 30 minutes of brisk walking 5 days per week can significantly reduce the risk of several cancers:

- breast and colon cancers: 25-30% reduction in risk.
- prostate cancer: 10-25% reduction in risk.
- endometrial cancer: 30-35% reduction in risk.

According to the largest study ever published on the subject of breast-cancer prevention with exercise, only women who worked up a sweat for at least 5 or more times per week appeared to get dramatic protection [2]. However, some other studies show that moderately intense exercise may offer as much benefit as vigorous exercise. For example, a 2018 study in the *Journal of Applied Physiology* reported that walking just an hour per day is associated with significantly lower breast-cancer risk [3].

Evidence backing both mild and vigorous exercise was nicely illustrated in a study investigating breast-cancer-survival rates in relation to the intensity of the exercise. In this study, they found that those who did one mile of brisk walking per day reduced their risk of dying from breast cancer by 24%. Those who stepped it up a notch and ran ⅔ of a mile daily reduced their risk of dying from breast cancer by 40%. Finally, the high achievers, who ran 2.3 miles per day, lowered their chance of recurrence by a spectacular 95%!

We are not 100% sure of the mechanism of how this works, but we do know that even just 6 minutes of aerobic exercise can increase natural killer cell immune activity by 50%. These natural killer cells are the immune cells that attack cancer cells during their deadly evolution.

We also know from mouse studies [3] that exercise does increase the oxygen content in the tumor microenvironment. If you remember in chapter 1, we discussed how cancer thrives in a microenvironment of high acidity and low oxygen. In several studies, exercise has been shown to increase the oxygen content in the microenvironment, making it harder for cancer to thrive. In one of these studies, published in the *Journal of Applied Physiology*, there was a verified 90% increase of the oxygen levels inside the tumors of rats that engaged in long-term, moderate-intensity treadmill exercise [4].

The beauty of exercise is that it does not cost one bloody cent. It doesn't require a prescription or an appointment with a doctor, but it is one of the most powerful stimulators of the immune system, and all that it requires is self-discipline.

EXERCISE AND EMOTIONS

In my daily review of the scientific literature, I have found numerous articles demonstrating that exercise works extremely well to counter depression and, in many studies, does it better than anti-depressants [5,6]. It is also a great way to reduce feelings of stress, which is critically important and discussed in the next chapter about "the power of stress reduction." Exercise is, therefore, an activity that I encourage all people who struggle with depression and anxiety to engage in because it is free, has only good side effects, and is highly effective. Some of my medical colleagues, however, push anti-depressants or anti-anxiety drugs on just about every patient complaining of even the slightest innuendo of depression or nervousness.

For instance, many doctors tout that anti-depressant drugs have many "published" studies that demonstrate that they are effective [7]. Notice how I have enclosed "published" in quotation marks. What if drug companies published only the studies that showed a positive effect but quietly hid from the public any studies showing that the drugs didn't work? To find out the truth, Dr. Michael Greger's research group applied to the Food and Drug Administration under the U.S. Freedom of Information Act (FOIA) to get access to the published and unpublished studies submitted by pharmaceutical companies. What they found was pretty unbelievable. The published literature reported that the results of nearly all anti-depressant trials were positive. In comparison, FDA scrutiny of trial data (published and unpublished studies) demonstrated that approximately half of the trials showed that the drugs didn't work. When all the data was joined, the anti-depressants failed to show a clinically convincing advantage over placebo sugar pills [8]. The result of this study demonstrated that the placebo effect may be the primary explanation of how anti-depressants may work. So it may be the power of the belief that the drug is going to work that is the primary mode of action [9].

What was even more appalling to Dr. Greger and his group was that the FOIA documents exposed that the FDA knew that drugs like Paxil and Prozac didn't work much better than placebo yet made a disgusting decision to protect drug companies by keeping this information from the general public and prescribing physicians [10]. How could the pharmaceutical companies get away with something like this? The drug industry is considered one of the most lucrative and politically influential industries in the United States, and depression is the golden goose because it is chronic, common, and frequently treated with multiple drugs [11]. Indeed, anti-depressants are taken by more than 8% of the US population [12].

So, if doctors are willing to give patients placebo-equivalent treatments, some contend that it would be better for them just to lie to patients and give them actual sugar pills [13]. Unlike the toxic drugs, sugar pills do not cause the multitude of side effects associated with anti-depressants. For instance, anti-depressants cause sexual dysfunction in up to 75% of users. Other side effects include long-term weight gain and insomnia. And about 20% of people have withdrawal symptoms when they try to quit taking the medications [14]. To me, the most alarming fact is that anti-depressants may make people more likely to become depressed in the future. Studies demonstrate that patients have a higher probability to become depressed again after anti-depressant use than after treatment by other means, including placebos [15].

So even if the mood-boosting benefit of exercise is also a placebo effect (which it isn't), at least it's one with benefits rather than risks. So we see that anti-depressants have many undesirable side effects such as weight gain, insomnia, decreased sex drive, anxiety and fatigue. Look at every one of those side effects. Exercise causes the exact opposite . . . weight loss, improved sleep, increased sex drive, diminished anxiety and higher energy levels. Why would anyone not want to try the power of exercise before ingesting toxic chemicals into their system on a daily basis? The only answer that I can think of is laziness and lack of self-discipline. I always say that if the benefits of exercise were in a pill—every single person in the world would would be taking it.

When cancer patients ask me for counsel . . . daily exercise and a whole food, plant-based diet are the 2 that I emphasize because they are highly effective and free. Many people incorporate the whole food, plant-based diet recommendation, but daily exercise is the one that many will not take up the sword and do. As I have shown above, even 150 minutes per week of simple, brisk walking has amazing cancer- and cardiovascular-protective effects, but, unfortunately, the majority of people in the United States do not do it. There are some people who love it—but for many, it is the bane of their existence.

WHY DON'T WE EXERCISE?

These are the 11 most common reasons that people do not exercise:

⊚ *It Is Uncomfortable*

I can understand this. When I begin my daily bike ride up a steep hill, I start to get a very uncomfortable feeling inside of me. This is when the body is using up the available oxygen and starting to use a no-oxygen (anaerobic) form of metabolism that creates lactic acid. This induces an uneasy feeling inside of you. Once you work through that initial period and the body adapts to the exercise, that feeling goes away fairly quickly. In fact, if you continue to exercise, you can get a mental high from the endorphin (narcotic-like chemicals) release from the brain. Furthermore, the more you exercise on a daily basis, the more fit you will become, and that lactic-acid-uneasy period may not even happen.

The memory of that uncomfortable feeling may be enough to stop someone from engaging in daily exercise.

⊚ *No Time*

People are busy. In this day and age, with work, family obligations, attending school, homework and other obligations, it is difficult to fit exercise into the daily schedule, but it certainly is not impossible. For busy people, the one recommendation that I always make is to do the exercise in the morning, do it in your house (not at a gym), and keep the sessions short (10–15 minutes).

The reason that I recommend short sessions at home and in the morning is that it is much easier to talk yourself out of driving to the gym, running into someone you know, working out, showering, and driving back home. That is at least a 2-hour endeavor.

Conversely, waking up, having a cup of coffee, with a short period of prayer, meditation, and gratitude, and then starting a 15-minute exercise routine before showering is not a monumental mountain that needs to be climbed every day. I personally do a 15-minute resistance-band routine every morning that hits every muscle group. By the end of the routine, I am very short of breath, because I do it quickly and vigorously.

As I previously stated, one study demonstrated that only 6 minutes of exercise increased natural killer cell activity by 50%, so you don't need to do long, laborious exercise routines to get immune stimulation. In fact, many studies indicate that, once you exercise beyond 45 minutes, the testosterone levels start to decline. Up to 45 minutes, they rise, but beyond that time, they gradually start declining.

The other way to get exercise throughout the day is to take the stairs when you can, walk on your lunch break, or park in the parking space the farthest distance away from the entrance to your destination. Other things you can do are to walk to the store instead of driving, walk to pick up your kids from school, or run around the backyard with your dog. In fact, they have found that people who own dogs actually walk a lot more than non-dog owners. So maybe buy yourself a cute little Frenchy!

I personally have an iWatch that measures the number of steps that I take in a day. Studies show that 10,000 steps should be a goal for maximum health. I feel that an iWatch or a FitBit will motivate you throughout the day to hit your goal.

⊚ *No Energy*

This is a very common excuse I get from cancer patients and an amazingly frequent excuse from people without health problems. I admit that a full day of work or school, taking care of kids, running errands, and meeting other obligations can be exhausting, but that is why the morning is the best time to schedule exercise. You are fresh, you have lots of energy, and there are no competing interests.

And one of the added benefits of daily exercise (that most people who refuse to do it don't realize) is that the energy you put into exercise actually creates more energy. Lack of energy is especially a problem with cancer patients. The chemo and radiation so wipes them out that they have no energy left for exercise. Also the chemo in most instances lowers the white-blood-cell counts that are so important to immunity. I find that, when these kinds of patients take my advice and force themselves to exercise, they actually feel more energetic and get improved white-blood-cell counts because exercise does stimulate stem cell growth in the bone marrow.

◉ *Competing Interests*

Let's face it, we live in a technological age where texting, emailing, doing Facebook, playing video games, or watching a movie takes up a large chunk of our time. To counter this, choose a social activity that doesn't require you to sit. Go bowling, play tennis, go shopping with a friend, or walk around the park with a relative. Also, while you are doing technologic activities like Facebook or watching a movie at home, try to get up and walk around the room every 10 minutes to help you hit your 10,000 steps per day.

Many scientists are calling "sitting" the new "smoking" because of extensive sitting's negative effect on health. So make a conscious effort to move throughout the day. Once again, the FitBit or iWatch will help keep you motivated as it has done for me.

◉ *Haven't Developed a Habit*

Self-discipline is something that is extremely difficult for most people. You must make a commitment to yourself that you are going to do this 15-minute, morning exercise program every day for a straight month. Most experts on habits espouse that, if you can do an activity regularly for a straight month, a habit has developed that has now become a regular part of your life. Constantly remind yourself why you are exercising . . . more energy, a better immune and cardiovascular system, better appearance and better psychological attitude. And if you have cancer, remind yourself that you are kicking the cancer in the butt every single day.

⊚ *No Motivation*

If you see no reason to exercise, then you are not going to do it. So, you need to get educated about the many positive benefits of exercising. Buying and reading this book is one step. You need to watch YouTube videos, read books, follow Facebook and Instagram sites that espouse the benefits of exercise, which are voluminous.

I tell people the same thing about a whole food, plant-based diet. If you don't know why it is very beneficial to your health to limit the consumption of animal products, why in the world would you give up that juicy hamburger or chicken wings? Constant education is key. That is why I constantly encourage people who come to my lectures to watch at least one 5-minute video every day on *nutritionfacts.org.*

⊚ *Too Overwhelming*

I will tell you that, in regard to writing this book . . . I procrastinated for a year because the task just seemed so overwhelming. That changed when I hired a writing coach, Lynda Goldman, who was able to get me motivated. I remember very vividly when I was able to break through this mind block. It was when Lynda told me that all I needed to do was to dedicate one hour every day for 2–3 months, and my book would be done. All of a sudden, a task that seemed insurmountable seemed easily achievable. I started this book on Memorial Day and finished it

THE POWER OF EXERCISE | 239

on Labor Day . . . exactly 3 months—just like Lynda promised! All I needed was a little motivation.

The same principle applies to exercise. You might be overwhelmed because you have never had an exercise routine in your entire life. So, take baby steps. Maybe just start parking in a more-distant parking spot or taking the stairs at work instead of the elevator. Buy a Fitbit to tempt you into getting more steps in per day. Watch some YouTube videos about the benefit of exercise or some different types of exercises that you might enjoy. Do some jumping jacks while watching a movie at home. Before you know it, exercising will not be such an overwhelming thought and will be a part of your daily life.

◉ *Poor Diet*

This is a big one. Most Westerners, as I have reiterated to you in this book, have a horrible diet. This fact is proven by the alarmingly rapid increase of obesity rates in Western cultures. The evidence illustrates that limiting animal products and increasing fruits, vegetables, whole grains, legumes, mushrooms, nuts and seeds will lead to an optimally functioning body.

So if your diet is lacking in the vitamins, minerals and phytonutrients that Nature requires for excellent health, you may not have enough mental energy to overcome some of the obstacles described above. So, educate yourself about the benefits of a whole food, plant-based diet. Follow my Instagram site *@cancerveggiedoc*. Watch 5-minute videos daily on Dr. Michael Greger's amazing website *nutritionfacts.org*. Watch the movie *Forks Over Knives*. Read the book *How Not to Die* by Dr. Michael Greger.

It's like with exercise . . . if you don't know why you should change your diet, why in the world would you give up that cheese pizza and French fries? Again . . . education is key.

⊚ *Current Physical Condition*

Many of you reading this book have cancer. Others may be morbidly obese, have a heart condition, or have a bad knee or hip. You may want to get approval from your doctor first, but I will tell you that almost every single person can do some type of exercise.

For example, if you have a bad knee or hip, there are a multitude of arm exercises that you can do with resistance bands or light weights. If you have a heart condition, start with some very light walking around the neighborhood. Buy a FitBit or iWatch to monitor your heart rate as you exercise. If you have cancer and have low energy levels, walk on your indoor treadmill for 5 minutes in the morning.

⊚ *No Access*

As I stated earlier, not having access to a fancy gym is actually an advantage, not a disadvantage. The drive to the gym, the workout, the after-shower, and the drive back home will stifle just about anyone's motivation to do that on an habitual basis.

You can have everything that you need at home. If you are just a walker or only do exercises that solely use your own body weight, then you need zero equipment. If you want to incorporate resistance bands, a full set of bands from *blackmountainproducts. com* will cost you $26 on Amazon. Light weights can be purchased at Walmart for a minimal cost. If you want to buy a treadmill or elliptical for use at home, that will be more expensive, but the cost over many years of use will be minimal in relation to the great health benefits that you will achieve. There are also many DVDs, books and online videos available on yoga, pilates and other forms of exercise. There really is no excuse here, because the options are limitless.

◉ *Lack of Results*

If you are exercising daily and you feel that you are not getting results, don't let that keep you from doing it. The evidence is enormous that exercise benefits your immune system, your mental well-being, your cardiovascular system, your endurance and your appearance. So even if you don't feel that you are getting results, you are most definitely helping your body.

SHOULD I EXERCISE DURING CHEMO AND RADIATION?

For sure!!! Exercise during cancer treatment is not only safe, but also beneficial for reducing fatigue, improving your physical function, and enhancing your overall sense of well-being. Studies show that exercise during cancer treatment reduces the occurrence of negative post-treatment outcomes, including loss of bone density, muscle mass and cardiovascular performance. It's important to keep in mind that exercise programs may need to be adapted, depending on your health status and medical treatments you have received (e.g., radiation therapy, surgery, hormonal therapy.) Low-intensity exercise programs, including walking, stretching and yoga are best suited for individuals who were sedentary prior to their cancer diagnosis. Individuals who are on bed rest can benefit greatly from physical therapy, which maintains strength and range of motion while also counteracting the effects of depression and fatigue.

DIET VERSUS EXERCISE

People often ask me, "What is more important . . . diet or exercise?" To try to figure this out, a UCLA research team compared 3 groups of men: a plant-based-diet-and-exercise group, an exercise-only group, and a control group of couch potatoes eating a Standard American Diet [16]. The diet-and-exercise group had been following a plant-based diet for

15 years, along with performing daily moderate exercise, such as a brisk daily walk. Conversely, the exercise-only group exercised strenuously 5X per week for at least an hour for 15 years, while eating the Standard American Diet.

To find out which group had the greatest cancer-fighting ability, the scientists took the blood from each group and dripped it onto human prostate-cancer cells growing in a petri dish to see whose blood would decimate cancer cells the best. The blood of the control group wasn't totally without cancer-fighting capability. The Dorito-eating couch potatoes were able to destroy 1%-2% of the cancer cells in the petri dish. On the other hand, those who exercised strenuously 5X per week for 15 years killed 2,000% more cancer cells than the control group. Those results were impressive, but not compared to the blood of those in the plant-based-diet-and-exercise group. That blood killed an incredible 4,000% more cancer cells than that of the Dorito-eating couch-potato group. Clearly exercise alone had a significant effect, but at the end of the day, many hours in the gym without the right diet appeared to be no match for a plant-based diet combined with exercise.

FASTING'S SIMILAR EFFECTS AS EXERCISE

The reason I have included fasting with exercise in this chapter is that fasting, in several studies, has been shown to induce many of the same positive effects as exercise. The benefits of fasting cannot be denied, and if you look at the history of fasting, it can't have a beginning point because there's no reason to think that early man did not fast in the normal course of his existence. In fact, every other animal in existence today will fast during times of stress or illness, and sometimes even at the slightest turmoil. It is a natural instinct for animals to seek rest and conserve energy at demanding times. Herbert Shelton (1895–1985), a doctor who looked after the fasts of more than 40,000 people in the

20th century, wrote, "Fasting must be recognized as a fundamental and radical process that is older than any other mode of caring for the sick organism, for it is employed on the plane of instinct."

Many of the early great thinkers, such as Hippocrates and Aristotle acclaimed the benefits of fasting. Paracelsus, one of the 3 fathers of Western medicine, stated emphatically that fasting was the greatest remedy—"the physician within." In fact, if you look throughout history almost all of the healing arts recognized the revitalizing power of fasting.

From a spiritual perspective, religious groups have used fasting as a part of ceremonies throughout history. A point of fact is that almost every major religion uses fasting in one form or another, whether for forgiveness, repentance or sacrifice. Many faiths recommend regular fasts to break the addiction to food, which we know especially plagues many people in Western culture.

In India, fasting dates back thousands of years. In present days, the old healing practice of Ayurveda involves fasting as a technique of physical cure, with its well-known method of utilizing kitchari (a dish of rice and beans).

Unfortunately, conventional medicine has not fully embraced natural remedies like fasting. But as Western medicine learns more and more about the body's ability to foster its own healing mechanisms, I believe that utilizing fasting as a treatment modality will become more a part of traditional medicine. Scientific research is proving that there are many mechanisms induced during fasting that bring the body toward balance and health. And any scientist will concede that only the body itself can restore tissues to their original state of perfection. Fasting is an ideal method of allowing the body to concentrate all of its energy on healing and not on the day-to-day activities of digestion and running hurriedly from place to place.

Even a one-day fast will bring subtle, and sometimes not-so-subtle, changes to the overall psyche. There are several ways to fast. There are prolonged fasts, which require medical supervision, and there are daily fasts, which can been done safely for the majority of people. If you are thinking about doing a prolonged fast, I would highly recommend going to *The True North Clinic* in California. There, they educate you on the benefits of a whole food, plant-based diet while you are undergoing a prolonged fast under medical supervision.

As science is investigating fasting, we are finding that the benefits are numerous . . . the purging of precancerous and cancer cells, a rapid shift into nutritional ketosis, decrease in fat tissue, increased sirtuit gene (longevity gene) expression, increase in cancer-cell suicide, repair of damaged cells, increase in autophagy (the cleaning up of unwanted cells and proteins), improved insulin sensitivity, decreased oxidative stress and inflammation, enhanced cognitive effects and protection of the nervous system.

I personally do nightly fasting because it is easy to do, and the science is starting to show that it is effective. Presently, the epidemiologic data on nightly fasting duration and clinical outcomes is not extensive. However, there are limited data from small trials in humans suggesting that many types of intermittent-fasting regimens positively affect risk factors for poor breast-cancer outcomes, such as glucose regulation, inflammation, obesity and sleep [17]. Two analyses have been published correlating nightly fasting duration with biomarkers of breast-cancer risk in women using US National Health and Nutrition Examination Survey data. In the first analysis, among 2,122 women without diabetes mellitus, longer nightly fasting was associated with significant improvements in biomarkers of blood-sugar control [18]. In the second analysis, a longer duration of nightly fasting was associated with significantly lower inflammatory biomarker C-reactive protein (CRP) concentrations in women who ate less than 30% of their total daily energy intake after 5 PM [19]. Taken together, the rodent and human data support the hypothesis that a prolonged nightly fasting interval could reduce cancer risk and improve cancer outcomes.

Because of this information, a research group performed a study of 2,413 patients with early-stage breast cancer and had them fast nightly for more or less than 13 hours. What they found was that nightly fasting less than 13 hours was associated with a statistically significant 36% increased risk of breast-cancer recurrence compared with nightly fasting more than 13 hours, which prevented that increased risk [20].

Because of this data I personally do a 15- to 16-hour fast every night. I usually eat my last food at 8:00 PM and don't eat until 11:00 AM or even noon the next day.

SUMMARY

Exercise and fasting are 2 activities that you can do that have tremendous health benefits and cost you zero money. It really is a matter of asking yourself . . . how much do I want to live a healthier life? If you are in a remission from cancer . . . how much do I want to lower my chances of getting a relapse? Or if you are battling cancer . . . do I want to improve my chances of defeating this cancer or, at the very minimum, keep it in a dormant state?

In this book, I present the scientific evidence that I have discovered in my research. You then need to decide whether or not you want to use this information and put in the effort to see significant change in your health, your mental outlook, your appearance and your future.

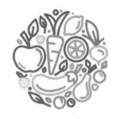

CHAPTER 9

The Power of Stress Reduction

Cancer is definitely one of the most dreaded diseases on the face of the Earth. When most of us think of cancer, we think of a long, drawn-out process of pain and suffering. That will stress anyone out. I personally can tell you that, when I was initially diagnosed with multiple myeloma, I experienced the highest stress and fear levels that I have ever felt in my life. It was not really the fear of dying but the fear of a long suffering.

Those extremely high stress and fear levels were what prompted me immediately, on the advice of a friend with myeloma, to see a psychologist who specialized in treating cancer patients and their caregivers. The psychologist gave me some excellent insight into how cancer patients emotionally deal with their cancer and how they cope with the final months of their life. I was quite surprised when she told me that 95% of her cancer patients are not depressed near the end, and they graciously accept what is before them. The other 5%, on the other hand, go down kicking, heading to Mexico for their Laetrile infusion, angry about their fate.

She let me know that, when her patients had a lot of social interaction with a strong family unit and lots of friends, and received much love and support during those final days, it helped many of them to keep a happy heart. That information, in itself, put my anxious and stressed mind at ease, and I noticed my sleeping patterns immediately improving. You will find in the next chapter that sleep is critical in the fight against cancer, and I just wasn't getting enough of it. Before my cancer diagnosis, when I was performing surgery day in and day out, my sleep patterns were already poor, but after my diagnosis, they further deteriorated, due to the fear of the unknown that lay before me.

Another stressor was the fear of severe pain for a prolonged period of time in my final days. In relation to the cancer patient's pain, my psychologist relayed to me that cancer patients can receive many variations of pain relief. If the pain is more intense, the better the chance of getting a pain-relief method that yield not only better pain relief but also greater sedation. Conversely, if the the pain is less, a milder pain medication is administered with less sedation. Bottom line, if you are really hurting, your medical professional can give you something that will totally wipe out the pain while totally wiping out your mind. That kind of pain is typically near the end of your life; so, if I get there and have made amends with all my family and friends . . . pour it on, baby! After 3 visits with my excellent psychologist, my sleep patterns improved tremendously, I felt at ease, and I was prepared for the battle that lay before me.

CHRONIC STRESS

As most of us know, chronic stress is a part of modern life. We live in a world of technology, where there is a constant barrage of text messages, social media, emails, spam, YouTube videos and advertisements coming across our screens. Simply buying a car is a major stressor because of the numerous choices before us. And most of us just don't take the time to stop to be quiet with our thoughts and prayers. We run from task to task, stressing over finances, relationships and our health.

Because of this chronic stress, it has become one of the most insidious health conditions in modern society and is linked to increased risk of developing nearly every chronic disease, including cancer. Researchers have found that chronic stress may promote cancer growth, metastasis (spread) and recurrence by causing changes in your body that make it more prone to cancer growth. Stress stimulates our adrenal glands to produce cortisol ("the stress hormone"), and if this cortisol release remains uncontrolled, your adrenal glands will continually produce cortisol, leading to the following disastrous physiologic changes:

- Reduced immune function
- Increased inflammation throughout the whole body
- Increased levels of free radicals in all tissues
- Genes being mutated from safe proto-oncogenes to dangerous oncogenes
- A diminished metabolism
- Increased abdominal fat that produces inflammatory chemicals called "cytokines"
- Increased production of growth factors that initiate cancer growth
- Insulin resistance
- Adrenal-gland exhaustion

I know this seems a bit overwhelming, but studies show that, if you learn techniques to reduce stress in your life, this will help you prevent and/or fight cancer. When you work with these cognitive-management methods, you can actually affect genetic expression (epigenetics) . . . something we have repeatedly talked about in this book. If you remember earlier in this book, we examined a Dr. Dean Ornish/Dr. Elizabeth Blackburn heat-map-analysis study of genetic expression in early-prostate-cancer patients who were eating a whole food, plant-based diet, along with exercise and stress management. In that study, the lifestyle changes up-regulated 48 good genes and down-regulated 453 bad genes. In other words . . . more than 500 genes were made to act in a more positive way.

In another study, using only stress management, by Antoni and group [1], 191 women undergoing treatment for breast cancer were randomly assigned to 2 groups . . . a cognitive-behavioral, stress-reduction-intervention group or to a control group, which had usual care, with no stress reduction. Amazingly, the individuals undergoing the stress-reduction techniques lowered the expression of their pro-inflammatory and metastasis-related genes and increased expression of interferon-related good genes as compared to the group that did no stress-reduction techniques. Interferons are proteins that allow communication between our cells to initiate the protective immune defenses against viruses, bacteria, and, most importantly, cancer cells. In other words, intensive mind-body, stress-reduction practices can reshape our bodies right down to our cellular and genetic responses.

In another important study published in the peer-reviewed journal *Cancer* in 2008, researchers found that breast-cancer patients who participated in techniques that reduced stress, improved mood, coping abilities and health behaviors had better survival rates 7 and 11 years later than patients who did not receive such intervention. Specifically, they found that patients in the stress-reduction group had about 55% less risk of recurrence compared to the group without stress reduction.

In patients who did suffer a relapse, those who used stress-reduction techniques remained cancer-free an average of 6 months longer than the non-stress-reduction group, which is a 45% improvement. Patients receiving the stress-reduction techniques also had a 45% less risk of death from breast cancer and a reduced risk of death from all causes, not just cancer. The results from this long-term study emphasize the importance of providing stress-modification programs for all patients diagnosed with cancer.

Another important 2008 study in *Nature Reviews Clinical Oncology* demonstrated the negative effects of chronic stress on cancer. Researchers in this group did a meta-analysis of 165 epidemiological studies investigating the associations between stress-related psychosocial factors and cancer outcomes [2]. The results of 165 studies indicated that stress-related psychosocial factors are associated with higher cancer incidence in initially healthy populations. In addition, there was poorer survival in cancer patients in 330 studies and higher cancer mortality in 53 studies. They concluded that a stress-prone personality or unfavorable coping styles and negative emotional responses are correlated with higher cancer incidence, poorer cancer survival and higher cancer mortality.

We know that chronic stress contributes to cancer formation and progression . . . so let's get those stress levels down! But the question is how? That is our next discussion.

STRESS REDUCTION TECHNIQUES

Laughter

It is so true that laughter is strong medicine. Laughter makes your immune system stronger, improves your mood, diminishes pain, and protects you from the damaging effects of stress. Nothing works quicker or more predictably to bring your mind and body back into balance than a good laugh. It lightens your burdens, releases anger, and gives us hope. With so much power to heal, the ability to laugh easily and frequently is a tremendous resource for solving problems, enhancing relationships, and supporting physical and emotional health. Best of all, laughter is fun and free.

As children, we would laugh thousands of times in a day, but as adults, life tends to be more grim, and laughter becomes less frequent. But by seeking out more opportunities for laughter in your life, you can improve your emotional health, strengthen your relationships with friends and family, find greater happiness—and add years to your life by helping your body fight cancer.

Physiologically, scientists have found that laughter relaxes the whole body. A hearty laugh relieves physical tension and has been found to relax your muscles for up to 45 minutes. There are several studies that show that laughter boosts the immune system. It decreases stress hormones and increases natural killer cell immune activity, thus improving your resistance to cancer. In 2 recent studies, mirthful laughter was found to have a very positive effect on the cardiovascular system [3,4].

In the previous chapter on exercise, we learned that exercise past a certain point can cause the brain to release narcotic-like chemicals that make us feel happy. Well, laughter triggers the same release of endorphins, the body's natural feel-good chemicals. These endorphins can even temporarily relieve pain.

Believe or not, laughter even burns calories. Of course, it's no replacement for doing your daily walk or bike ride, but one study found that laughing for 10 to 15 minutes per day can burn approximately 40 calories. Add that up over a year, and that could be 4–5 pounds.

I believe the most important thing about laughter is that it lightens anger's heavy load. Nothing gets rid of anger and conflict faster than a shared laugh. Looking at the funny side of any situation can put the problem into perspective and enable you to move on from confrontations without holding onto bitterness or resentment.

Lots of laughter may even help you to live longer. A study in Norway found that individuals with a strong sense of humor outlived those who didn't laugh as much. The difference was particularly observable for those battling cancer. It doesn't cure cancer, but it has long been regarded as an excellent coping mechanism for cancer patients dealing with the stress of their disease. In some American oncology settings, it has been accepted as an effective therapeutic tool. Those who believe in the benefits of laughter for cancer often point to the U.S. author Norman Cousins, who boasted that reruns of Candid Camera and the Marx Brothers helped him overcome cancer in the 1970s. A few belly laughs, he said, helped him enjoy a pain-free night of peace.

Deep, Slow Breathing

Slow, mindful deep breathing is one of the easiest stress-management techniques that can be done anywhere. You could be driving down the highway and perform deep, slow breathing, which calms you down by kicking in the parasympathetic nervous system. So to discover how this simple technique works, let's do a review of high school biology and review of the autonomic nervous system.

As you probably remember from high school science class, we all have a parasympathetic nervous system that controls the involuntary functions of our body such as breathing, digestion and excretion. Conversely, the sympathetic nervous system controls our fight-or-flight response. If a giant grizzly bear was in our sight, immediately our sympathetic nervous system would kick into gear. Our heart rate would increase, our breathing would be rapid and shallow, our muscles would tense, and digestion would halt in preparation for the possible confrontation ahead of us.

This sympathetic response is a requirement for our survival, but the problem with our modern society, with all of its chronic stressors, such as the barrage of technology, the inordinate amount of choices before us, relational difficulties, financial and work stress . . . many of us are in a constant state of sympathetic discharge, which is at the root of many of the chronic diseases prevalent in modern culture.

There is a constant discharge of epinephrine, norepinephrine, and cortisol from the adrenal gland, which can cause high blood pressure, atherosclerosis, kidney disease, immune dysfunction and even cancer. Epinephrine and norepinephrine cause our arteries to constrict, which can lead to chronic hypertension, which can lead to atherosclerosis, heart attacks and strokes. And chronic cortisol release can create a whole slew of problems, as we previously discussed.

So, how do we do these slow, mindful deep-breathing exercises? During my reading over the years, I have found that Dr. Andrew Weil's 4-7-8 breathing exercise is very effective and one of the easiest to do.

The 4-7-8 (or Relaxing Breath) Exercise

The 4-7-8 breathing exercise is utterly simple, takes almost no time, requires no equipment, and can be done anywhere. Although you can do the exercise in any position, while learning the exercise, you sit with your back straight. Place the tip of your tongue against the ridge of tissue just behind your upper front teeth, and keep it there through the entire exercise.

- Exhale completely through your mouth, making a *whoosh* sound.
- Close your mouth, and inhale quietly through your nose to a mental count of 4.
- Hold your breath for a count of 7.
- Exhale completely through your mouth, making a *whoosh* sound to a count of 8.
- This is one breath. Now inhale again, and repeat the cycle 3 more times for a total of 4 breaths.

Note that, with this breathing technique, you always inhale quietly through your nose and exhale audibly through your mouth. The tip of your tongue stays in position the whole time. Exhalation takes twice as long as inhalation. The absolute time you spend on each phase is not important . . . the ratio of 4:7:8 is important. If you have trouble holding your breath, speed up the exercise, but keep to the ratio of 4:7:8 for the 3 phases. With practice, you can slow it all down and get used to inhaling and exhaling more and more deeply.

This breathing exercise is a natural tranquilizer for the nervous system. Unlike tranquilizing drugs, which are often effective when you first take them but then lose their effectiveness over time, this exercise is subtle when you first try it, but gains power with repetition and practice. Do it when you feel even the least amount of stress. You cannot do it too frequently. If you feel a little lightheaded when you first breathe this way, do not be concerned; it will pass. Once you develop this technique by practicing it every day, it will be a very useful tool that you will always have with you. Use it whenever you get upset. Use it whenever you are aware of internal tension or stress. Use it to help you fall asleep. This exercise cannot be recommended too highly. Everyone can benefit from it.

Meditation

Meditation is another very common method to kick in your parasympathetic nervous system, getting you into a relaxed state. There are several ways to do this. I personally am a little ADD and have a difficult time being inactive, so I must trap myself into my portable infrared sauna to do my meditation. My meditation technique is simply to focus on deep breathing. I do this for a minimum of 10 minutes and try to get to 20 minutes every day. Additionally, the infrared sauna causes me to sweat, which helps release toxins from my body.

Other ways that people meditate is to keep repeating a phrase or sound, called a "mantra," over and over again, which forces their mind away from the problems of their life and gets them into a state of parasympathetic relaxation.

Mindfulness

This involves bringing your attention to the present moment. Too many of us fret about what is about to happen or what happened in the past.

Mindfulness involves focusing on your current surroundings and taking in all experiences in a nonjudgemental way, allowing for the release of tension. Doing this on a regular basis has been shown to improve immune function and focus, attention, sleep and feelings of overall well-being.

Personally, I have noticed, since having cancer, that I live much more in the moment. I notice the cloud formations and marvel at Nature's artistry every single day . . . something that I did infrequently before. I also do something fun every day and genuinely get into the moment, knowing that my days are numbered. In fact, we all should be doing this, because every one of us "is like a vapor that appears for a little while, then vanishes" (James 4:14).

Gentle Motion

The following is a good relaxing exercise that allows you to focus on your movement and postures and let all unwanted thoughts or feelings to pass away.

1. Stand with your feet shoulder-width apart and your arms relaxed by your side.
2. Take a deep breath in, and raise your arms up over your head.
3. As you exhale, gently lower your arms to the side, and bring your arms to the side; bring your right foot forward.
4. Take a deep breath in, and slowly shift your weight onto your right leg; bring both arms out in front of you, with the fingers extended and pointing forward.
5. As you exhale, return your right leg and arms back to the center, and bring your left foot forward.
6. Take a deep breath in, and slowly shift your weight onto your left leg; bring both arms out in front of you, with your fingers extended and pointing forward.
7. As you exhale, return your left leg and arms back to the center.

8. Take a deep breath in, and raise your arms up over your head.

9. As you exhale, slowly bend at the waist, and reach down to the ground.

10. Take a deep breath in, and gently bring your arms back up; reach up as high as you can.

11. As you exhale, bring your arms slowly back down to your sides.

Time Management

How many times have you planned way too many activities that a day could ever hold? Probably every one of you. Was that day a stressful day or a relaxed day? Were you late for any of your appointments? If you were late for your appointment, was your sympathetic nervous system in overdrive, or were you in a relaxed parasympathetic state?

You are probably getting the drift. Improper time management can cause a lot of detriment to your body. My recommendation is to make a list for the week on Sunday evening in preparation for the week. Not only will this help you with setting goals, but you will be able to postpone meetings or activities that might make your day overly busy. I also recommend making a nightly list to evaluate the following day. If the day seems like it will cause too much overactivity, move those meetings or appointments to another day. Bottom line is to not force too much activity into too small of a space so that you accomplish more than is reasonable. This was a problem I had and do believe was very detrimental to my health.

Exercise

Exercise is one of the scientifically proven natural ways to beat back cancer, and we dedicated a whole chapter to it. We talked about how it activates your immune system and how it causes endorphin release from your brain, which puts you in a relaxed state. Besides that, you end up looking better, which causes you to feel better about yourself, which puts you into a better frame of mind . . . something in the medical community we call "a state of psychological well-being." As I keep repeating . . . if exercise were a pill, every single person in the world would be taking it.

As I discussed in the last chapter, there are many studies demonstrating that exercise works extremely well to counter depression and, in some studies, does it better than anti-depressants [5,6]. Also, as I already communicated, anti-depressants have many undesirable side effects such as weight gain, insomnia, decreased sex drive, anxiety and fatigue. Look at every one of those side effects. Exercise causes the exact opposite . . . weight loss, better sleep, increased sex drive, less anxiety and higher energy levels. Why would anyone not want to try the power of exercise before ingesting toxic chemicals into their system on a daily basis? The only answer that I can think of is laziness and a lack of willpower.

Prayer

As I've already told you, when you are a cancer patient, your time is valued in a new and more urgent way, and you do not wish to waste a minute of it. If you are in treatment for cancer, you no doubt understand this very well. Like many cancer patients, you may also be feeling a greater-than-ever desire for a spiritual meaning in your life. Cancer often represents a spiritual turning point for many, leading them to seek out new sources of inner strength and purpose for living.

It really is regrettable that conventional treatments, while necessary for treating the disease, do little or nothing to address this inner spiritual longing that many patients have. The medical community is simply not equipped to help patients acquire a sense of spiritual well-being. Even many alternative therapies don't offer the kinds of support that cancer patients need to strengthen themselves mentally and spiritually. Fortunately, this doesn't stop the majority of them from seeking help anyway. In a 1999 study, breast-cancer patients were given a choice of 18 different alternative methods, of which 85% chose prayer [7].

In another study of religious and spiritual coping strategies among patients newly diagnosed with cancer, subjects reported that their religious and spiritual faith provided distinct benefits, most notably the emotional support necessary to deal with their cancer (91%), social support (70%), and the ability to derive purpose in their everyday life (64%), particularly during their cancer experience [8].

There have been thousands of anecdotal reports over thousands of years demonstrating the healing power of prayer, but it was not studied until the late 1980s. In 1988 cardiologist Randolph C. Byrd conducted a seminal, randomized, double-blind, prospective study to assess the effects of intercessory prayer on health outcomes in 393 patients admitted to the coronary-care unit [9]. Each patient was randomly assigned to a "prayed for" or "control" group while receiving the same-quality medical treatment. The people who would pray were chosen as "born again" Christians, defined by Byrd as people with an active Christian life demonstrated by daily devotional prayer and an active fellowship in a local church. Each of these "healers" prayed daily for a definitive outcome: rapid recovery, prevention of complications and death, and any other areas they felt would help the patient. The prayers had a positive outcome. Members of the group who received healing prayer were 5X less likely to need antibiotics and 3X less likely to develop pulmonary edema. Furthermore, fewer of them died than in the control group, and none of the prayed-for group required endotracheal intubation, whereas 12 in the "control" group did.

While these results are intriguing, the study was not definitive. Byrd did not, for instance, assess the mental health of those entering the study, which could have affected the study's interpretation. Nonetheless, the results of this well-known study have been quoted from pulpits to podiums and hailed energetically as proof that "prayer really works." Given the spiritual, social, and scientific relevance of Byrd's findings, it is remarkable that it took another 12 years for other researchers to conduct a similar study.

In 1999, Dr. Harris, working with 999 patients admitted to the coronary-care unit, also found that the medical course of his patients was better in those who were prayed for [10]. This study, unlike Byrd's, used "healers" from a variety of Christian traditions (35% were listed as nondenominational, 27% as Episcopalian, and the remainder as either Protestant or Roman Catholic). Dr. Harris also chose a more comprehensive score to assess the result of this prayer on coronary recovery. Like Byrd, Harris came to the conclusion that his patients benefited unquestionably from the intercessory prayer they received. Taken together, these 2 studies provide strong confirmation that people engaged in healing prayer can affect the physical well-being of people at a distance.

Yoga

Yoga is known for its ability to ease stress and promote relaxation. In fact, multiple studies have shown that it can decrease the secretion of cortisol, the primary stress hormone [11]. Another study demonstrated the powerful effect of yoga on stress by following 24 women who perceived themselves as emotionally distressed. After a 3-month yoga program, the women had significantly lower levels of cortisol. They also had lower levels of stress, anxiety, fatigue and depression [12]. Another study of 131 people had similar results, showing that 10 weeks of yoga helped reduce stress and anxiety. It also helped improve quality of life and mental health [13].

Guided Imagery

The first exercise in any group guided-imagery session is relaxation. This is accomplished through guided-breathing exercises, during which each participant is encouraged to focus on breathing slowly and to release any tension in the muscles, from the toes to the top of the head. The therapist then works with the group, assisting each person in mentally constructing relaxing scenes that are pleasant. These can be actual experiences from the past or entirely new ones created in the moment. Soft background music may be used. The task of the therapist is to encourage the participants to imagine the pleasure-giving scenes as vividly as possible to maximize the relaxation they produce.

The guide also encourages participants to mentally visualize as many details as possible in each scene and to actively intervene to banish any negative images that might present themselves. Groups that benefit from relaxation imagery include those suffering from stress and rehabilitation groups coping with anxiety. Guided imagery is both a technique and a therapeutic tool. It entails the use of the imagination to promote health, success and well-being. The first step in this process is achieving deep relaxation through breathing exercises. Once in a relaxed state, the main exercises involve mental visualization induced by a therapist.

Self Hypnosis

The process of self-hypnosis involves entering a trance, or a deeply relaxed but focused state (like that of daydreaming or meditation), and making suggestions for your subconscious mind to accept. You can go to a trained professional for hypnotherapy, and they will talk you through it. Or, you can employ the use of books, videos, or even short articles to learn what's involved and achieve effective results at home.

Biofeedback

Biofeedback is a way to measure the body's physiological responses in real time and a tool to learn to control them. Biofeedback generally relies on machines that measure heart rate, muscle tension or even brain waves, and usually requires a therapist or other health professional to operate the machine, explain what the readings mean, and work with clients to incorporate the information into lifestyle changes.

A Good Book

The most simple relaxation technique, besides deep breathing, is to escape into the world of a good book. It will help get your mind away from the stress of life, or, if you are battling cancer . . . the constant worry about your disease.

SUMMARY

As we have learned, chronic stress is one of the major factors that can cause cancer and allow it to kill us after contracting it. Look at each of the different stress-reduction methods that I have described, and see which one would fit with your personality and lifestyle best. Don't underestimate the importance of this natural power. It is just as important as what we eat, what supplements we take, how we exercise, and, as you will discover in the next chapter, how well we sleep.

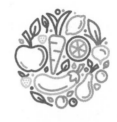

CHAPTER 10

The Power of Sleep

Sleep has been a source of obsession and perplexity since the beginning of time. Throughout history, scientists, physicians, spiritual healers and great thinkers have all tried to explain why we sleep. The compilation of all their contributions have given us what we know to be true today . . . sleep is essential to a healthy mind and body.

What is very interesting is that throughout history, many civilizations followed a sleep pattern very much different from our own. The invention of the light bulb was the striking change in the timing of sleep. This abrupt change allowed people to do activities much later than sunset, which developed later bedtimes. Generally, what many pre-lightbulb civilizations followed was a schedule whereby they slept for approximately 4 hours, woke up to carry out some light activities for an hour or 2, and then slept for another 4 hours until daylight. This type of sleep schedule was followed by many cultures until the 18th to

19th century, when an uninterrupted 6- to 8-hour slumber was more agreeable to the demands of society.

In regard to the usefulness of sleep, many early thinkers thought that sleep was just a passive process that involved our bodies merely switching off at night. During the late 1800s, this concept started to be questioned. In the mid-1900s, the understanding of the biological clock, the identification of the many different biochemicals involved and the diagnosis of various sleep disorders by EEG helped us to get a more profound comprehension of the "Why?" for sleep.

THE BODY CLOCK

Sleep and wakefulness merge to create what is known as the sleep-wake cycle. This is a 24-hour period in which we spend about ⅔ of the time awake and ⅓ of our time asleep. This circadian rhythm is governed by the section of the brain called the "suprachiasmatic nucleus" (SCN). The SCN identifies the light hitting the eye and then delivers a signal to the pineal gland (a tiny gland that sits at the base of the brain). This gland then secretes a hormone called "melatonin" that compels us to fall asleep.

What is utterly fascinating is that the circadian rhythm does not entirely mature until the third or fourth month of life. This is the reason that infants frequently wake up in the middle of the night, to the chagrin of their poor parents. Teenagers also have an odd sleep cycle, in that it changes over more toward night. This is why a lot of teenagers have a propensity to hit the sack late and get up late.

Another part of the normal sleep cycle that can play havoc with our workday is that we have an inclination to develop a drowsiness about 6 to 7 hours after waking. In many cultures throughout the world, this is when the "siesta" occurs. In America, where the siesta is not practiced, the ideal way to get through this portion of the day is to take a step outside for some fresh air and natural light, and take a short walk. When I performed surgery, I would take a short power nap for 10 minutes, and I would feel brand new after my mini-siesta. As most of you have experienced, this drowsiness is normally short-lived, and your alertness returns relatively quickly.

THE FOUR STAGES OF SLEEP

As I previously alluded to, sleep was once thought of as a time of total inactivity. Nowadays we understand that sleep is an extremely intricate series of stages that can be identified by EEG (electroencephalogram) brain activity in the form of certain types of wave forms.

Stage 1
At the kickoff of sleep, we enter into a light and slightly alert type of sleep. The body gets into a very tranquil state during this phase. The brain waves at the starting point of this phase are known as "alpha waves" and are slow and wide on the EEG. As we delve further into stage 1, the waves become even slower than the alpha waves and are called "theta waves." At the tail end of stage 1, the body is still in a period of very light sleep.

Stage 2
The individual can still be aroused without difficulty during this phase, but the EEG wave forms start transforming. The waves are more accelerated and rhythmic and are known as sleep spindles. These take place every 1–2 minutes during stage-2 sleep. Another type of wave observed on EEG is called a "k-complex," which crops up slightly before or after the sleep spindles.

During stage 2, the body temperature starts to plunge a bit, the heart rate diminishes, the breathing rate drops, and the body starts laying the groundwork to enter deep sleep.

Stage 3

This the stage that the extremely slow waves called the "delta waves" begin appearing. That is why stage 3 is often referred to as "delta sleep." This is the stage when the body is in a state of deep sleep, and sounds and surrounding activity go unnoticed by the brain. This is also the most important mode for our protection against cancer, because this is the stage when growth, DNA-mutation repair and autophagy (the cleaning up of unwanted proteins and cellular debris) occurs. It is also quite fascinating to note that sleepwalking and bed-wetting most commonly occur during this stage.

Stage 4

This stage is well known as "rapid eye movement (REM) sleep." This name was aquired from the fast movement of the eyes during this stage, which is calculated by an instrument called an "electro-oculogram" (EOG). Adults spend about 20% of their sleep time in REM, and it is during this period of time that your muscles are incapacitated, and you do the majority of your dreaming.

It is paramount to note that we typically do not progress through all of these stages in order. It is commonplace that after stages 2 and 3, we will backtrack to stage 2 and then to REM sleep. Once REM is accomplished, the individual will enter stage 2 again and the cycle continually repeats itself up to 5 times during the night. To put the times of these stages into perspective . . . it takes approximately 90 minutes to go from stage 1 to REM sleep.

Increasing Alpha Wave Activity

As we discussed, alpha-wave activity occurs at the beginning of sleep. Scientists are learning that increasing the alpha-wave activity is important to overall brain health, as it improves focus, attention span, and memorization capability. Also, when there is diminished alpha-wave activity, scientists are discovering that there is a tendency toward being more anxious and depressed.

So how do we increase alpha-wave activity to get us more quickly into an alpha-wave state? The 4 actions that we can do to increase this alpha activity are things that we actually learned about in the last chapter on stress reduction. That is to increase our mindfulness, meditate, concentrate on our breathing, and do gentle motion exercises before we go to bed. We will discuss these and more techniques at the end of this chapter.

THE BRAIN CHEMICALS RELEASED DURING SLEEP

The masterminding of the sleep cycles involves the hypothalamus, the thalamus, the brainstem, the basal forebrain and cerebral cortex. The intercommunication between these parts of the brain is achieved through the secretion of a multitude of hormones and neurotransmitters, which I am going to explain at this time.

Seratonin

This hormone is frequently called the "happy hormone" because of its capability to elevate our mood. It is manufactured in the part of the brainstem called the "raphe nuclei" and boosts your attentiveness while inhibiting the REM stage of sleep. If your seratonin levels are too low, you will have frequent nighttime awakenings. This hormone is enzymatically converted by the body to melatonin.

Melatonin

As we previously learned, melatonin is the most important hormone for maintaining the circadian rhythm. When it is secreted by the pineal gland, as night approaches, we get sleepy, and when its levels start to decline, we start to wake up. It is also the most powerful antioxidant secreted by our bodies. It is extremely important at night that harmful free-radical activity is in check, while the body is repairing DNA that was damaged throughout the day. That is one of melatonin's most critically imperative functions.

Melatonin is so important as a nighttime free-radical scavenger that I highly recommend taking 15 mg sublingually before bedtime. I use a GNC product called *Fast Dissolving Melatonin 5 mg*. I dissolve 3 of these under my tongue before bed, and, if I awake in the middle of the night, I will place an additional 5–10 mg lozenge under my tongue to get me through the night.

The reason I do this every night is that the studies have shown that an increased melatonin level sends signals to the body's cells and organs that it is nighttime, and it starts organizing target organs and organ systems into appropriate metabolic rhythms [2]. Therefore, too much light before bed could disrupt the circadian rhythm and the appropriate melatonin secretion by the pineal gland [3], which could contribute to the development, promotion, and progression of cancers. Because of all the technology that most of use in the way of television, cell phones and computers, I think that taking a melatonin supplement before bed makes certain that we are getting enough melatonin to carry out its anti-cancer functions.

In an important 2017 article in *Oncotarget*, it was shown how melatonin is an excellent candidate for the prevention and treatment of several cancers, such as breast cancer, prostate cancer, gastric cancer and colorectal cancer. The article reviewed the results of epidemiological, experimental and clinical studies which show clearly that melatonin has potent anti-cancer effects [4].

Other research papers demonstrate clearly that melatonin is not only a hormone that makes us go to sleep but is also a cell protector [5] and is involved with the modulation of the immune system, anti-oxidation and the production of white and red blood cells [6]. Its anti-cancer mechanisms are its antioxidant activity, regulation of cancer-cell suicide, tumor metabolism and cancer immunity, inhibition of angiogenesis (blood-vessel formation to the tumor), cancer-cell migration, and prevention of circadian disruption [7,8,9]. Melatonin has also shown the potential to be utilized as an addition to conventional cancer therapies, through reinforcing the therapeutic effects and reducing the side effects of chemotherapy or radiation [10]. We will look at more of these important studies near the end of this chapter.

Gamma-Aminobutyric Acid (GABA)

GABA is the key calming neurotransmitter in the brain and works by decreasing the liveliness of the excitatory nerve cells. It is theorized by many scientists that anxiety, insomnia and addiction is correlated with reduced GABA activity.

Acetylcholine

This neurotransmitter is secreted by a part of the brainstem and is responsible for the rapid eye movement that is characteristic of REM sleep.

Histamine

Histamine is emitted by a section of the hypothalamus and is a strong sleep-cycle regulator. It is at its highest levels during times of alertness and diminishes during sleep.

Norepinephrine

Norepinephrine is secreted near the end of sleep by the adrenal gland. It supports morning awakening and also the transition between REM and non-REM sleep.

Orexin

This chemical is also manufactured in the hypothalamus and activates attentiveness by forcing the body to secrete histamine, serotonin and norepinephrine. Some scientists have correlated orexin deficiency with narcolepsy.

Glutamate

Glutamate is actually made from GABA and is another extremely important excitatory neurotransmitter and works by stimulating the release of orexin. Portobello mushrooms are especially high in glutamate, so they should be avoided in the evening. MSG (monosodium glutamate) should also be avoided in the evening due to its excitatory activity. Glutamate should also be avoided in individuals with brain tumors, as it has been associated in a few studies with increased brain-cancer activity.

Cortisol

Cortisol (the stress hormone) is produced in the adrenal glands and is secreted in reaction to stress and in the morning to cause us to awake. Its levels are highest in the morning and lowest in the evening. Because many cancer patients take dexamethasone (a relative of cortisol) as a part of their chemotherapy regimens, I recommend taking this first thing in the morning, so that the diurnal rhythms are not too disrupted.

Because dexamethasone also causes severe insomnia the day of taking the medication, I strongly recommend asking your physician for a sleep medication for that night so that your diurnal rhythms can stay on track.

Corticotropin-Releasing Hormone (CRH)

This hormone is produced in the hypothalamus and is also released in times of stress. Its job is to stimulate the release of ACTH (see below) from the pituitary gland, which then triggers the release of cortisol from the adrenal gland. Like cortisol, it stimulates wakefulness and decreases the amount of time spent in REM sleep.

Adrenocorticotropic Hormone (ACTH)

CRH (hypothalamus) triggers the release of ACTH (pituitary gland), which triggers the release of cortisol (adrenal gland). As would be suspected, this hormone peaks in the morning and diminishes as the day progresses.

Growth Hormone-Releasing Hormone (GHRH)

GHRH is produced in the hypothalamus and functions to increase the length and depth of non-REM sleep. Its most important role, however, is to stimulate the release of human growth hormone from the pituitary gland.

Glycine

This is an amino acid that is manufactured by your body from the essential amino acids that you consume on a daily basis. It has a calming effect and helps to induce sleep by lowering your body temperature at night. Glycine is also responsible for the disappearance of muscle tone that happens during REM sleep.

Dopamine

Dopamine, synthesized in the brain and kidney, causes a decrease in melatonin production as the morning approaches. It, therefore, promotes wakefulness. It is also important in the establishment of REM sleep and in helping to create muscle immobility during this stage of sleep.

Neuropeptide S

This neurotransmitter stimulates the release of dopamine, so, therefore, is involved in stimulating wakefulness. It also has been shown to diminish anxious feelings during times of stress.

Neuropeptide Y

This neurotransmitter peptide promotes sleep by inhibiting the release of CRH from the hypothalamus. It also has been demonstrated to have the capability to shift the timing of the circadian rhythm.

Adenosine

Adenosine causes the brain to relax and helps you to establish non-REM sleep. Its level increases as the day progresses and peaks at night. One of the ways that caffeine actually works is by blocking the brain-relaxing action of adenosine.

HOW SLEEP FIGHTS CANCER

So we just saw just how intricate sleep really is. In many ways, it really is mind-blowing. Now let's see how this very complicated system helps us in our fight against cancer. These are the predominant anti-cancer activities going on while we are quietly asleep:

- It is the time that the body is repairing DNA mutations.
- It is the time that the body is getting rid of unwanted proteins and cellular debris (autophagy).
- It is the time that melatonin (the powerful anti-cancer antioxidant and inducer of sleep) is released by the pineal gland.
- It is the time that the immune system is being rejuvenated.
- It is the time that strong anti-inflammatory chemicals are being released.

Let's look at each one of these activities.

SLEEP REPAIRS DNA MUTATIONS

Several studies have demonstrated the detrimental health effects of night-shift work. The mechanisms through which acute sleep deprivation may lead to cancer and chronic diseases has not been totally made clear, but it is thought that increased DNA damage or decreased DNA-mutation repair caused by lack of sleep leads to diseases like cancer. In one objective study, the researchers examined the effects of acute sleep deprivation on DNA damage. This was a cross-sectional observational study on 49 healthy, full-time doctors. Baseline blood was sampled from each of the doctors after either 3 consecutive days of adequate sleep (the control) or 3 consecutive days of inadequate sleep. The 24 non-control participants were required to work overnight on-site and had additional blood drawn on a morning after acute sleep deprivation. DNA damage and expression of DNA-repair genes was quantified. What was discovered was quite interesting . . . the overnight on-site call participants had lower baseline DNA-repair gene expression and more DNA breaks than participants who did not work overnight [11].

Other studies show that people who work night shifts have significantly increased cancer risk. One of these studies looked at breast-cancer risk and found a 14%-60% increase over the control group that had regular diurnal sleep patterns [12]. Another study looked at colorectal-cancer risk in night-shift workers and demonstrated a 35% increase in the risk of cancer [13]. Still another study dealing with prostate cancer and night-shift work found that the increased prostate-cancer risk of night-shift work took 20 years to be completely wiped away [14]. Fascinating information.

SLEEP REJUVENATES THE IMMUNE SYSTEM

Sleep deprivation is considered to be a stress-causing factor and is associated with impaired immune activity. An interesting rodent study evaluated how sleep restriction affected lung-cancer metastasis and the tumor immune response. The results of sleep restriction showed that cancer-killing natural killer T-cells were reduced in number and that regulatory T-cells (inhibit the killing of cancer) were increased in the tumor microenvironment. Sleep-restricted mice also exhibited a reduced number of dendritic cells in their lymph nodes, which may have contributed to the ineffective activation of tumor-specific T-cells. Peripheral CD4+ and CD8+ T-cells were also reduced in the sleep-restricted mice, thus indicating an immunosuppressed status [15].

SLEEP COMBATS INFLAMMATION

The results of one study demonstrated significantly increased levels of the very inflammatory cytokine (interleukin-6) in the insomniac research participants when compared to those getting normal sleep [16]. This finding has been verified in many studies looking at the correlation between sleep deprivation and chronic inflammation in the body.

In fact, in a meta-analysis of 186 well-performed studies on the lack of sleep and its effects on inflammation, it was demonstrated clearly that sleep deprivation causes an increase in the inflammatory cytokine Interleukin-6 (IL-6), which then causes an increase in the biomarker for inflammation . . . C-reactive Protein (CRP) [17].

If any of you have ever had a poor night of sleep, I can almost guarantee you that the next day your muscles felt a little sore and tight. This is from the increased inflammation induced by these inflammatory cytokines.

As we have learned in this book . . . chronic inflammation is one of the primary drivers of cancer. And if you are chronically not getting enough sleep, you are indeed developing a state of chronic inflammation that is the perfect microenvironment for the initiation of cancer.

SLEEP RIDS US OF UNWANTED PROTEINS (AUTOPHAGY)

While you are asleep, there is a process going on called "autophagy," which involves getting rid of unwanted proteins, worn-out cells and cellular components. The word literally means "self-eating." It's one way your body cleans house. In this process, your cells create membranes that hunt down scraps of dead, diseased, or worn-out cells; gobble 'em up; strips 'em for parts; and use the resulting molecules for energy or to make new cell parts. Think of it as our body's innate recycling program.

If you are not getting adequate sleep, there is not enough autophagy going on, which can lead to cancer and many chronic diseases. Methods other than adequate sleep to increase autophagy are exercise and fasting. Both of these activities have been shown in clinical studies to increase this cleaning-up process.

MELATONIN HAS A POWERFUL ANTI-CANCER EFFECT

As you learned earlier in this chapter, as night approaches, there is a signal from the hypothalamus to the pineal gland to start secreting a hormone called "melatonin." Melatonin puts you to sleep, but it is also the body's most powerful antioxidant and fighter of cancer. As I alluded to earlier in this chapter, several epidemiological studies have indicated that melatonin has an anti-cancer effect against several different types of tumors. Furthermore, experimental studies have documented that melatonin exerts growth inhibition on some human tumor cells in people and in animal models. The underlying mechanisms appear to include antioxidant activity, stimulation of cancer-cell suicide (apoptosis), affecting tumor metabolism to make the tumor cell die, inhibition of angiogenesis (blood-vessel growth to the tumor), combating metastasis, and affecting our epigenetics (changing gene expression in a positive way to battle the cancer) [18,19,20]. Melatonin, as a supplement, is starting to be utilized as an adjunct to cancer therapies, through reinforcing the therapeutic effects and reducing the side effects of chemotherapies or radiation [21]. Because of the voluminous amount of scientific data, melatonin supplementation is being used by several practitioners as a prevention method and treatment adjunct for several cancers, such as breast cancer, prostate cancer, gastric cancer and colorectal cancer.

If you don't want to supplement, the easiest, least expensive and most effective way to get adequate melatonin levels is to get 8 hours of restful sleep. Also, you can eat a few pistachio nuts right before bed, as they have been shown to have the highest melatonin levels of any food. Believe it or not . . . just 2 pistachios give the equivalent of a person's nightly physiologic dose from the pineal gland.

SCARY SLEEP STATISTICS

I just told you that the best way to get adequate melatonin levels was to get 8 hours of restful sleep, but that is, indeed, a lot easier said than done.

Here are some scary statistics:

- People today sleep 20% less than they did 100 years ago.
- More than 30% of the population suffers from insomnia.
- One in three people suffer from some form of insomnia during their lifetime.
- More than half of Americans lose sleep due to stress and/or anxiety.
- Between 40%–60% of people older than 60 suffer from insomnia.
- Women are up to twice as likely to suffer from insomnia than men.
- Approximately 35% of insomniacs have a family history of insomnia.
- 90% of people who suffer from depression also experience insomnia.
- Approximately 10 million people in the U.S. use prescription sleep aids.
- People who suffer from sleep deprivation are 27% more likely to become overweight or obese.

- A National Sleep Foundation Poll shows that 60% of people have driven while feeling sleepy (and 37% admit to having fallen asleep at the wheel) in the past year.
- A recent Consumer Reports survey showed the top reason couples gave for avoiding sex was lack of sleep.

TECHNIQUES TO GET BETTER SLEEP

So how do we not become one of the above scary statistics? Here are some recommendations:

Increase Bright Light Exposure During the Day

As we have learned, your body has an extremely important internal clock known as your circadian rhythm. It affects your brain, body and hormones, helping you to stay alert during the day and making you sleepy as night approaches. Sunlight or other forms of bright light during the day is essential for keeping this circadian rhythm healthy and running smoothly. This improves your vigor during the day as well as improves the quality and length of your sleep [22].

In one study looking at people with insomnia, it was established that daytime bright-light exposure enhanced sleep quality and duration. It also diminished the time to fall asleep by a whopping 83% [23]. A similar study in older adults validated that 2 hours of bright-light exposure during the day improved sleep time by an impressive 2 hours and sleep quality by an equally impressive 80% [24]. While most of the scientific research on sleep has investigated people with serious insomnia problems, increased daily light exposure will most likely help all of us achieve a better sleep experience. It is best to get as much daily natural-sunlight exposure as possible each day. But if you can't get natural light, at least get as much bright artificial light as possible.

Reduce Blue Light Exposure in the Evening

As we just discovered, light exposure during the day is extremely important, but nighttime light exposure has the exact paradoxical effect [25]. This is due to its negative effect on our circadian rhythm, making our brains think that it is time to work and not time to sleep. This nighttime light exposure decreases melatonin secretion by the pineal gland, which causes us to not feel as sleepy as bedtime approaches. One of the main culprits causing nighttime light exposure is blue light. This is the kind of light that electronic devices like smartphones and computers emit in hefty amounts. There are many ways that you can use to decrease nighttime blue-light exposure. These include:

- Wear specially designed glasses that block blue light [26]. You can purchase these inexpensively on Amazon.
- Download an app such as F.lux, Redshift, Sunset Screen, Iris, Twilight or Night Shift that block blue light on your laptop or computer.
- Install an app that blocks blue light on your smartphone. I have an iPhone and the capability to block blue light is built right into my phone. All that I had to do was to enable it. Androids, on the other hand, from my research, do not have this built-in capability so you would need to purchase an app to perform that function.
- It is a good idea to stop watching your TV and turn off or dim all bright lights surrounding you 2 hours before bedtime.

Don't Consume Caffeine Late in the Day

Coffee and tea both have many health benefits and are consumed by the vast majority of the American population. A single dose of the caffeine in these drinks has been shown in several studies to enhance attention span, vigor and sports performance [27]. However, when you ingest caffeine late in the day, it will jack up your nervous system and will, in most of us, prevent our bodies from unwinding before bedtime. In one study, drinking caffeine up to 6 hours before bed dramatically deteriorated sleep quality [28]. Caffeine levels can remain elevated in your blood for up to 6–8 hours. I, therefore, do not recommend drinking large amounts of coffee after 3–4 p.m . . . especially if you are susceptible to caffeine or have difficulties with getting to sleep [29]. If you do crave a cup of coffee in the late afternoon or evening, make sure you drink a coffee or tea that is decaffeinated. I personally cannot drink any caffeinated products after 12 o'clock noon. My nighttime tea concoction consists of hibiscus, chamomile, dandelion and decaf green tea . . . all without even a hint of caffeine.

Reduce Irregular or Long Daytime Naps

While the short power naps that I used to take when I performed surgery are extremely beneficial, extended napping during the day can create problems getting to sleep later in the evening. Long daytime naps really screw up your internal clock, which then creates a struggle for you getting to sleep at nighttime [30]. In fact, in one study, participants wound up being drowsier during the day after taking long daytime naps [31]. Another research study observed that, while naps less than 30 minutes enhanced daytime brain function, longer naps, conversely, had a negative effect on sleep [32]. There are, however, some other studies that have established that there are some individuals who can regularly take long naps and not have it affect their sleep quality at all. The bottom line is . . . the effects of napping seem to be very individual [33]. Experiment and see what works best for you.

Try to Sleep and Wake at Consistent Times

Because your body's circadian rhythm is so critically important, being consistent with your sleep and waking times is equally as important [34]. One investigative study demonstrated that those who went to bed early during the workweek but went to bed late on the weekends developed overall poor sleep patterns over the course of the whole week [35]. Other studies have elucidated that irregular sleep patterns mess with your circadian rhythm and melatonin levels [36]. If you have sleep problems, get into a habit of waking up and going to bed at the same time each day. After several weeks, you may not even need an alarm clock. On the weekends, try not to get too far away from your normal "go to bed" time.

Take a Melatonin Supplement

As I previously discussed, melatonin is not only an excellent sleep aid but also a potent cancer fighter. And it has become the world's most popular sleep aid because it is so very effective. In one study, 2 mg of melatonin allowed people to fall asleep quicker and helped them get a better quality of sleep, which made the participants more energetic the following day [37]. In another quality study, the results were akin to the above study, with both demonstrating no side effects from the melatonin [38]. Another very positive characteristic about melatonin is that it can efficaciously help when traveling to a new time zone, as it assists you with getting back into a good circadian rhythm. You just need to cleverly figure out a way to manipulate the time zones [39]. Dr. Michael Greger actually has a good video on *nutritionfacts.org* to help you devise a plan on how to do this manipulation.

When first starting to use melatonin, it is best to first use 1–5 mg of melatonin 30–60 minutes before bed. It is best to initiate with a lower dose and gradually work your way up if you need a stronger strength. If you are thinking about using melatonin for your child, I would first consult with your healthcare provider, as this usage has not been well studied. You can buy melatonin supplements on Amazon very inexpensively. I personally use a peppermint-flavored, ***Fast Dissolving Melatonin 5 mg*** GNC sublingual (under the tongue) product. I use 15 mg for sleep and cancer treatment. If I wake up in the middle of the night, I use an additional 5–10 mg, which almost always gets me back to sleep.

Consider These Other Supplements

Several supplements can induce relaxation and help you sleep, including:

- Ginkgo biloba: This is a natural herb well known for its memory-enhancing properties, but it also has been discovered to assist with stress reduction and sleep. If you want to give it a try, take 250 mg 30–60 minutes before bed [40].
- Glycine: Remember how we discussed how the amino acid glycine (manufactured by the body) has a calming effect and helps to induce sleep by lowering your body temperature at night and is also responsible for the disappearance of muscle tone that happens during REM sleep? Well, you can take this as a supplement. There are a few studies in the scientific literature that demonstrate that 3 grams of the amino acid glycine can enhance the quality of sleep [41].
- Valerian root: This is another natural herb that has also been established in studies to improve the ability to get to sleep and stay asleep. Take 500 mg before you retire for the night [42].
- Magnesium: This common mineral not only helps you fall asleep, but helps you enjoy deeper, more restful sleep as well [43]. Take 100–350 mg before bed. This dose can vary widely due to the individual's magnesium levels. Many people in Western cultures have low magnesium levels due to poor diet, so get your levels checked by your doctor to see if you have a deficiency.
- L-theanine: This amino acid promotes relaxation and facilitates sleep by boosting GABA release by the brain and inducing the release of other calming brain neurotransmitters. Take 100–200 mg before bed [44].

⦿ Lavender: Researchers have found that lavender increases stage-3, slow-wave delta sleep . . . the very deep slumber in which the heartbeat slows and muscles relax [45]. Many people place the oil on their face or their pillow before bed. Other people place it in a diffuser and run it throughout the night.

⦿ Chamomile tea: I personally use this in my nightly tea concoction not only for its relaxing effects but also for the fact that it has high apigenin levels, which assist me in the fight against myeloma.

Other common sleep-inducing herbs found in many over-the-counter sleep-inducing herbal teas are passion flower, lemon balm, kava kava, and magnolia bark.

Don't Drink Alcohol

A stiff alcoholic drink right before bed is probably one of the best ways to guarantee a poor night's sleep, as it can unfavorably affect the proper secretion of many of your nighttime hormones. This bad habit can also increase sleep-apnea episodes, cause excessive snoring, and create very poor sleep patterns [46]. Alcohol before bed can also disturb melatonin secretion, which, I hope we all know by now, is so very important to maintaining the body's circadian rhythm [47]. Another study found that drinking alcohol right before bed decreased the normal nighttime release of human growth hormone (HGH), which plays an important role not only in keeping us in a steady diurnal rhythm but also in carrying out other essential duties in your body [48].

Optimize Your Bedroom Environment

Most sleep experts believe that the bedroom environment is critically important for you to get a good night's sleep. These factors include temperature of the room, extraneous noise, the amount of lighting and the way the furniture is arranged in your room [49]. Many studies demonstrate that external traffic noise can cause not only poor sleep but also long-term health issues [50]. In one study, 50% of the participants noticed better sleep quality when external noise and lights were decreased [51]. To optimize your bedroom environment, try to minimize artificial lights and noises from technologic devices, and make sure the room is clean, organized and peaceful. Trying to get to sleep in an extremely messy room is not a good way to begin your sleep journey.

Set Your Bedroom Temperature

As most of us probably know from experience, the room temperature can definitely play a role in our sleep quality. In fact, one analysis determined that bedroom temperature affected sleep quality more than external noise [52]. Another study illustrated that, when the temperature was too high, it created restless nights of wakefulness [53]. For most of us, 70°F seems to be the ideal temperature to get a good night's sleep, but that temperature can, of course, vary from person to person. You personally may have a spouse who likes the room warm to get to sleep, while you may prefer a cooler temperature. If you search the Internet, you will find quite a few mattresses that allow you to heat or cool each side independently.

Don't Eat Late in the Evening

Eating right before bed has been found to have a negative impact on melatonin release and the overall quality of sleep [54]. The type of food may also play a role. In one study, a high-carb meal 4 hours before bed helped people fall asleep faster [55], but in another study, a low-carb meal 4 hours before bed improved sleep. Therefore, if you are on a low-carb diet, carbs may not work as well for you [56]. In this regard, figure what type of food works best for you. Ideally, I would not recommend eating any food for at least 2 hours before bedtime. Your body needs to focus its energy on getting you to sleep and on repairing all the damage incurred to your DNA during the day . . . not on expending energy for digestion.

Relax and Clear Your Mind in the Evening

Many people have a pre-sleep routine that helps them unwind. Relaxation techniques before bed have been proven to improve sleep quality and are another common way to alleviate insomnia [57]. In one study, a calming massage enhanced sleep quality in people who were ill [58]. Other methods include listening to stress-reducing music, reading a good book, taking a nice, warm bath, meditating, deep breathing and guided imagery. Try out different methods, and find what works best for you. Many of these techniques we discussed at length in the previous chapter on "the power of stress reduction."

Take a Relaxing Bath or Shower

A stress-relieving bath or shower right before bed is an awesome way to get a better night's sleep. Studies have validated that it can enhance sleep quality and help you enter sleep more quickly [59]. In one study, a warm bath 90 minutes before bedtime caused people's brains to employ more time in that all-important, cancer-fighting, deep-sleep stage 3 that we learned about earlier [60]. Alternatively, if you don't want to take the time for a full bath at night, simply bathing your feet in hot water can help you wind down and better your sleep [61].

Rule Out a Sleep Disorder

Sleep apnea is a relatively common sleep disorder and may be the reason you can't sleep. This disorder causes people to stop breathing incessantly throughout the night [62]. This disorder is much more commonplace than you may think. One observational review published in the *New England Journal of Medicine* revealed that 24% of men and 9% of women have sleep apnea [63]. Other fairly prevalent sleep disorders include sleep-movement disorders and circadian-rhythm sleep/wake disorders, which are diagnosed more commonly in night-shift workers [64]. If you are someone who has always struggled with your sleep, you should seek out a medical doctor who specializes in sleep disorders.

Get a Comfortable Bed, Mattress, and Pillow

Did you ever question why you usually get better sleep in a 4- or 5-star hotel? Aside from getting away from all of the stressors in your life, the quality of the mattress in that better-quality hotel may be positively affecting your sleep [65]. One study published in the *Journal of Manipulative and Physiologic Therapeutics* examined the benefits of a new, high-quality mattress for 28 days and validated that a high-quality mattress diminished back pain by 57%, shoulder pain by 60% and back tightness by 59%. It also boosted the quality of sleep by 60% [66]. Another published study pointed out that brand-new, high-quality bedding can also improve sleep. Furthermore, poor-quality bedding can lead to increased lower-back pain [67]. From this scientific data, it is recommended by sleep authorities that you upgrade your mattress and bedding at least every 5–8 years [68].

Exercise Regularly—But Not Before Bed

Exercise is one of the best methods to improve your sleep and health. It can improve all parts of your sleep and has been used successfully to reduce insomnia [69]. One study published in the revered *Journal of the American Medical Association* analyzed sleep patterns in seniors and found that exercise nearly halved the amount of time to enter sleep and increased the overall sleep time by 41 minutes [70]. In individuals with severe insomnia, exercise delivered more benefits than almost every single drug tested. Exercise diminished the time to enter sleep by 55%; decreased the time awake during the night by 30%, and diminished a sense of anxiety by 15% while increasing the total time that these individuals were asleep by 18% [71]. Those are some impressive results!

Although daily exercise is extremely important for getting good sleep, performing it too late in the day is not a great idea. This is due to the fact that exercise increases hormones like epinephrine and norepinephrine, which are both excitatory. Conversely there are other studies showing that late exercise does not affect sleep, so it is really individual in nature [72]. I would, however, generally not recommend doing exercise too close to bedtime.

Don't Drink Any Liquids Before Bed

If you are urinating too much during the night, this certainly can affect the quality of your sleep [73]. Drinking large amounts of liquids before bed can be a major cause of this problem. On the other hand, there are some individuals who can drink a lot before bed and not have an issue. Even though good hydration is necessary for good health, it makes good sense to limit the amount of fluid you drink 1–2 hours before bedtime. It is also makes good sense to urinate right before going to bed, as this will certainly decrease the probability of you needing to wake up in the middle of the night to do your business.

SUMMARY

In summary, I hope I have elucidated how critical adequate sleep is to your overall good health and, for those of you battling cancer—how essential it is against a formidable enemy. I have shown you simple and applicable ways that can help you achieve better overall sleep quality. Implement these tools, and watch your mood, your productivity, your appearance and your health improve dramatically. And beat back cancer naturally!

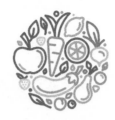

CHAPTER 11

How to Incorporate a Plant-Based Diet

As I speak at various meetings about "The 5 Natural Ways to Beat Back Cancer," I always start my lecture realizing that, if 100 people are in the audience, there might be 5 at most who are going to make an immediate change to a whole food, plant-based diet. There might be another 5 who slowly incorporate it into there life. The remaining 90 will keep eating the way they were eating regardless of how dire their health situation is.

I have learned not to take it personally, but to realize that what people eat day in and day out is very difficult to change. Our diets are influenced by so many factors over so many years. And discussing it with someone can be as tense as discussing religion or politics. There are the fond memories of your mother's favorite recipes, which might have been laden with creams, cheeses and meats. There are the family food traditions that you have enjoyed your entire life. There are the parties with friends laughing together, drinking beer, eating pizza and chicken wings. There is the fact that most people in Western culture eat a very unhealthy diet. We look around, and everyone else is eating lots of animal products and processed foods . . . so how unhealthy can it be? Many of these foods most likely are filled with tons of saturated fats and sugar, which are tasty and create a dopamine surge in our brain. Some individuals with a more addictive personality will have a more difficult time weaning themselves away from these kinds of foods. People with this genetic makeup will also have difficulty getting through the withdrawal period that is commonly experienced when transitioning to a whole food, plant-based diet. I highly recommend that you read *The Pleasure Trap*, by Dr. Douglas Lisle and Dr. Alan Goldhamer, if you feel that you are in this category. In fact, I think it is a good idea that everyone read that extremely well-written book.

What most people in Western culture don't realize is that half the world actually eats a whole food, plant-strong diet. In fact, if you read the highly recommended book *The Blue Zones*, by Dan Buettner, which analyzes the 5 areas of the world that have the longest longevity, you will see that those cultures eat primarily a plant-strong diet. They also have healthy social ties, live relatively stress-free lives, and exercise regularly.

So, what are the different ways to incorporate a whole food, plant-based diet? These are 3 primary methods that I have seen people use:

- Just jump in and do it. This is what I did, and it goes along with my personality. When I want to do something, I just put my head down and go at it.
- Start it after a week of research. This is the way Dr. Neal Barnard recommends people make the change. I would recommend reading his book *The Vegan Starter Kit*. He recommends that during the first week you go to Italian, Mexican, Indian, Chinese, and Thai restaurants and take a look at the menus to see the plant-based dishes that you would enjoy. During that week, you also

purchase cookbooks like the *How Not to Die Cookbook*, by Michael Greger, MD, *The Whole Foods Cookbook*, by John Mackey, the *Forks Over Knives Cookbook*, by Del Sroufe and the *Engine 2 Cookbook*, by Rip Esselstyn and see what recipes you could use to replace the meals that you are eating during that first week. I also highly recommend the *The Forks Over Knives Food Planner App*. After intense research the first week, you just jump in full force the following week.

⊙ You purchase the cookbooks and check out the above restaurants, and then start adding one whole food, plant-based meal per week. For example, during week one, you maybe do a plant-based breakfast. The next week, a plant-based breakfast and dinner. The third week, a plant-based breakfast, lunch, and dinner, etc., etc. With this approach, it will take you 21 weeks to be eating totally whole food, plant-based. Or you may choose to do add one whole food, plant-based day per week. This approach will get you to your goal in only 7 weeks.

I have found that, when people use the third approach, they rarely ever get to eating a strictly whole food, plant-based diet. I think the reason is that you don't allow yourself to get over the addictive nature of the Western diet. In fact, Dr. Neal Barnard has written about caseomorphine molecules in dairy products that actually attach to the narcotic receptors in the brain.

Another thing to look into is a free online program called *21-Day Vegan Kickstart* that has helped more than 600,000 people regain control of their health. Dr. Neal Barnard started the program in 2010. In 2018, he and The Physicians Committee for Responsible Medicine redesigned the website and created a new mobile app which will reach even more people through hundreds of healthy recipes with step-by-step photos, meal plans, grocery lists, cooking demonstrations, updated nutrition tips highlighting the latest in scientific research, and a clean design that is easy to navigate. The new program features leading nutrition experts, including Neal Barnard, M.D., Susan Levin, M.S., R.D., and Jill Eckart, C.H.H.C., of the Physicians Committee for Responsible Medicine; Tracy McQuirter, M.P.H., public health nutritionist and author of *Ageless Vegan*; Aurora Leon, M.D.; and Joaquin Carral, M.D.

Another good book is Dr. Sally Lipsky's *Beyond Cancer*. She very nicely shows you how to simply incorporate whole food, plant-based recipes into your daily life.

If, after trying one of these approaches, you still feel that you can't make the change to a whole food, plant-based diet, then at least shoot for a plant-strong diet. One of your goals should be to aim for The National Cancer Institute's recommended 9 servings of fruits and vegetables for the prevention of cancer. And if you have cancer, shoot for 12 servings.

The other point that I stress at every lecture that I give is that you need to be constantly educating yourself to keep yourself pointed in the right direction. Again, the easiest way to do this is to watch one to two 5-minute videos on *nutritionfacts.org* on a daily basis or at least a weekly basis. As I already mentioned, every morning I do a 15-minute band-resistance workout, and, during the workout, I watch or listen to 3 of Dr. Greger's videos. When you sign up for a free subscription, you will get a video emailed to you daily. Those emailed videos are a constant reminder that eating a whole food, plant-based diet is the secret for optimal health. If you are fighting cancer, it's an absolute essential.

A reminder . . . Dr. Greger has a team of 20 scientists who review every single article in the clinical nutritional literature, collate the studies, and then produce amazing, information-packed videos. In 2018 they reviewed 190,000 articles. I divided that by 52 weeks and came up with approximately 3,600 articles per week! That is mind-blowing. There is no way that any one of us could achieve that feat. Dr. Greger's group is doing it for us. So, take advantage of this free opportunity. His website has more than 4,000 videos for you to take advantage of.

Right now, go to *nutritionfacts.org* on your smartphone. Put it on your home screen as an icon. Order the free subscription. Start watching at least one video or at least listen to one while driving in your car every single day. The key is to put invaluable information into your head on a daily basis so that you know exactly why you are making this significant lifestyle change. Why would you want to give up pizza and chicken wings if you don't know why you are doing it? That is why, at the beginning of all my lectures, I have everyone in the audience go to their smartphone and put the website icon on their smartphones. At least I had them take the first step.

There are also several books that I recommend that you start reading. I have placed some of them in the selected bibliography at the end of this book. Also watch the movies *Forks over Knives* and *What the Health* and *Game Changers* on Netflix.

If you would like me to do one-on-one sessions on Facetime, Facebook Messenger, Snapchat, or Whats App, I do these for a reasonable fee. I offer 1- to 2-hour face-to-face virtual sessions, which allow you and your family members to ask me as many questions as you would like. Contact me at *info@naturalinsightsintocancer.com* to set up this face-to-face session.

So, start getting educated, start incorporating more plants into your diet, and enjoy a healthy, long life. And for those of you battling cancer, improve your chances of winning your battle against a tough enemy . . . but an enemy that you can beat.

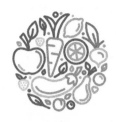

CHAPTER 12

My Daily Regimen

This is what I do on a day-in-and-day-out basis. As I have stated previously, very few of you are going to take as many supplements as I do. I have asterisked the supplements, drink concoctions and activities that I think are the most important. Every single supplement that I take is backed by either petri-dish, animal, or human studies—and lots of them. I am not going to waste my hard-earned money on supplements that have no value. So here we go!

MORNING ROUTINE

I usually do a nighttime fast greater than 13 hours (usually 15–16 hours) which has shown health benefits in several studies.

* ◎ ***ORGANIC CAFFEINATED LIGHT ROAST COFFEE CONCOCTION.*** Every morning I start off with a cup of organic caffeinated coffee with an added one tablespoon of *Organic Cacao Powder*, one teaspoon of *Organic Goji Powder*, one teaspoon of *Organic Pomegranate Powder*, ¼ teaspoon of *Thrive 6* mushroom powder, one teaspoon of *Organic Açaí Powder*, one teaspoon of *Organic Mangosteen Fruit Powder*, 10 shakes of *Organic Ceylon Cinnamon*, ⅛ teaspoon of baking soda to neutralize the acidity of coffee and cacao, *Organic Stevia* for taste, and soy milk (you can substitute almond milk). You can get all of the powders on Amazon.

I use a Keurig coffee maker. All the powders are in place before I hit the "On" switch. I then continuously stir as the coffee comes in contact with the powders. I also keep a spoon in my cup as I sip during my morning work. The mixture needs to be stirred occasionally as you are drinking, because some of it will precipitate to the bottom if you just let it sit dormant.

✱ ◎ *ORGANIC DECAF LIGHT ROAST COFFEE CONCOCTION.* I work as soon as I wake up and drink my organic caf coffee as I work. When I am finished with my caffeinated coffee, I make a cup of organic decaf light roast coffee with all of the above powders added.

✱ ◎ *BREAKFAST SMOOTHIE.* At around 11:00 AM, I break my fast and do a breakfast smoothie. I use ½ bag of *Trader Joe's Frozen Fancy Berry Medley* (strawberries, raspberries, blackberries, blueberries), 4 cubes of frozen organic mango, ¼ bag of frozen organic cranberries, some frozen organic grapes, an organic banana, an organic apple and a cup of organic kale.

I add one tablespoon of *Organic Ground Flaxseeds*, one tablespoon of *Organic Ground Chia Seeds*, one teaspoon of *Organic AMLA Powder*, one teaspoon of *Organic Guava/Matcha Powdered Green Tea*, one teaspoon of *Organic Dragon Fruit*

Powder, one teaspoon of *Organic Noni Fruit Powder* and one tea-spoon of *Organic Camu Camu Powder* (3,000 mg of vitamin C).

I add one cup of organic soy milk, one cup of filtered water, one ml of *Liquid Vitamin D3* from Douglas Labs (10,000 IU), and one drop of *Iodine Edge Nascent Iodine* (Amazon).

This will usually make two 12-ounce glasses of smoothie. I drink one and give one to my wife, Trina.

I take my supplements with the smoothie. I start with 2 organic walnuts, 2 organic pecans, 2 organic almonds, a few organic pumpkin seeds for zinc, a brazil nut for selenium, a few organic raw peanuts, a few organic pistachios and a few organic cashews. I then take 3 **OMAX3 PROFESSIONAL STRENGTH ULTRA-PURE* omega-3 essential-fatty-acid supplements (Amazon) and 2 **OMAX COGNITIVE* for more DHA. You will be amazed how the nuts and seeds will curb your appetite for a long while.

Remember that you must ingest fat before taking supplements so that you can absorb your fat-soluble vitamins and phytonutrients.

The following are my 31 morning supplements after the nuts, seeds, and my *OMAX3* supplements. Remember that the most important are asterisked.

* 1. *TURMERIC CURCUMIN WITH PIPERINE* (aSquared Nutrition from Amazon) 5 capsules for cancer
* 2. *BIOPERINE* (Source Naturals from Amazon) 5 tablets to improve turmeric's bioavailability
3. *ULTRA I-3-C* (Douglas Labs from Amazon) 1 capsule for cancer
* 4. *METHYLATED RESVERATROL PLUS* (Douglas Labs from Amazon) 1 capsule for cancer
5. *BENI KOJI RYR* (Douglas Labs from Amazon) 2 capsules for cancer and cardiovascular health
6. *UBIQUINOL-QH* (Douglas Labs from Amazon) 2 soft gels for cancer and cardiovascular health

* 7. *GARLIC* (Douglas Labs from Amazon) 2 tablets for cancer/ cardiovascular health

8. *K2-D3* (Douglas Labs from Amazon) 1 capsule for bone health, cancer, and cardiovascular health

* 9. *QUERCIPLEX* (Douglas Labs from Amazon) 1 capsule for cancer

10. *CAL/MAG 2001* (Douglas Labs from Amazon) 2 tablets for bone health

11. *TRI-EN-ALL 400* (Douglas Labs from Amazon) 1 softgel capsule for neuropathy

* 12. *METHYL B12 PLUS* (Douglas Labs from Amazon) dissolve 1 tablet under the tongue for red blood cell production

* 13. *ZINC LOZENGE* (Douglas Labs from Amazon) chew 1 lozenge for the immune system

14. *METATROL* (American Biosciences from Amazon) 1 capsule for cancer

15. *GFS-2000* (Douglas Labs on Amazon) 4 capsules for cancer

16. *GRAVIOLA 2000 mg* (Horbaach from Amazon) 1 capsule for cancer

17. *PURE PREMIUM MORINGA* (Fresh Healthcare from Amazon) 1 capsule for cancer

18. *NONI CONCENTRATE* (Doctor's Best from Amazon) 1 capsule for cancer

19. *MANGOSTEEN* (Solaray from Amazon) 1 capsule for cancer

* 20. *GINGER ROOT MAX-V* (Douglas Labs from Amazon) 1 capsule for cancer

21. *AYUR-ASHWAGANDHA* (Douglas Labs from Amazon) 1 capsule for cancer

* 22. *BERBERINE 1200 mg* (Naturulse from Amazon) 1 capsule for cancer and blood sugar control

23. *ASTRAGALUS* (Douglas Labs from Amazon) 1 capsule for the immune system

* 24. **MILK THISTLE** (Douglas Labs from Amazon) 1 capsule for cancer and the liver

25. **BLACK SEED OIL** (Healths Harmony from Amazon) 1 capsule for cancer

* 26. **MYOCEUTICS** (Douglas Labs from Amazon) 1 capsule for cancer

* 27. **GYMNEMA SYLVESTRE 400 mg** (Now Foods from Amazon) 1 capsule for cancer and blood sugar control

* 28. **PECTASOL** (Douglas Labs from Amazon) 1 capsule for cancer/metastasis control

29. **FULL SPECTRUM CAROTENE** (Source Naturals from Amazon) 1 gel cap for cancer

* 30. **LIQUID VITAMIN D-3** (Douglas Labs from Amazon) 1 cc in my smoothie for bone health and immune function

* 31. **KELP** (Nature's Way from Amazon) 1 capsule to maintain iodine levels

If you are not eating a whole food, plant-based diet, I would recommend taking a multivitamin. I recommend **ULTRA PREVENTIVE X** (Douglas Labs from Amazon) 4 capsules in the morning. I personally do not take a multivitamin because I know that I am getting all the basic nutrients that I need from all of the plants that I eat on a daily basis.

If you are having difficulty keeping your urine pH between 6.5 and 7.5, using **HYDRION pH 5.5-8.0 STRIPS** (Amazon), you can add an **ALKASELTZER GOLD** tablet (Amazon) to your drinking water to help you accomplish this goal. After following the **Alkaline/Base Food Chart** that I have included in the addendum for about a month, it will be a rare occasion that your urine pH is not between 6.5 and 7.5. I also use an alkalinizing water purifier on my kitchen faucet. You can purchase these from *www.alkalinepgh.com*.

*MORNING EXERCISE . . . 15 MINUTE RESISTANCE BAND TRAINING

Remember that the first 6 minutes gives you a 50% increase in immune function!

✱ ◎ *LUNCH AND DINNER* . . . Trina and I follow the **Daily Dozen App** to get 9 servings of fruits and vegetables with as many different colors (phytonutrients) as possible and 3 bean servings. Remember that you get a lot of your servings in your smoothies and salads.

Learn as many different recipes as possible from the books and websites that I've recommended in this book. Before you know it, you won't be craving a hamburger . . . you will be craving one of your new favorites!

Also, just about every Italian, Indian, Middle Eastern, Chinese, Thai, and Mexican restaurant has a lot of vegan choices. Panera, Corelife, Whole Foods, Chipotle, Blaze Pizza, Olive Garden (whole-wheat pasta), and Subway (all vegetable spinach wrap) are good choices. If you ask . . . almost every restaurant has a vegan option, or they can make one for you. You just need to ask.

✱ ◎ *EVENING EXERCISE . . . 30 MINUTES OF BIKING OR ELLIPTICAL MACHINE*

Remember that exercise significantly lowers the incidence and recurrence of cancer. The more vigorous, the better. Think of it as your medication. Would you miss taking your meds?

EVENING SUPPLEMENTS

My evening supplements are exactly the same as the morning supplements except that I eliminate the following:

1. No *CAL/MAG 2001*
2. No *OMAX COGNITIVE*
3. No *ASTRAGALUS*
4. No *AYUR-ASHWAGHANDA*
5. No *TRI-EN-ALL 400*
6. No *FULL SPECTRUM CAROTENE*
7. No *GFS 2000*
8. No *METHYL 12 PLUS*
9. No *ZINC LOZENGE*
10. No *LIQUID VITAMIN D*
11. No *KELP*

I do, however, add these:

* 1. *FAST-DISSOLVING MELATONIN 5MG* (GNC on Amazon) 3 under the tongue before sleep.
2. *STRONTIUM* (Douglas Labs from Amazon) 3 capsules for bone health.

* ◉ *NIGHTTIME TEA CONCOCTION.* I use one hibiscus tea bag, one chamomile tea bag, one decaf green-tea tea bag and one dandelion tea bag with one wedge of lemon and lime. I use this tea for my nighttime supplements.
* ◉ *DON'T EAT LATE SO THAT YOU CAN HAVE A NIGHTTIME FAST GREATER THAN 13 HOURS.* You do not want high sugar and insulin in the middle of the night

causing tumor growth when your body could be fighting tumors and repairing mutated genes and cells.

In regard to the fat-soluble vitamins *TRI-EN-ALL 400* (mixed natural vitamin E), *FULL SPECTRUM CAROTENE* (mixed carotenoids), *LIQUID VITAMIN D-3* (vitamin D), *UBIQUINOL-QH* (coenzyme Q10) and *K2-D3* (vitamin K), I would strongly recommend finding a doctor who can evaluate those blood levels with a blood test. I personally use a test from Genova Labs to check vitamins E, K, D, beta-carotene and coenzyme Q10 levels every 6-12 months. Remember fat-soluble vitamins dissolve into the fat tissues, so toxicity can develop if you don't keep an eye on the levels.

It is also a good idea to ask your doctor to check your omega-6 to omega-3 essential-fatty-acid ratio measured with an inexpensive test from Quest Labs. This will help you keep this ratio around 2:1. Most Westerners are anywhere from 20:1 to 40:1.

Food and Chemical Effect on Acid / Alkaline Body Chemical Balance

Natural Insights Into Cancer

Most Alkaline	More Alkaline	Low Alkaline	Lowest Alkaline	Food Category	Lowest Acid	Low Acid	More Acid	Most Acid
*Baking Soda Sea Salt	Spices/Cinnamon	Herbs (most)	Sulfite	Spices/Herbs Preservative	Curry MSG	Vanilla Benzoate	Nutmeg Aspartame	Pudding/Jam/Jelly Table Salt (NaCl)
Mineral Water	*Kombucha	*Green or Mu Tea	Ginger Tea	Beverages	Kona Coffee	Alcohol Black Tea	Coffee	Beer Yeast/Hops/Malt
	Molasses Soy Sauce	Rice Syrup Apple Cider Vinegar	*Sucanat *Umeboshi Vinegar	Sweeteners Vinegar	Honey/Maple Syrup Rice Vinegar	Balsamic Vinegar	Saccharin	Sugar/Cocoa White/Acetic Vinegar
*Umeboshi Plums		*Sake	*Algae, Blue Green	Therapeutics		*Antihistamines*	*Psychotropics*	*Antibiotics*
			*Ghee (Clarified Butter)	Processed Dairy	Cream/Butter	Cow Milk	*Casein, Milk, Protein Cottage Cheese	Processed Cheese
				Cow/Human Soy Goat/Sheep	Yogurt Goat/Sheep Cheese	Aged Cheese Soy Cheese Goat Milk	New Cheeses Soy Milk	Ice Cream
		*Quail Eggs	*Duck Eggs	Eggs	Chicken Eggs			
				Meat Game Fish/Shellfish	Gelatin/Organs *Venison Fish	Game Meat Lamb/Mutton Boar/Elk Shellfish/Mollusks	Pork/Veal Bear *Mussels/Squid	Beef Lobster
				Fowl	Wild Duck	Goose/Turkey	Chicken	*Pheasant
			Oats Grain Coffee *Quinoa Wild Rice Japonica Rice	Grains Cereal Grass	*Triticale Millet Kasha *Amaranth Brown Rice	Buckwheat Wheat *Spelt/Teff/Kamut Farina/Semolina White Rice	Maize Barley Groats Corn Rye Oat Bran	Barley
Pumpkin Seed Hydrogenated oil	Poppy Seed Cashews Chestnuts Pepper	Primrose Oil Sesame Seed Cod Liver Oil Almonds *Sprouts	Avocado Oil Seeds (Most) Coconut Oil Olive Oil Linseed/Flax Oil	Nuts Seeds/Sprouts Oils	Pumpkin Seed Oil Grape Seed Oil Sunflower Oil Pine Nuts Canola Oil	Almond Oil Sesame Oil Safflower Oil Tapioca *Seitan	Pistachio Seed Chestnut Oil Lard Pecans Palm Kernel Oil	Cottonseed Oil/Meal Hazelnuts Walnuts Brazil Nuts Fried Foods
Lentils Broccoflower *Seaweed: Nori, Kombu, Wakame, Hijiki Onion/Miso *Daikon/Taro Root *Sea Vegetables (other) *Burdock/Lotus Root Sweet Potato/Yam	Kohlrabi Parsnip/Taro Garlic Asparagus Kale/Parsley Endive/Arugula Mustard Green Ginger Root Broccoli	Potato/Bell Pepper Mushroom/Fungi Cauliflower Cabbage Rutabaga *Salsify/Ginseng Eggplant Pumpkin Collard Green	Brussel Sprout Beet Chive/Cilantro Celery Okra/Cucumber Turnip Greens Squashes Lettuces Jicama	Beans Vegetables Legume Pulses Roots	Spinach Fava Beans Kidney Beans Black-eyed Peas String/Wax Zucchini Chutney Rhubarb	Tofu Pinto Beans White Beans Stevia Navy/Red Beans Aduki Beans Lima Beans Chard	Green Pea Peanut Snow Pea Legumes (Other) Carrots Chickpeas/Garbanzo	Soybean Carob
Lime	Grapefruit	Lemon	Orange	Citrus Fruits	Coconut Guava	Plum	Cranberry	
Nectarine Persimmon Raspberry Watermelon Tangerine Pineapple	Cantaloupe Honeydew Citrus Olive *Dewberry Loganberry Mango	Pear Avocado Apple Blackberry Cherry Peach Papaya	Apricot Banana Blueberry Pineapple Juice Raisin, Currant Grape Strawberry	Fruits	*Pickled Fruit Dry Fruit Figs Persimmon Juice *Cherimoya Dates	Prune Tomatoes	Pomegranate	

*Therapeutic, gourmet, or exotic items   TRY TO KEEP YOUR URINE pH BETWEEN 6.5 AND 7.5 WITH HYDRION pH STRIPS (AMAZON).

Prepared by Dr. Russell Jaffe, Fellow, Health Studies Collegium. Sources include USDA food data zone (Box 9 & 10), Food & Nutrition Encyclopedia, Nutrition Applied Personally by M Walczak, Acid & Alkaline by H Albara. Food growth, transport, storage, processing, preparation, combination, and assimilation influence effect inherent.

Thanks to Hank Liers for his original work, Nov 1998

REFERENCES

Chapter 1: The Way Cancer Starts and Progresses

1. Wilbur B, ed. 2009 *The World of the Cell* (7th ed.) San Francisco,Calif.
2. Kimball's Biology Pages *Oncogenes* Free full text
3. The Nobel Prize in Physiology or Medicine 2002 Illustrated presentation
4. Croce CM (January 2008). "Oncogenes and cancer." *The New England Journal of Medicine.* 358 (5):502-11.
5. Yokota J (March 2000). "Tumor progression and metastasis" (PDF). *Carcinogenesis.* 21(3)497-503
6. The Nobel Prize in Physiology or Medicine 1989 to J Michael Bishop and Harold E Varmus for their discovery of *The Cellular Origin of Retroviral Oncogenes.*
7. Negrini M, Ferracin, Sabbioni S, Croce CM (June 2007). "MicroRNAs in human cancer: from research to therapy." *Journal of Cell Science.* 120 (Pt 11):1833-40.
8. Esquela-Kerscher A, Slack FJ (April 2006) "Oncomirs-microRNAswith a role in cancer." *Nature Reviews Cancer.* 6(4):259-69.

9. Hekimi S, Lapointe J, Wen Y. Taking a "good" look at free radicals in the aging process. *Trends in Cell Biology*. 2011;21(10) 569-76.

10. Erbas M, Sekerci H. Importance of free radicals and occurring food processing. *Serbest Radikallerin Onemi Ve Gida Isleme Sirasinda Olusumu*. 2011; 36(6) 349-56.

11. Halliwell B. Superoxide dismutase, catalase and glutathione peroxidase: solutions to the problems of living with oxygen. *New Physiologist*. 1974. 1469-8137.

12. Ames BN, Shigenaga MK, Hagen TM. Oxidants, antioxidants and the degenerative diseases of aging. 1993. *Proc Natl Acad Sci* 90:7915-7922.

13. Ogle KS, Swanson GM, Woods N, Azzouz F. Cancer and comorbidity: redefining chronic disease. *Cancer* 2000 Feb 1;88(3):653-63.

14. Prasad KN, Cole W, Hovland P. Cancer prevention studies: past, present and future directions. *Nutrition* 14:197-210, 1998.

15. Bishoff FZ, Hansen MF. Genetics of familial breast cancer. *Cancer Bull* 45:476-482, 1993.

16. Pace LE, Keatong NL. A systematic assessment of benefits and risks to guide breast cancer screening decisions. *JAMA* 2014 Apr 2;311(13):1327-35.

17. Heyes GJ et al. Enhanced biological effectiveness of low energy X-rays and implications for the UK breast screening program. *Br J Radiol*. 2006 Mar;79(939):195-200.

18. Hellegass JM, Shukla A, Lathrop SA, MacPherson MB, Beuschel SL, Butnor KJ et al. Inflammation precedes the development of human malignant mesotheliomas in a SCID mouse xenograft. *Ann NY Acad Sci* 2010;1203-14.

19. Demaria S, Pikarsky E, Karin M, Coussens LM, chen YC, El-Omar EM et al. Cancer and inflammation: Promise for biological therapy. *J Immunother* 2010;33:335-51.

20. Ames BN, Gold LS, Willett WC. The causes and prevention of cancer. *Proc Natl Sci* USA 92:5258-5265, 1995.

21. Martin-Green M, Boudreau N, Bissel MJ. Inflammation is responsible for the development of wound-induced tumors in chickens infected with Rous sarcoma virus. *Cancer Res* 1994;54:4334-41.

22. Boccardo E, Lepique AP, Villa LL. The role of inflammation in HPV carcinogenesis. *Carcinogenesis* 2010;31:1905.

23. Sinkovics JG. Molecular biology of oncogenic inflammatory processes. Non-oncogenic and oncogenic pathogens, intrinsic inflammatory reactions without pathogens, and microRNA/DNA interactions (review). *Int J Oncol* 2012;40:305-49.

24. Ishioka T, Kuwabara N et al. Induction of colorectal tumors in rats by sulfinated polysaccharides. *CRC Crit Rev Toxicol* 17:215-244, 1987.

25. Colotta F, Allavena P, Sica A, Garlanda C, Mantovani A. Cancer related inflammation, the seventh hallmark of cancer: Links to genetic instability. *Carcinogenesis* 2009;30:1073-81.

26. Crawford S. Anti-inflammatory/antioxidant use in long-term maintenance cancer therapy: A new therapeutic approach to disease progression and recurrence. *Ther Adv Med Oncol* 2014;6:52-68.

27. Sparmann A, Bar-Sagi D. Ras-induced interleukin-8 expression plays a critical role in tumor growth and angiogenesis. *Cancer Cell* 2004;6:447-58.

28. Allavena P, Garlanda C, Borrello MG, Sica A, Mantovani SJ, Clarke MF. Pathways connecting inflammation and cancer. *Curr Opin Genet Dev* 2008;18:3-10.

29. Keibel A, Singh V, Sharma MC,. Inflammation, microenvironment, and the immune system in cancer progression. *Curr Pharm Des* 2009;15:1949-55.

30. Phillips SL et al. Connexin 43 in the development and progression of breast cancer: What's the connection? (Review). *Int J Oncol.* 2017 Oct;51(4):1005-1013.

31. Hann HI et al. Antitumor effect of deferoxamime on human hepatocellular carcinoma growing in athymic mice. *Cancer* 70:2051-2056, 1992.

32. Bajbouj K, Shafarin J, Hamad M. High dose deferoxamine treatment disrupts intracellular homeostasis, reduces growth, and induces apoptosis in metastatic and nonmetastatic breast cancer cell lines. *Technol Cancer Res Treat* 2018 Jan 1;17:1533033818764470.

33. Jiang XP, Elliott RL. Decreased iron in cancer cells and their microenvironment improves cytolysis of breast cancer cells by natural killer cells. *Anticancer Res* 2017 May;37(5):2297-2305.

34. Kuban-Jankowska A, Sahu KK, Gorska-Ponikowska M, Tuszynski JA, Wozniak M. Inhibitory activity of iron chelators ATA and DFO on MCF-7 breast cancer cell lines and phosphatases PTP1B and SHP2. *Anticancer Res* 2017 Sept;37(9):4799-4806.

35. Takami T, Yamasaki T, Saeki I, Matsumoto T, Suehiro Y, Sakaida I. Supportive therapies for prevention of hepatocellular carcinoma recurrence and preservation of liver function. *World J Gastrooenterol* 2016 Aug 28;22(32):7252-63.

36. Chan JM et al. Plasma insulin-like growth factor 1 and prostate cancer risk: a prospective study. *Science* 1998 January (279):563-66.

37. LeRoith D et al. The role of insulin-like growth factor 1 receptor in cancer. *Ann NY Acad Sci* 1995, Sept 7(766):402-08.

38. Mantzoros CS et al. Insulin-like growth factor 1 in relation to prostate cancer and benign prostatic hyperplasia. *Brit J Cancer.* 1997 9(76):1115-18.

39. Halpern BC, Clark BR, Hardy DN, Smith RA. The effect of replacement of methionine by homocystine on survival of malignant and normal adult mammalian cells in culture. *Proc Natl Acad Sci USA*. 1974 Apr;71(4):1133-36.

40. Guo Hy, Herrara H, Hoffman RM. Expression of the biochemical defect of methionine dependence and fresh patient tumors and primary histoculture. *Cancer Res* 1993 Jun 1;53(11):2479-83.

41. Epner EE. Can dietary methionine restriction increase the effectiveness of chemotherapy in treatment of advanced cancer? *J Amer Coll Nutri* 2001 Oct;20(5 Suppl):473S-475S.

42. Hoffman RM. Development of recombinant methioninase to target the general cancer-specific metabolic defect of methionine dependence: a 40 year odyssey. *Expert Opin Biol Ther* Jan;15(1):21-31.

43. Dirks AJ et al. Caloric restriction in humans: potential pitfalls and health concerns. *Mech Ageing Dev* 2006 Jan;127(1):1-7.

44. Shinichi N et al. Comparative and meta-analytic insights into life extension via dietary restriction. *Aging Cell* 2012 (11):401-409.

45. Fontana L et al. Extending healthy lifespan—from yeast to humans. *Science* 2010 April 16;328:321-6.

46. Warburg O (24 February 1956). "On the Origin Of Cancer Cells." *Science*. 123 (3191):309-14.

47. Chia-Jui W, Gow-Chin Y. Flavonoids, a ubiquitous dietary phenolic subclass, exert extensive in vitro anti-invasive and in vivo anti-metastatic activities. *Cancer Metastasis Rev* 2012 31:323-351.

48. Tariq A et al. Fisetin inhibits various attributes of angiogenesis in vitro and in vivo-implications for angioprevention. *Carcinogenesis* 2012 33(2):385-393.

49. Danilo C, Frank PG. Cholesterol and breast cancer development. *Curr Opin Pharmacol* 2012 Dec;12(6):677-82.

50. Kitahara CM et al. Total cholesterol and cancer risk in a large prospective study in Korea. *J Clin Oncol* 2011 Apr 20;29(12):1592-8.

51. Mei Z et al. Effects of statins on cancer mortality and progression: a systematic review and meta-analysis of 95 cohorts including 1,111,407 individuals. *Int J Cancer* 2017 Mar 1;140(5):1068-1081.

52. Nelson ER et al. 27-Hydroxycholesterol links hypercholesterolemia and breast cancer pathophysiology. *Science* 29 Nov 2013 342(6162)a:1094-1098.

53. Balkwill F et al. Smoldering and polarizing inflammation in the initiation and promotion of malignant disease. *Cancer Cell* 2005;7:211-217.

54. McCullough DJ et al. Effects of exercise training on tumor hypoxia and vascular function in the rodent preclinical orthotopic prostate cancer model. *J Appl Physiol* (1985). 2013 Dec;115(12):1846-54.

55. Glunde K et al. Extracellular acidification alters lysosomal trafficking in human breast cancer cells. *Neoplasia* 2003 Nov-Dec;5(6):533-45.

56. Rozhin H et al. Pericellular pH affects distribution and secretion of cathepsin B in malignant cells. *Cancer Res* 1994 Dec 15;54(24):6517-25.

57. Rofstad EK et al. Acidic extracellular pH promotes experimental metastasis of human melanoma cells in athymic nude mice. *Cancer Res* 2006 Jul 1;66(13):6699-707.

58. Turner GA. Increased release of tumour cells by collagenase at acid pH: a possible mechanism for metastasis. *Experientia* 1979 Dec 15;35(12):1657-8.

59. Fukumara D et al. Hypoxia and acidosis independently upregulate vascular endothelial growth factor transcription in brain tumors in vivo. *Cancer Res* 2001 Aug 15;61(16):602 Acidic environment causes apoptosis by increasing caspase activity.

60. Park HJ et al. Acidic environment causes apoptosis by increasing caspase activity. *Br J Cancer* 1999 Aug;80(12):1892-7.

61. Gatenby RA et al. Acid-mediated tumor invasion: a multidisciplinary study. *Cancer Res* 2006 May 15;66(10):5216-23

Chapter 2: Chemotherapy . . . The Pros and the Cons

1. Block KI et al. Impact of antioxidant supplementation on chemotherapeutic toxicity: a systematic review of the evidence of randomized controlled trials. *Int J Cancer* 2008 Sept 15;123(6):1227-39.

2. Simone CB 2nd et al. Antioxidants and other nutrients do not interfere with chemotherapy or radiation therapy and can increase kill and increase survival, part 1. *Altern Ther Health Med.* 2007 Jan-Feb;13(1):22-8.

3. Levine EG, Bloomfield CD. Leukemias and myelodysplastic syndromes secondary to drug, radiation and environmental exposure. *Semin Oncolo* 1992. 19:47-84.

4. Moss RW. *Questioning Chemotherapy.* Brooklyn, NY: Equinox Press, 1995.

5. Fields KK et al. Maximum-tolerated doses of ifosfamide, carboplatin and etoposide given over 6 days followed by autologous stem-cell rescue: toxicity profile. *J Clin Oncol* 1995. 13:323-332.

6. Houston SJ et al. The influence of adjuvant chemotherapy on outcome after relapse in patients with breast cancer. *Proc Ann Meet ASCO* 1992. 11; A108.

7. McMillian TJ, Hart IR. Can cancer chemotherapy enhance the malignant behavior of tumors? *Cancer and Metastasis Rev* 1987. 6:503-520.

8. Fuge O, Vasdev N, Allchorne P, Green JS. Immunotherapy for bladder cancer. *Research and Reports in Urology* 2015 7:65-79.

9. Eggermont AM, Schadendorf D. Melanoma and immunotherapy. *Hematol Oncol Clini.* 2009 June 23(3):547-64.

10. Brandhorst S, Choi I et al. A Diet Mimicking Fasting Promotes Regeneration and Reduces Autoimmunity and Multiple Sclerosis Symptoms. *Cell Rep.* 2016 Jun 7;15(10):2136-2143.

11. Grevelman, EG; Breed, WP (March 2005). "Prevention of chemotherapy-induced hair loss by scalp cooling." *Annals of Oncology.* 6(3): 352–8.

12. Lenzhofer R et al. Acute cardiotoxicity in patients after doxorubicin treatment and the effect of combined tocopherol and nifedipine pretreatment. *J Cancer Res Clin Oncol* 1983 106:143-147.

13. Iarussi D et al. Protective effect of coenzyme Q10 on anthacyclines cardiotoxicity: controlled study in children with acute lymphoblastic leukemia and non-Hodgkin's lymphoma. *Mol Aspects Med* 1994 15:s207-212.

14. Sleijfer S. Bleomycin-induced pneumonitis. *Chest.* 2001;120 (2):617.

15. Fantone JC, Phan SH. Oxygen metabolite detoxifying enzyme levels in bleomycin-induced fibrotic lungs. *Free Radic Biol Med.* 1988;4(6):399.

16. Martin WJ 2nd, Kachel DL. Bleomycin-induced pulmonary endothelial cell injury: evidence for the role of iron-catalyzed toxic oxygen-derived species. *J Lab Clin Med.* 1987;110(2):153.

17. Chandler DB et al. Effect of iron deficiency on bleomycin-induced lung fibrosis in the hamster. *Am Rev Respir Dis.* 1988;137(1):85.

18. Jules-Elysee K, White DA. Bleomycin-induced pulmonary toxicity. *Clin Chest Med.* 1990;11(1):1.

19. Senior JR. Unintended hepatic adverse events associated with cancer chemotherapy. *Toxicol Pathol.* 2010;38:142–147.

20. Bosch-Barrera J et al. Targeting STAT3 with silibinin to improve cancer therapeutics. *Cancer Treat Rev.* 2017 Jul;58:61-69.

21. Kitchlu A et al. Acute Kidney Injury in Patients Receiving Systemic Treatment for Cancer: A Population-Based Cohort Study. *J Natl Cancer Inst.* 2018 Nov 13. doi: 10.1093.

22. Ali Karakuş, Yeter Değer & Serkan Yıldırım (2017) Protective effect of Silybum marianum and Taraxacum officinale extracts against oxidative kidney injuries induced by carbon tetrachloride in rats, *Renal Failure*, 39:1, 1-6.

23. Steinberg, JA et al. Alpha Lipoic Acid (ALA) Inhibits the Anti-Myeloma Effects of Bortezomib. *Blood* 2009 114:3832.

24. Steinberg JA et al. Alpha Lipoic Acid (ALA) Inhibits the Anti-Myeloma Effects of Bortezomib. *Blood* 2009 114:3832.

25. Guido S et al. Influence of piperine on the pharmacokinetics of curcumin in animals and human volunteers. *Planta Med* 1998;64(4):353-356.

26. Ghoreishi et al. Omega-3 fatty acids are protective against paclitaxel-induced peripheral neuropathy: a randomized double-blind placebo controlled trial. *BMC Cancer.* 2012 Aug 15;12:355.

27. Pace A et al. Vitamin E neuroprotection for cisplatin neuropathy: a randomized, placebo-controlled trial. *Neurology.* 2010 Mar 2;74(9):762-6.

28. Eum S et al. Protective effects of vitamin E on chemotherapy-induced peripheral neuropathy: a meta-analysis of randomized controlled trials. *Int J Vitam Nutr Res.* 2013;83(2):101-11.

Chapter 3: Radiation therapy . . . The Pros and the Cons

1. Pusey W Allen (1900), Roentgen rays in the treatment of skin diseases and for the removal of hair. *J Cutan Disease Ind Syphilis* 18: 3021318.

2. Squibb, E. H. (1900). *Transactions of the New York State Medical Association for the Year 1884–1899. 16:*710–731.

3. Simone CB 2nd et al. Antioxidants and other nutrients do not interfere with chemotherapy or radiation therapy and can increase kill and increase survival, part 1. *Altern Ther Health Med.* 2007 Jan-Feb;13(1):22-8.

4. Block K et al. Impact of antioxidant supplementation on chemotherapeutic toxicity: a systematic review of the evidence from randomized controlled trials. *Int J Cancer.* 2008 Sep 15;123(6):1227-39.

5. Levenson SM, Rettira G, Seifer E. Effects of supplemental dietary vitamin A and B-carotene on experimental tumors: local tumor excision, chemotherapy, radiation injury and radiotherapy. In Butterworth CE, Hutchenson ML. *Nutritional Factors in the Induction and Maintenance of Malignancy.* New York: Academic Press Inc, 1983, pp. 169-203.

6. Jatoi A et al. voluntary vitamin and mineral supplementation associated with better outcome in non-small cell lung cancer patients? Results from the Mayo Clinic lung cancer cohort. *Lung Cancer.* 2005 Jul;49(1):77-84.

7. Blot WJ et al. Nutrition intervention trials in Linxian, China: supplementation with specific vitamin/mineral combinations, cancer incidence, and disease-specific mortality in the general population. *J Natl Cancer Inst.* 1993 Sep 15;85(18):1483-92.

8. Alpha-tocopherol, beta-carotene cancer prevention study group. The effect of vitamin E and beta carotene on the incidence of lung cancer and other cancers in male smokers. *New Engl J Med.* 1994 Apr 14;330(15):1029-35.

9. Omenn GS et al. Effects of a combination of beta carotene and vitamin A on lung cancer and cardiovascular disease. *New Eng J Med.* 1996 May 2;334(18):1150-5.

10. Hennekens CH et al. Lack of effect of long-term supplementation with beta carotene on the incidence of malignant

neoplasms and cardiovascular disease. *New Eng J Med.* 1996 May 2;334(18):1145-9.

11. Lee IM et al. Beta-carotene supplementation and incidence of cancer and cardiovascular disease: the Women's Health Study. *J Natl Cancer Inst.* 1999 Dec 15;91(24):2102-6.

12. Hercberg S et al. The SU.VI.MAX Study: a randomized, placebo-controlled trial of the health effects of antioxidant vitamins and minerals. *Arch Int Med.* 2004 Nov 22;164(21):2335-42.

13. Sesso HD et al. Effects of long-term vitamin E supplementation on cardiovascular events and cancer: a randomized controlled trial. *JAMA.* 2008 Nov 12;300(18):2123-33.

14. Lippman SM et al. Effect of selenium and vitamin E on risk of prostate cancer and other cancers: the Selenium and Vitamin E Cancer Prevention Trial (SELECT). *JAMA.* 2009 Jan 7;301(1):39-5.

15. Gaziano GM et al. Vitamins E and C in the prevention of prostate and total cancer in men: the Physicians' Health Study II randomized controlled trial. *JAMA.* 2009 Jan 7;301(1):52-62.

16. Milas L, Nishiguchi I et al. Radiation protection against early and late effects of ionizing irradiation by prostaglandin inhibitor indomethacin. *Adv Space Res* 1992. 12:275-271.

17. Guido S et al. Influence of piperine on the pharmacokinetics of curcumin in animals and human volunteers. *Planta Med* 1998; 64(4):363-3659.

18. Fang F et al. A potential role for resveratrol as a radiation sensitizer for melanoma treatment. *J Surg Res* 2013 Aug 183(2):645-53.

Chapter 5: Common Myths

1. Werner H, Bruchim I. The insulin-like growth factor-1 receptor as an oncogene. *Arch Physiol Biochem* 2009; 115:58-71.

2. Chitnis MM, Yuen JS, Protheroe AS et al. The type 1 insulin-like growth factor receptor pathway. *Clin Cancer Res* 2008 14:6364-70.

3. Wang Z et al. mTOR co-targeting strategies for head and neck cancer therapy. *Cancer Metastasis Rev.* 2017 Sep;36(3):491-502.

4. Helal I et al. Glomerular hyperfiltration: definitions, mechanisms and clinical implications. *Nat Rev Nephrol.* 2012 Feb 21;8(5):293-300.

5. Huang S et al. Acidic extracellular pH promotes prostate cancer bone metastasis by enhancing PC-3 stem cell characteristics, cell invasiveness and VEGF-induced vasculogenesis of BM-EPCs. *Oncol Rep.* 2016 Oct;36(4):2025-32.

6. Arguin H et al. Impact of adopting a vegan diet or an olestra supplementation on plasma organochlorine concentrations: results from two pilot studies. *Br J Nutr.* 2010 May;103(10): 1433-41.

7. Golden EB et al. Green tea polyphenols block the anticancer effects of bortezomib and other boronic acid-based proteasome inhibitors. *Blood.* 2009 Jun 4;113(23):5927-37.

8. Steinberg J et al. Alpha Lipoic Acid (ALA) Inhibits the Anti-Myeloma Effects of Bortezomib. *Blood* 2009 114:3832.

9. Perrone G et al. Dietary Supplement Vitamin C Significantly Abrogates Bortezomib-Induced Multiple Myeloma (MM) Cell Growth Inhibition. *Blood* 2008 112:3687.

10. Block K et al. Impact of antioxidant supplementation on chemotherapeutic toxicity: a systematic review of the evidence from randomized controlled trials. *Int J Cancer.* 2008 Sep 15;123(6):1227-39.

11. Fillmore KM et al. Moderate alcohol use and reduced mortality risk: systematic error in prospective studies and new hypotheses. *Ann Epidemiol.* 2007 May;17(5 Suppl):S16-23.

12. Bagnardi V et al. Alcohol consumption and site-specific cancer risk: a comprehensive dose-response meta-analysis. *Br J Cancer.* 2015 Feb 3;112(3):580-93.

13. Bischoff-Ferrari HA et al. Milk intake and risk of hip fracture in men and women: a meta-analysis of prospective cohort studies. *J Bone Min Res* 2011;26(4):833-9.

14. Feskanich D et al. Milk consumption during teenage years and risk of hip fractures in older adults. *JAMA Pediatr* 2014;168(1):54-60.

15. Michaelsson K et al. Milk intake and risk of mortality and fractures in men and women: cohort studies. *BMJ* 2014;349:g6015.

16. Schooling CM. Milk and mortality. *BMJ* 2014;346:g6205.

17. Richmond EL et al. Intakes of fish, poultry and eggs and the risk of prostate cancer progression. *Am J Clin Nutr* 2010;91(3):712-21.

18. Johansson M et al. One-carbon metabolism and cancer risk: prospective investigation of seven circulating B vitamins and metabolites. *Cancer Epidemiol Biomarkers Prev* 2009;18(5): 1538-43.

19. Richmond EL et al. Intakes of fish, poultry and eggs and the risk of prostate cancer progression. *Am J Clin Nutr* 2010;91(3):712-21.

20. Richmond EL et al. Choline intake and risk of lethal prostate cancer: incidence and survival. *Am J Clin Nutr* 2012;96(4):855-63.

21. Richmond EL et al. Egg, red meat and poultry intake and risk of lethal prostate cancer in the prostate-specific antigen era: incidence and survival. *Cancer Prev Res* (Phila) 2011;4(12):2110-21.

22. Tang WH et al. Intestinal microbial metabolism of phosphatidylcholine and cardiovascular risk. *N Eng J Med* 2013;368(17):1575-84.

23. Koeth RA et al. Intestinal microbiota metabolism of L-carnitine, a nutrient in red meat, promotes atherosclerosis. *Nat Med* 2013;19:576-85.

24. Tang WH et al. Intestinal microbial metabolism of phos-phatidylcholine and cardiovascular risk. *N Eng J Med* 2013;368(17):1575-84.

25. Choline: there's something fishy about this vitamin. *Harv Health Lett*. 2004;30(1):3.

26. Mitch Kanter PhD. E-mail communication. January 6, 2010.

27. Bergeron N et al. Effects of red meat, white meat, and non-meat protein sources on atherogenic lipoprotein measures in the context of low compared with high saturated fat intake: a randomized controlled trial. *The American Journal of Clinical Nutrition*, Volume 110, Issue 1, July 2019, Pages 24–33.

28. Oseni T et al. Select estrogen receptor modulators and phytoestrogen. *Planta Med* 2008;74(13):1656-65.

29. Nagata C et al. Soy intake and breast cancer risk: an evaluation based on a systematic review of the epidemiological evidence among the Japanese population. *Jpn J Clin Oncol* 2014;44(3):282-95.

30. Chen MN et al. Effect of phytoestrogens on menopausal symptoms: a meta-analysis and systematic review. *Climateric* 2015;18(2):260–9.

31. Chi F et al. Post-diagnosis soy intake and breast cancer survival: a meta-analysis of cohort studies. *Asian Pac J Canc Prev* 2013;14(4):2407-12.

32. Nechuta SG et al. Soy food intake after diagnosis of breast cancer and survival: an in-depth analysis of combined evidence from cohort studies of US and Chinese women. *Am J Clin Nutr* 2012 96(1):123-32.

33. Kang HB et al. Study on soy isoflavone consumption and the risk of breast cancer and survival. *Asian Pac J Cancer Prev* 2012;13(3):995-8.

34. Bosviel R et al. Can soy phytoestrogens decrease DNA methylation in BRCA1 and BRCA2 oncosuppressor genes in breast cancer? *OMICS* 2012;16(5):235-44.

35. Bal A et al. BRCA1-methylated sporadic breast cancers are BRCA1-like in showing a basal phenotype and absence of ER expression. *Virchows Arch* 2012;461(3):305-12.

36. Bosviel R et al. Can soy phytoestrogens decrease DNA methylation in BRCA1 and BRCA2 oncosuppressor genes in breast cancer? *OMICS* 2012;16(5):235-44.

37. Rozati M et al. Cardio-metabolic and immunological impacts of extra virgin olive oil consumption in overweight and obese older adults: a randomized controlled trial. *Nutrition and Metabolism* 12(2015):28.

38. Bonura A et al. Hydroxytyrosol modulates par j1-induced IL-10 production by PBMCs in healthy subjects. *Immunobiology* 221 no.12(2016):1374-77.

39. C. Romero and M. Brenes, "Analysis of Total Contents of Hydroxytyrosol and Tyrosol in Olive Oils," *Journal of Agricultural and Food Chemistry* 60, no. 36 (2012): 9017–9022.

40. S. Silva et al., "High Resolution Mass Spectrometric Analysis of Secoiridoids and Metabolites as Biomarkers of Acute Olive Oil Intake—An Approach to Study Interindividual Variability in Humans," *Molecular Nutrition and Food Research* 62, no. 2 (2018).

41. B. Corominas-Faja et al., "Extra-Virgin Olive Oil Contains a Metabolo-Epigenetic Inhibitor of Cancer Stem Cells," *Carcinogenesis* 39, no. 4 (2018): 601–613.

42. C. Bosetti, C. Pelucchi, and C. La Vecchia, "Diet and Cancer in Mediterranean Countries: Carbohydrates and Fats," *Public Health Nutrition* 12, no. 9A (2009): 1595–1600.

43. M-P. St-Onge; P.J.H. Jones (2003). "Greater rise in fat oxidation with medium-chain triglyceride consumption relative to long-chain triglyceride is associated with lower initial body weight and greater loss of subcutaneous adipose tissue." *International Journal of Obesity.* 27(12): 1565–1571.

44. Clegg, ME (2010). "Medium-chain triglycerides are advantageous in promoting weight loss although not beneficial to exercise performance." *International Journal of Food Sciences and Nutrition.* 61(7): 653–679.

45. Talbott, Shawn M. and Kerry Hughes. (2006). *The Health Professional's Guide to Dietary Supplements.* Lippincott Williams & Wilkins. pp. 60-63.Clegg, ME (2010).

46. "Medium-chain triglycerides are advantageous in promoting weight loss although not beneficial to exercise performance." *International Journal of Food Sciences and Nutrition.* 61(7): 653–679.

47. Rego Costa, AC; Rosado, EL; Soares-Mota, M (2012). "Influence of the dietary intake of medium chain triglycerides on body composition, energy expenditure and satiety: a systematic review." *Nutr Hosp.* 27(1): 103–138

48. Chazelas E et al. Sugary drink consumption and risk of cancer: results from NutriNet-Santé prospective cohort. *BMJ* 2019; 366.

49. Craig WJ et al. Position of the American Dietetic Association: vegetarian diets. *J Am Diet Assoc.* 2009;109(7):1266-82.

50. Pan A et al. Red meat consumption and mortality: results from two prospective cohort studies. *Arch Int Med.* 2012;172(7):555-63.

51. Sinha R et al. Meat intake and mortality: a prospective study of over half a million people. *Arch Int Med.* 2009;169(6):562-71.

52. Ornish D, Blackburn E et al. Changes in prostate gene expression in men undergoing intensive nutrition and lifestyle alterations. *Proc Natl Acad Sci USA.* 2008 Jun 17;105(24):8369-74.

53. Svilaas A et al. Intakes of antioxidants in coffee, wine, and vegetables are correlated with plasma carotenoids in humans. *J Nutr.* 2004 Mar;134(3):562-7.

54. Pulido R et al. Contribution of beverages to the intake of lipophilic and hydrophilic antioxidants in the Spanish diet. *Eur J Clin Nutr.* 2003 Oct;57(10):1275-82.

55. Freedman ND et al. Association of Coffee Drinking with Total and Cause-Specific Mortality. *N Engl J Med.* 2012 May 17; 366(20): 1891–1904.

Chapter 6: The Power of a Whole food, plant-based Diet

1. Liu PH et al. Expected years of life lost for six potentially preventable cancers in the United States. *Prev Med.* 2013;56(5):309-13.
2. Bertram et al. Rationale and strategies for chemoprevention of cancer in humans. *Cancer Res* 1987;47(11):3012-31.
3. Key TJ et al. Cancer incidence in British vegetarians. *Br J Cancer.* 2009; 101(1):192-7.
4. Suppipat K et al. Sulphorane induces cell cycle arrest and apoptosis in acute lymphoblastic leukemia cells. *PLoS One.* 2012 7(12):e51251.
5. Han X et al. Vegetable and fruit intake and non-Hodgkin's lymphoma survival in Connecticut women. *Leuk Lymphoma.* 2010;51(6):1047-54.
6. Thompson CA et al. Fruit and vegetable intake and survival from non-Hodgkin's lymphoma: does an apple a day keep the doctor away? *Leuk Lymphoma.* 2010;51(6):963-4.
7. Thompson CA et al. Antioxidant intake from fruits, vegetables and other sources and risk of non-Hodgkin's lymphoma: the Iowa Women's Health Study. *Int J Cancer.* 2010;126(4):992-1003. Açaí
8. Del Pozo-Insfran D et al. Açaí (Euterpe oleracea Mart.) polyphenolics in their glycoside and aglycone forms induce apoptosis of HL-60 leukemia cells. *J Agric Food Chem.* 2006;54(4):1222-9.
9. Schauss et al. Antioxidant capacity and other bioactivities of freeze dried Amazonian palm berry, Euterpe oleraceae mart. *J Agric Food Chem.* 2006;54(22):8604-10.

10. Jahn JL et al. The high prevalence of prostate cancer at autopsy: implications for epidemiology and treatment of prostate cancer in the Prostate-specific Antigen-era. *Int J Cancer* 2014 Dec;29.

11. Draisma G et al. Lead time and over-diagnosis in prostate-specific antigen screening: importance of methods and context. *J Natl Cancer Inst* 2009;101(6):374-83.

12. Melnik BC et al. Milk is just not food but most likely a genetic transfection system activating mTORC1 signaling for post natal growth. *Nutr J* 2013;12:103.

13. Ludwig DS, Willett WC. Three daily servings of reduced fat milk: an evidence based recommendation? *JAMA Pediatr* 2013;167(9):788-9.

14. Ludwig DS, Willett WC. Three daily servings of reduced fat milk: an evidence based recommendation? *JAMA Pediatr* 2013;167(9):788-9.

15. Tate PL et al. Milk stimulates the growth of prostate cancer cells in culture. *Nutr Cancer* 2011;63(8):1361-6.

16. Piantanelli L. Cancer and aging: from the kinetics of biological parameters to cancer incidence and mortality. *Ann NY Acad Sci* 1988;521:99-109.

17. Savioli S et al. Why do centenarians escape or postpone cancer? The role of IGF-1, inflammation and p53. *Cancer Immunol Immunother* 2009;58(12):1909-17.

18. Rowlands MA et al. Circulating insulin-like growth factor peptides and prostate cancer risk: a systematic review and meta-analysis. *Int J Cancer* 2009;124(10):2416-29.

19. Guevara-Aguirre J et al. Growth hormone receptor deficiency is associated with a major reduction in pro-aging signaling, cancer and diabetes in humans. *Sci Transl Med* 2011;3(70):70ra13.

20. Allen NE et al. The association of diet with serum insulin growth factor 1 and its main binding proteins in 292 women

meat eaters, vegetarians and vegans. *Cancer Epidemiol Biomarkers Prev.* 2002;11(11):1441-8.

21. Soliman S et al. Analyzing serum-stimulated prostate cancer cell lines after low fat, high fiber diet and exercise intervention. *Evid Based Complement Alternat Med* 2011;2011:529053.

22. Ngo TH et al. Effect of diet and exercise on serum insulin, IGF-1, IGFBP-1 levels and growth of LNCaP cells in vitro (United States). *Cancer Causes Control* 2002;13(10)929-35.

23. Enos WF et al. Coronary disease among United States soldiers killed in Korea: a preliminary report. *JAMA* 1953;152: 190-193.

24. McNamara JJ et al. Coronary artery disease in combat casualties in Vietnam. *JAMA* 1971;216;1185-1187.

25. Stacy HC. Evolution and progression of atherosclerotic lesions in children and young adults. *Atherosclerosis* 1989;9 Suppl I:I;19-132.

26. Ornish D et al. Intensive lifestyle changes for reversal of coronary heart disease. *JAMA* 1999 Apr 21;281(5):1380.

27. Ornish D et al. Intensive lifestyle changes may affect the progression of prostate cancer. *J Urol.* 2005 Sep;174(3):1065-9; discussion 1069-70.

28. Ornish D, Blackburn E et al. Changes in prostate gene expression in men undergoing intensive nutrition and lifestyle intervention. *Proc Natl Acad Sci USA* 2008 Jun 17;105(24):8369-74.

29. Ornish D, Blackburn E et al. Effect of comprehensive lifestyle changes on telomerase activity and telomere length in men with biopsy-proven low-risk prostate cancer: a 5 year followup of a descriptive pilot study. *Lancet Oncol* 2013 Oct;14(11):1112-1120.

30. American Cancer Society. Breast cancer facts and figures 2013-2014.

31. Sanders ME et al. The natural history of low grade ductal carcinoma in situ of the breast in women treated by biopsy

only revealed over 30 years of long-term follow-up. *Cancer* 2005;103(12):1481-4.

32. Nielsen M et al. Breast cancer and atypia among young and middle aged women: a study of 110 medicolegal autopsies. *Br J Cancer.* 1987;56(6):814-9.

33. American Institute for Cancer Research. *AICR, the China study, and Forks over Knives.* January 9, 2015.

34. Hastert TA et al. Adherence to WCRF/AICR cancer prevention recommendations and risk of postmenopausal breast cancer. *Cancer Epidemiol Biomarkers Prev.* 2013;22(9): 1498-508.

35. Barnard RJ et al. Effects of a low fat, high fiber and exercise on breast cancer risk factors in vivo and tumor cell growth and apoptosis in vitro. *Nutr Cancer* 2006;55(1):28-34.

36. Bagnardi V et al. Light alcohol drinking and cancer: a meta-analysis. *Ann Oncol* 2013;24(2):301-8.

37. Chen WY et al. Moderate alcohol consumption during adult life, drinking patterns, and breast cancer risk. *JAMA* 2011;306(17)1884-90.

38. American Cancer Society. *Cancer Facts and Figures* 2014. Atlanta: American Cancer Society 2014.

39. Doll R. The geographical distribution of cancer. *Br J Cancer.* 1969;23(1):1-8.

40. Burkitt DP. Epidemiology of cancer of the colon and rectum. 1971 *Dis Colon Rectum* 1993;36(11):1071-82.

41. Englyst HN et al. Non-starch polysaccharide consumption in four Scandinavian populations. *Nutr Cancer.* 1982;4(1): 50-60.

42. Fonseca-Nunes A et al. Iron and cancer risk—a systematic review and meta-analysis of the epidemiological evidence. *Cancer Epidemiol Biomarkers.* 2014;23(1):12-31.

43. Vucenik I et al. Cancer inhibition by inositol hexaphosphate (IP6) and inositol: from laboratory to clinic. *J Nutr.* 2003;133(11 Suppl 1):3778S-84S.

44. Ogawa S et al. Sentinel node detection with (99m)Tc phytate alone is satisfactory for cervical cancer patients undergoing radical hysterectomy and pelvic lymphadenectomy. *Int J Clin Oncol.* 2010;15(1):52-8.

45. Vucenik I et al. Protection against cancer by dietary IP6 and inositol. *Nutr Cancer* 2006;55(2):109-25.

46. Vucenik I et al. Anti-angiogenic activity of inositol hexaphosphate (IP6). *Carcinogenesis.* 2004;25(11):2015-23.

47. Li Y et al. Sulforaphane, a dietary component of broccoli/broccoli sprouts, inhibits breast cancer stem cells. *Clin Cancer Res.* 2010 May 1;16(9):2580-90.

48. Singh AV et al. Sulforaphane induces caspase-mediated apoptosis in cultured PC-3 human prostate cancer cells and retards growth of PC-3 xenografts in vivo. *Carcinogenesis.* 2004 Jan;25(1):83–90.

49. Wu QJ et al. Cruciferous vegetables intake and the risk of colorectal cancer: a meta-analysis of observational studies. *Ann Oncol.* 2013 Apr;24(4):1079-87.

50. Fallahzadeh H et al. Effect of Carrot Intake in the Prevention of Gastric Cancer: A Meta-Analysis. *J Gastric Cancer.* 2015 Dec;15(4):256-61.

51. Xu X et al. Dietary carrot consumption and the risk of prostate cancer. *Eur J Nutr.* 2014 Dec;53(8):1615-23.

52. Pisani P et al. Carrots, green vegetables and lung cancer: a case-control study. *Int J Epidemiol.* 1986 Dec;15(4):463-8.

53. Yao Y et al. Dietary fibre for the prevention of recurrent colorectal adenomas and carcinomas. *Cochrane Database Syst Rev.* 2017 Jan 8;1:CD003430.

54. Lanza E et al. High Dry Bean Intake and Reduced Risk of Advanced Colorectal Adenoma Recurrence among Participants in the Polyp Prevention Trial. *The Journal of Nutrition*, Volume 136, Issue 7, July 2006, Pages 1896–1903.

55. Hangen L, Bennink MR. Consumption of black beans and navy beans (Phaseolus vulgaris) reduced azoxymethane-induced colon cancer in rats. *Nutr Cancer.* 2002;44(1):60-5.

56. Thomasset S et al. Pilot study of oral anthocyanins for colorectal cancer chemoprevention. *Cancer Prev Res* (Phila). 2009 Jul;2(7):625-33.

57. Knobloch TJ et al. Suppression of Proinflammatory and Prosurvival Biomarkers in Oral Cancer Patients Consuming a Black Raspberry Phytochemical-Rich Troche. *Cancer Prev Res* (Phila). 2016 Feb;9(2):159-71.

58. Kresty LA et al. Chemoprevention of esophageal tumorigenesis by dietary administration of lyophilized black raspberries. *Cancer Res.* 2001 Aug 15;61(16):6112-9.

59. Lala G et al. Anthocyanin-rich extracts inhibit multiple biomarkers of colon cancer in rats. *Nutr Cancer.* 2006;54(1):84-93.

60. Allen RW et al. Cinnamon use in type 2 diabetes: an updated systematic review and meta-analysis. *Ann Fam Med.* 2013 Sep-Oct;11(5):452-9.

61. Kwon HK et al. Cinnamon extract induces tumor cell death through inhibition of NFkappaB and AP1. *BMC Cancer.* 2010 Jul 24;10:392.

62. Yang QX et al. Essential oil of Cinnamon exerts anti-cancer activity against head and neck squamous cell carcinoma via attenuating epidermal growth factor receptor-tyrosine kinase. *J BUON.* 2015 Nov-Dec;20(6):1518-25.

63. Kwon HK et al. Cinnamon extract induces tumor cell death through inhibition of NFκB and AP1. *BMC Cancer.* 2010; 10: 392.

64. Bonaccio M et al. Nut consumption is inversely associated with both cancer and total mortality in a Mediterranean population: prospective results from the Moli-sani study. *Br J Nutr.* 2015 Sep 14;114(5):804-11.

65. Wu L et al. Nut consumption and risk of cancer and type 2 diabetes: a systematic review and meta-analysis. *Nutr Rev* 2015 Jul;73(7):409-25.

66. Fritz H et al. Selenium and Lung Cancer: A Systematic Review and Meta Analysis. *PLoS One.* 2011; 6(11): e26259.

67. Hardman WE. Walnuts have potential for cancer prevention and treatment in mice. *J Nutr.* 2014 Apr;144(4 Suppl): 555S-560S.

68. Psaltopoulouil T et al. Olive oil intake is inversely related to cancer prevalence: a systematic review and a meta-analysis of 13800 patients and 23340 controls in 19 observational studies. *Lipids Health Dis.* 2011; 10: 127.

69. Stoneham M et al. Olive oil, diet and colorectal cancer: an ecological study and a hypothesis. *J Epidemiol Community Health.* 2000 Oct;54(10):756-60.

70. Carroll RE et al. Phase IIa clinical trial of curcumin for the prevention of colorectal neoplasia. *Cancer Prev Res* (Phila). 2011 Mar;4(3):354-64.

71. Lim TG et al. Curcumin suppresses proliferation of colon cancer cells by targeting CDK2. *Cancer Prev Res* (Phila). 2014 Apr;7(4):466-74.

72. Amin AR et al. Curcumin induces apoptosis of upper aerodigestive tract cancer cells by targeting multiple pathways. *PLoS One.* 2015 Apr 24;10(4):e0124218.

73. Tsai JR et al. Curcumin Inhibits Non-Small Cell Lung Cancer Cells Metastasis through the Adiponectin/NF-κb/MMPs Signaling Pathway. *PLoS One.* 2015 Dec 10;10(12):e0144462.

74. Foschi R et al. Citrus fruit and cancer risk in a network of case-control studies. *Cancer Causes Control.* 2010 Feb;21(2):237-42.

75. Bae JM et al. Citrus fruit intake and pancreatic cancer risk: a quantitative systematic review. *Pancreas.* 2009 Mar;38(2):168-74.

76. Bae JM et al. Citrus fruit intake and stomach cancer risk: a quantitative systematic review. *Gastric Cancer.* 2008;11(1):23-32.

77. Thompson LU et al. Dietary flaxseed alters tumor biological markers in postmenopausal breast cancer. *Clin Cancer Res.* 2005 May 15;11(10):3828-35.

78. Demark-Wahnefried W et al. Flaxseed supplementation (not dietary fat restriction) reduces prostate cancer proliferation rates in men presurgery. *Cancer Epidemiol Biomarkers Prev.* 2008 Dec;17(12):3577-87.

79. Yao Y et al. Dietary fibre for the prevention of recurrent colorectal adenomas and carcinomas. *Cochrane Database Syst Rev.* 2017 Jan 8;1:CD003430.

80. Chen J et al. Lycopene/tomato consumption and the risk of prostate cancer: a systematic review and meta-analysis of prospective studies. *J Nutr Sci Vitaminol* (Tokyo). 2013;59(3):213-23.

81. Giovannucci E et al. A prospective study of tomato products, lycopene, and prostate cancer risk. *J Nat Cancer Inst.* 2002 Mar 6;94(5):391-8.

82. Bat-Chen W et al. Allicin purified from fresh garlic cloves induces apoptosis in colon cancer cells via Nrf2. *Nutr Cancer.* 2010;62(7):947-57.

83. Zhou Y et al. Consumption of large amounts of Allium vegetables reduces risk for gastric cancer in a meta-analysis. *Gastroenterology.* 2011 Jul;141(1):80-9.

84. Hsing AW et al. Allium vegetables and risk of prostate cancer: a population-based study. *J Natl Cancer Inst.* 2002 Nov 6;94(21):1648-51.

85. Millen AE et al. Fruit and vegetable intake and prevalence of colorectal adenoma in a cancer screening trial. *Am J Clin Nutr.* 2007 Dec;86(6):1754-64.

86. Fernandez E et al. Fish consumption and cancer risk. *Am J Clin Nutr.* 1999 Jul;70(1):85-90.

87. Norat T et al. Meat, fish, and colorectal cancer risk: the European Prospective Investigation into cancer and nutrition. *J Natl Cancer Inst.* 2005 Jun; 97(12): 906–916.

88. Garland CF et al. The Role of Vitamin D in Cancer Prevention. *Am J Public Health.* 2006 February; 96(2): 252–261.

89. Jing K et al. Omega-3 polyunsaturated fatty acids and cancer. *Anticancer Agents Med Chem.* 2013 Oct;13(8):1162-77.

Chapter 7: The Power of Targeted Supplements

1. Dashwood et al. Quantitative inter-relationships between afla-toxin B1 carcinogen dose, indole-3-carbinol anti-carcinogen dose, target organ DNA adduction and final tumor response. *Carcinogenesis* 1989 10(1):175-81.

2. Jing-Ru et al. Indole-3-Carbinol as a chemopreventive and anti-cancer agent. *Cancer Lett.* 2008 Apr 18;262(2):153.

3. Langcake P, Pryce RJ. Production of resveratrol by vitis-vinifera and other members of vitaceae as a response to infection or injury. *Physiological Plant Pathology.* 1976;9:77-86.

4. Fang F et al. A potential role for resveratrol as a radiation sensitizer for melanoma treatment. *J Surg Res* 2013 Aug 183(2):645-53.

5. Xiong Z et al. An overview of the bioactivity of monacolin K/lovastatin. *Food Chem Toxicol* 2019 Jun 14:110585.

6. Pandyra et al. Immediate utility of two approved agents to target both the metabolic mevolanate pathway and its restorative feedback loop. *Cancer Tes* 2014 Sep 1;74(17):4772-82. Minutes

7. Rusciani L et al. Low plasma coenzyme Q10 levels as an independent prognostic factor for melanoma progression. *J Am Acad Dermatol.* 2006 Feb;54(2):234-41.

8. Bauman-Fortin J et al. The association between omega-6/omega-3 ratio and anthropometrictraits differs by racial/ethnic groups and NFKB1 genotypes in healthy adults. *J Pers Med* 2019 Feb 16;9(1). pii E13.

9. Newell M et al. A critical review of the effect of docosahexaenoic acid (DHA) on cancer cell cycle progression. *Int J Mol Sci.* 2017; 18(8). Pii E1784.

10. Gutierrez-Orozco F, Failla ML. Biological activities and bioavailability of mangosteen xanthones: a critical review of the current evidence. *Nutrients.* 2013 Aug 13;5(8):3163-83.

11. Golombick T et al. The potential role of curcumin in patients with monoclonal gammopathy of undefined significance—its effect on paraproteinemia and the urinary N-telopeptide of type I collagen bone turnover marker. *Clin Cancer Res.* 2009 Sep 15;15(18):5917-22.

12. Golombick T et al. Monoclonal gammopathy of undetermined significance, smoldering multiple myeloma, and curcumin: a randomized, double-blind placebo-controlled cross-over 4g study and an open-label 8g extension study. *Am J Hematol.* 2012 May;87(5):455-60.

13. Guido S et al. Influence of Piperine on the Pharmacokinetics of Curcumin in Animals and Human Volunteers. *Planta Med* 1998; 64(4): 353-356.

14. Aggarwal BB et al. Curcumin-free turmeric exhibits anti-inflammatory and anticancer activities: Identification of novel components of turmeric. *Mol Nutr Food Res.* 2013 Sep;57(9): 1529-42.

15. lmatroudi A et al. Ginger: A Novel Strategy to Battle Cancer through Modulating Cell Signaling Pathways: A Review. *Curr Pharm Biotechnol.* 2019;20(1):5-16.

16. Saxena R et al. Ginger augmented chemotherapy: A novel multitarget nontoxic approach for cancer management. *Mol Nutr Food Res.* 2016 Jun;60(6):1364-73.

17. Bosch-Barrera J et al. Targeting STAT3 with silibinin to improve cancer therapeutics. *Cancer Treat Rev.* 2017 Jul;58:61-69.

18. Huang C et al. Reversal of P-glycoprotein-mediated multidrug resistance of human hepatic cancer cells by Astragaloside II. *J Pharm Pharmacol* 2012 Dec;64(12):1741-50.

19. McCulloch M et al. Astragalus-based Chinese herbs and platinum-based chemotherapyfor advanced non-small-cell lung cancer: meta-analysis of randomized trials. *J Clin Oncol* 2006; 24(3):419–430.

20. McQuistan TG et al. Cancer chemoprevention by dietary chlorophylls: A 12,000-animal dose-dose matrix biomarker and tumor study. *Food Chem Toxicol.* 2012 Feb; 50(2): 341–352.

21. Jubert C et al. Effects of Chlorophyll and Chlorophyllin on Low-Dose Aflatoxin B1 Pharmacokinetics in Human Volunteers. Doi: 10.1158/1940-6207.CAPR-09-0099 Published December 2009.

22. de Vogel J et al. Green vegetables, red meat and colon cancer: chlorophyll prevents the cytotoxic and hyperproliferative effects of haem in rat colon. *Carcinogenesis.* 2005 Feb;26(2):387-93

23. Lan J et al. Meta-analysis of the effect and safety of berberine in the treatment of type 2 diabetes mellitus, hyperlipemia and hypertension. *J Ethnopharmacol* 2015 Feb 23;161:69-81.

24. Tillhon M et al. Berberine: new perspectives for old remedies. *Biochem Pharmacol* 2012 Nov 15;84(10):1260-7.

25. Yao J et al. Learning from berberine: Treating chronic diseases through multiple targets. *Sci Chi Life Sci.* 2015 Sep;58(9):854-9.

26. 26. Yun S et al. Berberine, a Natural Plant Product, Activates AMP-Activated Protein Kinase With Beneficial Metabolic Effects in Diabetic and Insulin-Resistant States. *Diabetes* 2006 Aug; 55(8): 2256-2264.

27. Winder WW, Hardie DJ. AMP-activated protein kinase, a metabolic master switch: possible roles in type 2 diabetes. *Am J Physiol* 1999 Jul;277(1):E1-10.

28. Stapleton D et al. Mammalian AMP-activated protein kinase subfamily. *J Biol Chem.* 1996 Jan 12;271(2):611-4.

29. Yao J et al. Learning from berberine: Treating chronic diseases through multiple targets. *Sci Chin Life Sci.* 2015 Sep;58(9):854-9.

30. Chang W et al. Berberine as a therapy for type 2 diabetes and its complications: From mechanism of action to clinical studies. *Biochem Cell Biol.* 2015 Oct;93(5):479-86.

31. Lan J et al. Meta-analysis of the effect and safety of berberine in the treatment of type 2 diabetes mellitus, hyperlipemia and hypertension. *J Ethnopharmacol.* 2015 Feb 23;161:69-81.

32. Pang B et al. Application of berberine on treating type 2 diabetes mellitus. *Int J Endocrinol.* 2015;2015:905749.

33. Ortiz LM et al. Berberine, an epiphany against cancer. *Molecules.* 2014 Aug 15;19(8):12349-67.

34. Sun Y et al. A systematic review of the anticancer properties of berberine, a natural product from Chinese herbs. *Anti-Cancer Drugs.* 20(9):757-769, October 2009.

35. Wang MY et al. Morinda citrifolia (Noni): a literature review and recent advances in Noni research. *Acta Pharmacol Sin.* 2002 Dec;23(12):1127-41.

36. Furusawa E et al. Antitumour potential of a polysaccharide-rich substance from the fruit juice of Morinda citrifolia (Noni) on sarcoma 180 ascites tumour in mice. *Phytother Res.* 2003 Dec;17(10):1158-64.

37. Taskin EI et al. Apoptosis-inducing effects of Morinda citrifolia L. and doxorubicin on the Ehrlich ascites tumor in Balb-c mice. *Cell Biochem Func.* 2009 Dec;27(8):542-6.

38. Dussossoy E et al. Characterization, anti-oxidative and anti-inflammatory effects of Costa Rican noni juice (Morinda citrifolia L.). *J Ethnopharmacol.* 2011 Jan 7;133(1):108-15.

39. Syed Najmuddin SU et al. Anti-cancer effect of Annona Muricata Linn Leaves Crude Extract (AMCE) on breast cancer cell line. *BMC Complement Altern Med.* 2016 Aug 24;16(1):311.

40. Pieme CA et al. Antiproliferative activity and induction of apoptosis by Annona muricata (Annonaceae) extract on human cancer cells. *BMC Complement Altern Med.* 2014; 14: 516.

41. Zamudio-Cuevas Y et al. The antioxidant activity of soursop decreases the expression of a member of the NADPH oxidase family. *Food Funct.* 2014 Feb;5(2):303-9.

42. Chan P et al. Anti-arthritic activities of Annona muricata L. leaves extract on complete Freund's adjuvant (CFA) – induced arthritis in rats. *Planta Med* 2010; 76 - P166.

43. Adeyemi DO et al. Anti hyperglycemic activities of Annona muricata (Linn). *Afr J Tradit Complement Altern Med.* 2008 Oct 25;6(1):62-9.

44. Patchen ML, MacVittie TJ et al. Radioprotection by polysaccharides alone and in combination with aminothiols. *Adv Space Res* 1992 12:233-248.

45. Alonso EN et al. Antitumoral Effects of D-Fraction from Grifola Frondosa (Maitake) Mushroom in Breast Cancer. *Nutr Cancer.* 2017 Jan;69(1):29-43.

46. Tiloke C et al. The Antiproliferative Effect of Moringa oleifera Crude Aqueous Leaf Extract on Human Esophageal Cancer Cells. *J Med Food.* 2016 Apr;19(4):398-403.

47. Al-Asmari AK et al. Moringa oleifera as an Anti-Cancer Agent against Breast and Colorectal Cancer Cell Lines. *PLoS One.* 2015 Aug 19;10(8):e0135814.

48. Stan SD et al. Withaferin A causes FOXO3a- and Bim-dependent apoptosis and inhibits growth of human breast cancer cells in vivo. *Cancer Res.* 2008 Sep 15;68(18):7661-9.

49. Mohan R et al. Withaferin A is a potent inhibitor of angiogenesis. *Angiogenesis.* 2004;7(2):115-22.

50. Kuttan G. Use of Withania sominefera Dunal ad an adjuvant during radiation therapy. *Indian J Acp Res.* 1996. 34:275-271.

51. Maschio M et al. Prevention of Bortezomib-Related Peripheral Neuropathy With Docosahexaenoic Acid and α-Lipoic Acid in Patients With Multiple Myeloma: Preliminary Data. *Integr Cancer Ther.* 2018 Dec;17(4):1115-1124.

52. Steinberg JA et al. Alpha Lipoic Acid (ALA) Inhibits the Anti-Myeloma Effects of Bortezomib. *Blood* 2009 114:3832.

53. Pey HY et al. Vitamin E therapy beyond cancer: Tocopherol versus tocotrienol. *Pharmacol Ther.* 2016 Jun;162:152-69.

54. Argyriou AA et al. A randomized controlled trial evaluating the efficacy and safety of vitamin E supplementation for protection against cisplatin-induced peripheral neuropathy: final results. *Support Care Cancer.* 2006 Nov;14(11):1134-40.

55. Colin-Gonzales AL et al. The antioxidant mechanisms underlying the aged garlic extract- and S-allylcysteine-induced protection. *Oxid Med Cell Longev.* 2012;2012:907162.

56. Sharmila G et al. Hemopreventive effect of quercetin, a natural dietary flavonoid on prostate cancer in in vivo model. *Clin Nutr.* 2014 Aug;33(4):718-26.

57. Lamson DW, Brignall MS. Antioxidants and cancer, part 3: quercetin. *Altern Med Rev.* 2000 Jun;5(3):196-208.

58. Tiwari P et al. Gymnema sylvestre for Diabetes: From Traditional Herb to Future's Therapeutic. *Curr Pharm Dev.* 2017;23(11):1667-1676.

59. Effect of Extended Release Gymnema Sylvestre Leaf Extract (Beta Fast GXR). *Diabetes In Control Newsletter,* Issue 76 (1): 30 Oct 2001.

60. Xiangwang WU et al. Isolation, purification, immunological and anti-tumor activities of polysaccharides from Gymnema sylvestre. *Food Research International.* Volume 48, Issue 2, October 2012, Pages 935-939.

61. Qadi SA et al. Thymoquinone-Induced Reactivation of Tumor Suppressor Genes in Cancer Cells Involves Epigenetic Mechanisms. *Epigenet Insights.* 2019 Apr 4;12:2516865719839011.

62. Tibullo D et al. Anti-proliferative and Antiangiogenic Effects of Punica granatum Juice (PGJ) in Multiple Myeloma (MM). *Nutrients.* 2016 Oct 1;8(10). pii: E611.

63. Kao TH et al. Preparation of carotenoid extracts and nano-emulsions from Lycium barbarum L. and their effects on growth of HT-29 colon cancer cells. *Nanotechnology.* 2017 Mar 7;28(13):135103.

64. Wawruszak A et al. Anticancer effect of ethanol Lycium barbarum (Goji berry) extract on human breast cancer T47D cell line. *Natl Prod Res.* 2016 Sep;30(17):1993-6.

65. Wang Y et al. Lycium barbarum polysaccharides grafted with doxorubicin: An efficient pH-responsive anticancer drug delivery system. *Int J Biol Macromol.* 2019 Jan;121:964-970.

66. Alessandra Perini J et al. Anticancer potential, molecular mechanisms and toxicity of Euterpe oleracea extract (açaí): A systematic review. *PLoS One.* 2018 Jul 2;13(7):e0200101. doi: 10.1371/journal.pone.0200101. eCollection 2018.

67. Sadeghi S et al. Anti-cancer effects of cinnamon: Insights into its apoptosis effects. *Eur J Med Chem*. 2019 Sep 15;178:131-140. doi: 10.1016/j.ejmech.2019.05.067. Epub 2019 Jun 1.

68. Patra K et al. The inhibition of hypoxia-induced angiogenesis and metastasis by cinnamaldehyde is mediated by decreasing HIF-1α protein synthesis via PI3K/Akt pathway. *Biofactors*. 2019 May;45(3):401-415. doi: 10.1002/biof.1499. Epub 2019 Mar 10.

69. Lu T et al. Cinnamon extract improves fasting blood glucose and glycosylated hemoglobin level in Chinese patients with type 2 diabetes. *Nutr Res*. 2012 Jun;32(6):408-12. doi: 10.1016/j.nutres.2012.05.003. Epub 2012 Jun 14.

70. Martin MA et al. Potential for preventive effects of cocoa and cocoa polyphenols in cancer. *Food Chem Toxicol*. 2013 Jun;56:336-51. doi: 10.1016/j.fct.2013.02.020. Epub 2013 Feb 22.

71. Martin MA et al. Preventive Effects of Cocoa and Cocoa Antioxidants in Colon Cancer. *Diseases*. 2016 Jan 22;4(1). pii: E6. doi: 10.3390/diseases4010006.

72. Martin MA et al. Potential for preventive effects of cocoa and cocoa polyphenols in cancer. *Food Chem Toxicol*. 2013 Jun;56:336-51. doi: 10.1016/j.fct.2013.02.020. Epub 2013 Feb 22.

73. De Araujo QR et al. Cocoa and Human Health: From Head to Foot—A Review. *Crit Rev Food Sci Nutr*. 2016;56(1):1-12. doi: 10.1080/10408398.2012.657921.

74. Baliga MS, Dsouza JJ. Amla (Emblica officinalis Gaertn), a wonder berry in the treatment and prevention of cancer. *Eur J Cancer Prev*. 2011 May;20(3):225-39.

75. Sharma N et al. In vitro inhibition of carcinogen-induced mutagenicity by Cassia occidentalis and Emblica officinalis. *Drug Chem Toxicol*. 2000 Aug;23(3):477-84.

76. de Munter L et al. Vitamin and carotenoid intake and risk of head-neck cancer subtypes in the Netherlands Cohort Study. *Am J Clin Nutr.* 2015 Aug;102(2):420-32.

77. Azeredo H. Betalains: properties, sources, applications, and stability – a review. *Int J Food Sci Technol.* November 2009 https:// doi.org/10.1111/j.1365-2621.2007.01668.x

78. Ekou VU, Brown AK. Functional foods and their role in cancer prevention and health promotion: a comprehensive review. *Am J Cancer Res.* 2017 Apr 1;7(4):740-769.

79. Langley PC et al. Antioxidant and Associated Capacities of Camu Camu (Myrciaria dubia): A Systematic Review. *J Altern Complement Med* 2015 Jan 1;21(1):8-14.

80. Chen K C et al. Brain derived metastatic prostate cancer DU-145 cells are effectively inhibited in vitro by guava (Psidium gujava L.) leaf extracts. *Nutr Cancer.* 2007;58(1):93-106.

81. Ryu NH et al. A hexane fraction of guava Leaves (Psidium guajava L.) induces anticancer activity by suppressing AKT/mammalian target of rapamycin/ribosomal p70 S6 kinase in human prostate cancer cells. *J Med Food.* 2012 Mar;15(3):231-41.

82. Manosroi J et al. Anti-proliferative activity of essential oil extracted from Thai medicinal plants on KB and P388 cell lines. *Cancer Lett.* 2006 Apr 8;235(1):114-20.

83. Weiss DJ, Anderton CR et al. Determination of catechins in matcha green tea by micellar electrokinetic chromatography. *J Chromatogr A.* 2003 Sep 5;1011(1-2):173-80.

84. Siddiqui IA et al. Green tea polyphenol EGCG sensitizes human prostate carcinoma LNCaP cells to TRAIL-mediated apoptosis and synergistically inhibits biomarkers associated with angiogenesis and metastasis. *Oncogene.* 2008 Mar 27;27(14):2055-63.

85. Mantena SK et al. Epigallocatechin-3-gallate inhibits photocarcinogenesis through inhibition of angiogenic factors and

activation of CD8+ T cells in tumors. *Photochem photobiol.* 2005 Sep-Oct;81(5):1174-9.

86. Fogelman I et al. Bone mineral density in premenopausal women treated for node-positive early breast cancer with 2 years of goserelin or 6 months of cyclophosphamide, methotrexate and 5-fluorouracil (CMF). *Osteoporosis Inter.* 2003 Dec;14(12):1001-6.

87. Effect of anastrozole on bone mineral density: 5-year results from the anastrozole, tamoxifen, alone or in combination trial 18233230. *J Clon Oncol.* 2008 Mar 1;26(7):1051-7.

88. Practical guidance for the management of aromatase inhibitor-associated bone loss. *Ann Oncol.* 2008 Aug;19(8):1407-16.

89. Spronk GM et al. Tissue-specific utilization of menaquinone-4 results in the prevention of arterial calcification in warfarin-treated rats. *J Vasc Res.* 2003 Nov-Dec;40(6):531-7.

90. Schwalfenberg GK. Vitamins K1 and K2: The Emerging Group of Vitamins Required for Human Health. *J Nutr Metab.* 2017;2017:6254836.

91. Marie, P.J., Skoryna, S.C., Pivon, R.J., Chabot, G., Glorieux, F.H., Stara, J.F. Histomorphometry of bone changes in stable strontium therapy. In: *Trace Substances in Environmental Health XIX*, edited by D.D. Hemphill, University of Missouri, Columbia, Missouri, 1985, 193-208.

92. Meunier, P.J., Roux, C., Seeman, E., Ortolani, S., Badurski, J.E., Spector, T.D., Cannata, J., Balogh, A., Lemmel, E.M., Pors-Nielsen, S., Rizzoli R., Genant, H.K., Reginster J.Y. The effects of strontium ranelate on the risk of vertebral fracture in women with postmenopausal osteoporosis, *N Engl J Med*, 2004, Jan 29;350(5):459-68.

93. Skoryna, S.C., 1981. Effects of oral supplementation with stable strontium. *Can Med Assoc J*, 125: 703-712.

94. Bicarbonate increases tumor pH and inhibits spontaneous metastases. *Cancer Res.* 2009 Mar 15;69(6):2260-8.

95. Comin-Anduix B et al. Fermented wheat germ extract inhibits glycolysis/pentose cycle enzymes and induces apoptosis through poly(ADP-ribose) polymerase activation in Jurkat T-cell leukemia tumor cells. *J Biol Chem.* 2002 Nov 29;277(48):46408-14.

96. Fajka-Boja R et al. Fermented wheat germ extract induces apoptosis and downregulation of major histocompatibility complex class I proteins in tumor T and B cell lines. *Int J Oncol.* 2002 Mar;20(3):563-70.

97. Mechanism of the anti-angiogenic effect of Avemar on tumor cells. *Oncol Lett.* 2018 Feb;15(2):2673-78.

98. Mueller T et al. Promising cytotoxic activity profile of fermented wheat germ extract (Avemar®) in human cancer cell lines. *J Exp Clin Cancer Res.* 2011 Apr 16;30:42.

99. Marczek Z et al. The efficacy of tamoxifen in estrogen receptor-positive breast cancer cells is enhanced by a medical nutriment. *Cancer Biother Radiopharm.* 2004 Dec;19(6):746-53.

100. Effect of fermented wheat germ extract with lactobacillus plantarum dy-1 on HT-29 cell proliferation and apoptosis. *J Agric Food Chem.* 2015 Mar 11;63(9):2449-57.

101. Tai CJ et al. Fermented wheat germ extract induced cell death and enhanced cytotoxicity of Cisplatin and 5-Fluorouracil on human hepatocellular carcinoma cells. *Evid Based Complement Alternat Med.* 2013;2013:121725.

102. Hwalla N et al. The Prevalence of Micronutrient Deficiencies and Inadequacies in the Middle East and Approaches to Interventions. *Nutrients.* 2017 Mar; 9(3): 229.

103. Nangia-Makker P et al. Inhibition of human cancer cell growth and metastasis in nude mice by oral intake of modified citrus pectin. *J Natl Cancer Inst.* 2002 Dec 18;94(24):1854-62.

104. Huang ZL, Liu HY. Expression of galectin-3 in liver metastasis of colon cancer and the inhibitory effect of modified citrus pectin. *Nan Fang Yi Ke Da Xue Xue Bao.* 2008 Aug;28(8):1358-61.

105. Chauhan D et al. A Novel Carbohydrate-Based Therapeutic GCS-100 Overcomes Bortezomib Resistance and Enhances Dexamethasone-Induced Apoptosis in Multiple Myeloma Cells. *Cancer Res.* 2005 Sep 15;65(18):8350-8.

106. Malacrida A et al. Anti-tumoral Effect of Hibiscus sabdariffa on Human Squamous Cell Carcinoma and Multiple Myeloma Cells. *Nutr Cancer.* 2016 Oct;68(7):1161-70.

107. Nguyen C et al. Hibiscus flower extract selectively induces apoptosis in breast cancer cells and positively interacts with common chemotherapeutics. *BMC Complement Altern Med.* 2019 May 6;19(1):98.

108. Zhu H et al. Dandelion root extract suppressed gastric cancer cells proliferation and migration through targeting lncRNA-CCAT1. *Biomed Pharmacother.* 2017 Sep;93:1010-1017.

109. Dandelion root extract affects colorectal cancer proliferation and survival through the activation of multiple death signaling pathways. *Oncotarget.* 2016 Nov 8;7(45):73080-73100.

110. Shukla S, Gupta S. Apigenin: A Promising Molecule for Cancer Prevention. *Pharm Res.* 2010 Jun; 27(6): 962–978.

111. Patel, D et al. Apigenin and cancer chemoprevention: progress, potential and promise (review). *Int J Oncol.* 2007 Jan;30(1):233-45.

112. Riza E et al. The effect of Greek herbal tea consumption on thyroid cancer: a case-control study. *Eur J Pub Health.* 2015 Dec;25(6):1001-5.

113. Ogunleye AA et al. Green tea consumption and breast cancer risk or recurrence: a meta-analysis. *Breast Cancer Res Treat.* 2010 Jan;119(2):477-84.

114. Kurahashi N et al. Green tea consumption and prostate cancer risk in Japanese men: a prospective study. *Am J Epidemiol.* 2008 Jan 1;167(1):71-7.

115. Chen Y et al. An inverse association between tea consumption and colorectal cancer risk. *Oncotarget.* 2017 Jun 6;8(23): 37367-37376.

116. Hemila H. Zinc lozenges and the common cold: a meta-analysis comparing zinc acetate and zinc gluconate, and the role of zinc dosage. *JRSM Open.* 2017 May 2;8(5):2054270417694291.

117. Haase H, Rink L. The immune system and the impact of zinc during aging. *Immun Ageing.* 2009; 6:9.

Chapter 8: The Power of Exercise

1. Peters TM et al. Intensity and timing of physical exercise in relation to post menopausal breast cancer risk: the prospective NIH-AARP diet and health study. *BMC Cancer* 2009;9:349.

2. Hildebrand JS et al. Recreational physical activity and leisure time sitting in relation to postmenopausal breast cancer risk. *Cancer Epidemiol Biomarkers Prev.* 2013;22(10):1906-12.

3. Buss LA, Dachs GU. Voluntary exercise slows breast tumor establishment and reduces tumor hypoxia in ApoE-/- mice. *J Appl Physiol.* 2018 Apr 1;124(4):938-949.

4. McCullough DJ et al. Effects of exercise training on tumor hypoxia and vascular function in the rodent preclinical orthotopic prostate cancer model. *J Appl Physiol.* 2013 Dec;115(12):1846-54.

5. Abdollahi A et al. Effect of exercise augmentation of cognitive behavioural therapy for the treatment of suicidal ideation and depression. *J Affect Disord.* 2017 Sep;219:58-63.

6. Carek PG et al. Exercise for the treatment of depression and anxiety. *Int J Psychiatry Med.* 2011;41(1):15-28.

7. Penn E, Tracy DK. The drugs don't work? Antidepressants and the current and future pharmacological management of depression. *Ther Adv Psychopharmacol.* 2012;2(5): 179–88.

8. Turner EH, Matthews AM, Linardatos E, Tell RA, Rosenthal R. Selective publication of antidepressant trials and its influence on apparent efficacy. *N Engl J Med.* 2008;358(3): 252–60.

9. Kirsch I. Antidepressants and the placebo effect. *Z Psychol* 2014; 223(3):128-34.

10. Kirsch I. Antidepressants and the placebo response. *Epidemiol Psychiatr Soc* 2009; 18(4):318-22.

11. Spence D. Are antidepressants overprescribed? Yes. *BMJ* 2013; 346:f191

12. Sugarman MA et al. The efficacy of paroxetine and placebo in treating anxiety and depression: a meta-analysis of change on the Hamilton Rating Scales. *PLos One* 2014;9(8):e106337.

13. Blease C. Deception as treatment: the case of depression. *J Med Ethics* 2011;37(1):13-6.

14. Kirsch I. Antidepressants and the placebo effect. *Z Psychol* 2014; 223(3):128-34.

15. Kirsch I. Antidepressants and the placebo effect. *Z Psychol* 2014; 223(3):128-34

16. Barnard RJ et al. A low fat diet and/or strenuous exercise alters the IGF axis in vivo and reduces prostate tumor cell growth in vitro. *Prostate* 2003;56(3):201-6.

17. Patterson RE, Laughlin GA, LaCroix AZ, et al. Intermittent fasting and human metabolic health. *J Acad Nutr Diet.* 2015;115(8):1203-1212.

18. Marinac CR, Natarajan L, Sears DD, et al. Prolonged nightly fasting and breast cancer risk: findings from NHANES (2009-2010). *Cancer Epidemiol Biomarkers Prev.* 2015;24(5):783-789.

19. Marinac CR, Sears DD, Natarajan L, Gallo LC, Breen CI, Patterson RE. Frequency and circadian timing of eating may influence biomarkers of inflammation and insulin resistance associated with breast cancer risk. *PLoS One.* 2015;10(8):e0136240.
20. Marinac CR et al. Prolonged nightly fasting and breast cancer prognosis. *JAMA Oncol.* 2016 Aug 1;2(8):1049-55.

Chapter 9: The Power of Stress Reduction

1. Antoni MH et al. Cognitive-behavioral stress management reverses anxiety-related leukocyte transcriptional dynamics. *Biol Psychiatry.* 2012 Feb 15;71(4):366-72.
2. Chida Y et al. Do stress-related psychosocial factors contribute to cancer incidence and survival? *Nat Clin Pract Oncol.* 2008 Aug;5(8):466-75.
3. Sugawara J et al. Effect of mirthful laughter on vascular function. *Am J Cardiol.* 2010 Sep 15;106(6):856-9.
4. Miller M, Fry WF. The effect of mirthful laughter on the human cardiovascular system. *Med Hypotheses.* 2009 Nov;73(5):636-9
5. Abdollahi A et al. Effect of exercise augmentation of cognitive behavioural therapy for the treatment of suicidal ideation and depression. *J Affect Disord.* 2017 Sep;219:58-63. doi: 10.1016/j.jad.2017.05.012. Epub 2017 May 8.
6. Carek PG et al. Exercise for the treatment of depression and anxiety. *Int J Psychiatry Med.* 2011;41(1):15-28.
7. Vandecreek L, Lester J. Use of alternative therapies among breast cancer outpatients compared with the general population. *Alternative Ther* 1999; 5:71-76.
8. Feher S, Maly RC. Coping with breast cancer later in life: the role of religious faith. *Psychology* 1999; 8:408-16.

9. Byrd R. Positive therapeutic effects of intercessory prayer in a coronary care unit population. *South Med J* 1988; 81:826-829.

10. Harris W et al. A randomized, controlled trial of the effects of remote intercessory prayer on outcomes in patients admitted to the coronary care unit. *Arch Int Med* 1999;159:2273-78

11. Vedamurthachar A et al. Antidepressant efficacy and hormonal effects of Sudarshana Kriya Yoga (SKY) in alcohol dependent individuals. *J Affect Disord.* 2006 Aug;94(1-3):249-53.

12. Michelsan A et al. Rapid stress reduction and anxiolysis among distressed women as a consequence of a three-month intensive yoga program. *Med Sci Monit.* 2005 Dec;11(12):CR555-561.

13. Smith C et al. A randomised comparative trial of yoga and relaxation to reduce stress and anxiety. *Complement Ther Med.* 2007 Jun;15(2):77-83.

Chapter 10: The Power of Sleep

1. Slominski RM, Reiter RJ, Schlabritz-Loutsevitch N, Ostrom RS, Slominski AT. Melatonin membrane receptors in peripheral tissues: Distribution and functions. *Mol Cell Endocrinol.* 2012; 351:152-166.

2. Stevens RG, Brainard GC, Blask DE, Lockley SW, Motta ME. Breast cancer and circadian disruption from electric lighting in the modern world. *CA Cancer J Clin.* 2014; 64:207-218.

3. Luchetti F, Canonico B, Betti M, Arcangeletti M, Pilolli F, Piroddi M, Canesi L, Papa S, Galli F. Melatonin signaling and cell protection function. *Faseb J.* 2010; 24:3603-3624.

4. Li Y et al. Melatonin for the prevention and treatment of cancer. *Oncotarget.* 2017 Jun 13;8(24):39896-39921.

5. Vijayalaxmi, Thomas CR, Reiter RJ, Herman TS. Melatonin: From basic research to cancer treatment clinics. *J Clin Oncol.* 2002; 20:2575-2601.

6. Cutando A, Lopez-Valverde A, Arias-Santiago S, De Vicente J, De Diego RG. Role of melatonin in cancer treatment. *Anticancer Res.* 2012; 32:2747-53.

7. Srinivasan V, Spence DW, Pandi-Perumal SR, Trakht I, Cardinali DP. Therapeutic actions of melatonin in cancer: Possible mechanisms. *Integr Cancer Ther.* 2008; 7:189-203.

8. Sainz RM, Mayo JC, Rodriguez C, Tan DX, Lopez-Burillo S, Reiter RJ. Melatonin and cell death: Differential actions on apoptosis in normal and cancer cells. *Cell Mol Life Sci.* 2003; 60:1407-1426.

9. Hill SM, Belancio VP, Dauchy RT, Xiang S, Brimer S, Mao L, Hauch A, Lundberg PW, Summers W, Yuan L, Frasch T, Blask DE. Melatonin: An inhibitor of breast cancer. *Endocr Relat Cancer.* 2015; 22:R183-R204.

10. Sanchez-Barcelo EJ, Mediavilla MD, Alonso-Gonzalez C, Reiter RJ. Melatonin uses in oncology: Breast cancer prevention and reduction of the side effects of chemotherapy and radiation. *Expert Opin Inv Drug.* 2012; 21:819-831.

11. Chueng V et al. The effect of sleep deprivation and disruption on DNA damage and health of doctors. *Anaesthesia.* 2019; 74: 417–419.

12. Davis S et al. Night shift work, light at night, and risk of breast cancer. *J Natl Cancer Inst* 2001;93:1557-62.

13. Schernhammer ES et al. Night shift work and risk of colorectal cancer in the nurses' health study, *J Natl Cancer Inst* 2003;95:825-8.

14. Kogevinas M et al. Prostate cancer risk decreases following cessation of night shift work. *Int J Cancer* doi:10.1002/ijc.32528.

15. DeLorenzo BHP et al. Chronic Sleep Restriction Impairs the Antitumor Immune Response in Mice. *Neuroimmunomodulation.* 2018;25(2):59-67.

16. Burgos I et al. Increased nocturnal interleukin-6 excretion in patients with primary insomnia: a pilot study. *Brain Behav Immun* 2006 May;20(3):246-53.

17. Irwin MR et al. Sleep Disturbance, Sleep Duration, and Inflammation: A Systematic Review and Meta-Analysis of Cohort Studies and Experimental Sleep Deprivation. *Biol Psychiatry* 2016 Jul 1;80(1):40-52.

18. Srinivasan V et al. Therapeutic actions of melatonin in cancer: possible mechanisms. *Integ Cancer Therap* 2008 Sep;7(3):189-203.

19. Sainz RM et al. Melatonin and cell death: differential actions on apoptosis in normal and cancer cells. *Cell Mol Life Sci* 2003 Jul;60(7):1407-26.

20. Hill SM et al. Melatonin: an inhibitor of breast cancer. *Endocr Rel Cancer* 2015 Jun;22(3):R183-204.

21. Sanchez-Barcelo EJ et al. Melatonin uses in oncology: breast cancer prevention and reduction of the side effects of chemotherapy and radiation. *Expert Opin Investig Drugs.* 2012 Jun;21(6):819-31.S

22. Sanassi LA. Seasonal affective disorder: is there light at the end of the tunnel? *JAAPA* 2014 Feb;27(2):18-22.

23. Campbell SS et al. Alleviation of sleep maintenance insomnia with timed exposure to bright light. *J Am Geriatr Soc* 1993 Aug;41(8):829-36.

24. Fetveit A et al. Bright light treatment improves sleep in institutionalized elderly—an open trial. *Int J Geriatr Psychiatry.* 2003 Jun;18(6):520-6.

25. Fonken LK et al. Light at night increases body mass by shifting the time of food intake. *Proc Nat Acad Sci USA.* 2010 Oct 26;107(43):18664-9.

26. Figuero MG et al. The impact of light from computer monitors on melatonin levels in college students. *Neuro Endocrinol Lett.* 2011;32(2):158-63.

27. Fredholm BB et al. Actions of caffeine in the brain with special reference to factors that contribute to its widespread use. *Pharmacol Rev.* 1999 Mar;51(1):83-133.

28. Drake C et al. Caffeine effects on sleep taken 0, 3, or 6 hours before going to bed. *J Clin Sleep Med.* 2013 Nov 15;9(11):1195-200.

29. FredholmBB et al. Actions of caffeine in the brain with special reference to factors that contribute to its widespread use. *Pharmacol Rev.* 1999 Mar;51(1):83-133.

30. Groeger JA et al. Effects of sleep inertia after daytime naps vary with executive load and time of day. *Behav Neurosci.* 2011 Apr;125(2):252-60.

31. McDevitt EA et al. The effect of nap frequency on daytime sleep architecture. *Physiol Behav.* 2012 Aug 20;107(1):40-4.

32. Dhand R, Sohal H. Good sleep, bad sleep! The role of daytime naps in healthy adults. *Curr Opin Pul Med.* 2006 Nov;12(6):379-82.

33. Pilcher JJ et al. The prevalence of daytime napping and its relationship to nighttime sleep. *Behav Med.* 2001 Summer;27(2):71-6.

34. Van Dongen HP, Dinges DF. Investigating the interaction between the homeostatic and circadian processes of sleep-wake regulation for the prediction of waking neurobehavioural performance. *J Sleep Res.* 2003 Sep;12(3):181-7.

35. Giannotti F et al, Circadian preference, sleep and daytime behaviour in adolescence. *J Sleep Res.* 2002 Sep;11(3):191-99.

36. Baehr EK et al. Individual differences in the phase and amplitude of the human circadian temperature rhythm: with an emphasis on morningness-eveningness. *J Sleep Res.* 2000 Jun;9(2):117-27.

37. van Geijlswijk IM et al. Evaluation of sleep, puberty and mental health in children with long-term melatonin treatment for chronic idiopathic childhood sleep onset insomnia. *Psychopharmacology* (Berl). 2011 Jul;216(1):111-20.

38. Lemoine P et al. Prolonged-release melatonin improves sleep quality and morning alertness in insomnia patients aged 55 years and older and has no withdrawal effects. *J Sleep Res.* 2007 Dec;16(4):372-80.

39. Tortorolo F et al. Is melatonin useful for jet lag? *Medwave.* 2015 Dec 21;15 Suppl 3:e6343.

40. Hemmeter U et al. Polysomnographic effects of adjuvant ginkgo biloba therapy in patients with major depression medicated with trimipramine. *Pharmacopsychiatry.* 2001 Mar;34(2):50-9.

41. Bannai M, Kawai N. New therapeutic strategy for amino acid medicine: glycine improves the quality of sleep. *J Pharmacol. Sci.* 2012;118(2):145-8.

42. Fernandex-San-Martin MI et al. Effectiveness of Valerian on insomnia: a meta-analysis of randomized placebo-controlled trials. *Sleep Med.* 2010 Jun;11(6):505-11.

43. de Baaij JH et al. Magnesium in man: implications for health and disease. *Physiol Rev.* 2015 Jan;95(1):1-46.

44. Lu K et al. The acute effects of L-theanine in comparison with alprazolam on anticipatory anxiety in humans. *Human Psychopharmacol.* 2004 Oct;19(7):457-65.

45. Sayorwan W et al. The effects of lavender oil inhalation on emotional states, autonomic nervous system, and brain electrical activity. *J Med Assoc Thai7.* 2012 Apr;95(4):598-606.

46. Issa FG, Sullivan CE. Alcohol, snoring and sleep apnea. *J Neurol Neurosurg Psychiatry.* 1982 Apr;45(4):353-9.

47. Ekman AC et al. Ethanol inhibits melatonin secretion in healthy volunteers in a dose-dependent randomized double blind crossover study. *J Clin Endocrinol Metab.* 1993 Sep;77(3):780-3.

48. Ekman AC et al. Ethanol decreases nocturnal plasma levels of thyrotropin and growth hormone but not those of thyroid hormones or prolactin in man. *J Clin Endocrinol Metab.* 1996 Jul;81(7):2627-32.

49. Libert JP et al. Relative and combined effects of heat and noise exposure on sleep in humans. *Sleep.* 1991 Feb;14(1):24-31.

50. Waye KP et al. Effects of nighttime low frequency noise on the cortisol response to awakening and subjective sleep quality. *Life Sci.* 2003 Jan 10;72(8):863-75.

51. Lee KA, Gay CL. Can modifications to the bedroom environment improve the sleep of new parents? Two randomized controlled trials. *Res Nurse Health.* 2011 Feb;34(1):7-19.

52. Libert JP et al. Relative and combined effects of heat and noise exposure on sleep in humans. *Sleep.* 1991 Feb;14(1):24-31.

53. Okamoto -Mizuno K et al. Effects of mild heat exposure on sleep stages and body temperature in older men. *Int J Biometereol.* 2004 Sep;49(1):32-6.

54. Jalilolghadr S et al. Effect of low and high glycaemic index drink on sleep pattern in children. *J Pak Med Assoc.* 2011 Jun;61(6):533-6.

55. Afaghi A et al. High-glycemic-index carbohydrate meals shorten sleep onset. *Am J Clin Nutr.* 2007 Feb;85(2):426-30.

56. Afaghi A et al. Acute effects of the very low carbohydrate diet on sleep indices. *Nutr Neurosci.* 2008 Aug;11(4):146-54.

57. Coursey RD et al. A comparison of relaxation techniques with electrosleep therapy for chronic, sleep-onset insomnia a sleep-EEG study. *Biofeedback Self Regul.* 1980 Mar;5(1):57-73.

58. Richards KC. Effect of a back massage and relaxation intervention on sleep in critically ill patients. *Am J Crit Care.* 1998 Jul;7(4):288-99.

59. Liao WC et al. Effect of foot bathing on distal-proximal skin temperature gradient in elders. *Int J Nurs Stud.* 2005 Sep;42(7):717-22.

60. Kanda K et al. Bathing before sleep in the young and in the elderly. *Eur J Appl Physiol Occup Physiol.* 1999 Jul;80(2):71-5.

61. Liao WC et al. A warm footbath before bedtime and sleep in older Taiwanese with sleep disturbance. *Res Nurs Health.* 2008 Oct;31(5):514-28.

62. Phillipson EA. Sleep apnea—a major public health problem. *New Eng J Med.* 1993 Apr 29;328(17):1271-3.

63. Young T et al. The occurrence of sleep-disordered breathing among middle-aged adults. *New Eng J Med.* 1993 Apr 29;328(17):1230-5.

64. Aurora RN et al. The Treatment of Restless Legs Syndrome and Periodic Limb Movement Disorder in Adults—An Update for 2012: Practice Parameters with an Evidence-Based Systematic Review and Meta-Analyses. *Sleep.* 2012;35(8): 1039-1062.

65. Jacobson BH et al. Effect of prescribed sleep surfaces on back pain and sleep quality in patients diagnosed with low back and shoulder pain. *Appl Ergon.* 2010 Dec;42(1):91-7.

66. Jacobson BH et al. Effectiveness of a selected bedding system on quality of sleep, low back pain, shoulder pain, and spine stiffness. *J Manipulative Physiol Ther.* 2002 Feb;25(2):88-92.

67. Jacobson BH et al. Grouped comparisons of sleep quality for new and personal bedding systems. *Appl Ergon.* 2008 Mar;39(2):247-54.

68. Jacobson BH et al. Changes in back pain, sleep quality, and perceived stress after introduction of new bedding systems. *J Chiropr Med.* 2009 Mar; 8(1): 1–8.

69. Reid KJ et al. Aerobic exercise improves self-reported sleep and quality of life in older adults with insomnia. *Sleep Med.* 2010 Oct;11(9):934-40.

70. King AC et al. Moderate-intensity exercise and self-rated quality of sleep in older adults. A randomized controlled trial. *JAMA.* 1997 Jan 1;277(1):32-7.

71. Passos GS et al. Effect of acute physical exercise on patients with chronic primary insomnia. *J Clin Sleep Med.* 2010 Jun 15;6(3):270-5.

72. Myllymaki T et al. Effects of vigorous late-night exercise on sleep quality and cardiac autonomic activity. *J Sleep Res.* 2011 Mar;20(1 Pt 2):146-53.

73. Marschall-Kehrel D. Update on nocturia: the best of rest is sleep. *Urology.* 2004 Dec;64(6 Suppl 1):21-4.

SELECTED BIBLIOGRAPHY
OF BOOKS AND MOVIES

Barnard, Neal. *The Vegan Starter Kit*. New York-Boston: Grand Central Life and Style. 2018

Blaylock, Russell L. *Natural Strategies for Cancer Patients*. New York: Twin Stream Books. 2003

Buettner, Dan. *The Blue Zones*. Washington DC: National Geographic Society. 2012

Campbell, T. Colin and Thomas Campbell. *The China Study*. Dallas: BenBella Books. 2006

Chang, Raymond. *The Anti-Cancer Cocktail*. Garden City Park, NY: Square One Publishers. 2012

Esselstyn, Caldwell. *Prevent and Reverse Heart Disease*. New York. The Penguin Group. 1995

Esselstyn, Rip. *Plant-Strong*. Hachette Book Group. New York. 2015.

Forks Over Knives, Monica Beach Media. Directed by Lee Fulkerson. 2011.

Fuhrman, Joel. *Super Immunity*. New York: St. Martin's Griffin. 2011

Goldhamer, Alan and Lisle, Douglas J. *The Pleasure Trap*. Summertown, TN: Healthy Living Publications. 2003

Greger, Michael. *How Not to Die*. New York: Flatiron Books. 2015

Li, William. *Eat to Beat Disease*. New York: Grand Central Publishing. 2019

Lipsky, Sally. *Beyond Cancer*. Wellness Ink Publishing. 2018

McDougall, John A and McDougall Mary. *The Starch Solution*. New York: Rodale. 2012

McLelland, Jane. *How to Starve Cancer*. United Kingdom: Agenor Publishing. 2018

Tagliaferri, Mary and Cohen, Isaac and Tripathy, Debu. *Breast Cancer Beyond Convention*. New York: Simon and Schuster. 2002

Varadi, Lisa. *Sleep*. London: Hardy Grant Publishing

ABOUT THE AUTHOR

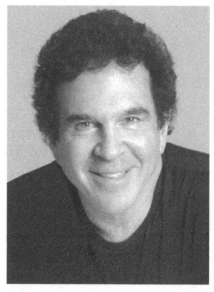

D OMINIC A BRANDY, MD is a medical doctor, thriving with myeloma, who has practiced anti-aging and aesthetic medicine for over 38 years. He has published over 70 articles and 9 textbook chapters in the peer reviewed scientific literature; given over 200 lectures at major physician conferences; is the author of a booked called *Head Start* and has written many lay articles in consumer magazines. He is the founder and president of the non-profit LLC, Natural Insights into Cancer, LLC.

Discover more on his website, *naturalinsightsintocancer.com* and his Instagram site *@cancerveggiedoc.*

INDEX

CPSIA information can be obtained
at www.ICGtesting.com
Printed in the USA
LVHW091052251119
638421LV00005B/27/P